Cardiac Pacing

Diagnostic and Therapeutic Tools

Edited by B. Lüderitz

With 75 Figures

Springer-Verlag
Berlin Heidelberg New York 1976

Privatdozent Dr. med. BERNDT LÜDERITZ
Oberarzt der Medizinischen Klinik I der Universität München, Klinikum Großhadern.

The papers contained in this book were presented at the international symposium on 'Diagnostic and Therapeutical Tools of Cardiac Pacing' held at Munich (G. F. R.) on November 7 and 8, 1975.

ISBN-13: 978-3-642-66358-1 e-ISBN-13: 978-3-642-66356-7
DOI: 10.1007/978-3-642-66356-7

Library of Congress Cataloging in Publication Data. Main entry under title: Cardiac pacing. "The papers contained in this book were presented at the international symposium on 'Diagnostic and Therapeutical Tools of Cardiac Pacing' held at Munich (G. F. R.) on November 7 and 8, 1975." Includes index. 1. Arrhythmia — Congresses. 2. Heart conduction system — Congresses. 3. Tachycardia — Congresses. 4. Pacemaker, Artificial (Heart) — Congresses. I. Lüderitz, Berndt, 1940– [DNLM: 1. Heart conduction system — Congresses. 2. Arrhythmia — Diagnosis — Congresses. 3. Arrhythmia — Therapy — Congresses. 4. Electrical stimulation — Congresses. 5. Pacemaker, Artificial — Congresses. WG26 C269 1975] RC685.A65C29 616.1'28 76-9755.

Softcover reprint of the hardcover 1st edition 1976

Contents

Introduction
G. RIECKER 1

I. Sinus Node

The Sinoatrial Node Function
F. I. M. BONKE 5
Clinical Aspects of the Sick Sinus Syndrome
H. P. GURTNER, H. R. LENZINGER, and M. DOLDER 12
The Significance of the Sinus Node Recovery Time in the Sick Sinus Syndrome
W. DELIUS and A. WIRTZFELD 25
Premature Atrial Stimulation for Evaluation of Sinoatrial Conduction in Man
H. C. STRAUSS and A. G. WALLACE 33
Sinus Node Recovery Time and Sinoatrial Conduction Time
G. STEINBECK and B. LÜDERITZ 45
The Influence of Drugs on Sinoatrial Conduction Time in Man
G. BREITHARDT and L. SEIPEL 58
Evaluation of Suction Electrode Recording
J. CABASSON and P. PUECH 73
The Recording of the Human Right Atrial Monophasic Action Potential
T. POP, D. FLEISCHMANN, and S. EFFERT 80

II. Atrioventricular Conduction

Contributions of Intracardiac Electrography to the Understanding of Normal and Disturbed AV Conduction
M. SCHLEPPER 87
Clinical Significance of AV Conduction Disturbances
K. LANG 99
Fascicular Block Patterns – Observations on Differential Diagnosis
M. GERTSCH and D. BERNOULLI 111
AV Nodal Tachycardias
PH. COUMEL 119

Drug Effects on AV Conduction
H. NEUSS, H.-J. SCHAUMANN, and B. STEGARU . . . 132
Split His
M. RUNGE and O. S. NARULA 142
Atrioventricular (AV) and Ventriculoatrial (VA) Conduction Pattern in Patients with Short P-R Interval and Normal QRS Complex
L. SEIPEL, G. BREITHARDT, and A. BOTH 152
The Wolff-Parkinson-White Syndrome
H. J. J. WELLENS 164

III. Supraventricular and Ventricular Tachycardias

An in Vitro Model of Circulating Excitation in the Absence of an Anatomic Obstacle
M. A. ALLESSIE, F. I. M. BONKE, F. J. G. SCHOPMAN, and W. J. E. P. LAMMERS 175
Clinical and Electrocardiographic Features of Supraventricular and Ventricular Tachycardias
D. M. KRIKLER 185
Reentry-Mechanism within the His-Purkinje-System in Man During Extrasystolic Stimulation of the Right Ventricle
D. FLEISCHMANN, T. POP, and J. M. A. DEBAKKER 194
Patient Initiated Rapid Atrial Pacing to Manage Supraventricular Tachycardia
A. R. KAHN and P. CITRON 205
Fundamentals of Orthorhythmic Pacing
F. I. ZACOUTO and L. J. GUIZE 212
Orthorhythmic Stimulation and Endocardial Detection as a Diagnostic Tool
K. THEISEN and H. JAHRMÄRKER 219
The Use of Programmed Rate-Related Premature Stimulation in Managing Tachyarrhythmias
B. LÜDERITZ and G. STEINBECK 227
Future Aspects of Cardiac Pacing
R. A. J. SPURRELL 235

Subject Index 241

List of Contributors

Allessie, M. A., M. D., Medical Faculty Maastricht, Department of Physiology, Biomedical Center, Beeldsnijdersdreef 101, NL Maastricht

Bernoulli, D., Dr. med., Medizinische Klinik der Universität Inselspital, Kardiologische Abteilung, CH-3008 Bern

Bonke, F. I. M., M. D., Medical Faculty, Department of Physiology, Biomedical Center, Beeldsnijdersdreef 101, NL Maastricht

Both, A., Doz. Dr. med., 1. Medizinische Klinik B der Universität Düsseldorf, Moorenstraße 5, D-4000 Düsseldorf 1

Breithardt, G., Dr. med., 1. Medizinische Klinik B der Universität Düsseldorf, Moorenstraße 5, D-4000 Düsseldorf 1

Cabasson, J., M. D., Service de Cardiologie, Centre Hospitalier, F-3000 Nimes

Citron, P., MSEE, 3055 Old Highway Eight, P. O. Box 1453, Minneapolis, Minnesota 55418/USA

Coumel, P., M. D., Hôpital Lariboisière, 2, Rue Ambroise-Paré, F-75475 Paris Cedex 10

de Bakker, J. M. T., Dr., Helmholtz-Institut für Biomedizinische Technik, Rheinisch-Westfälische Technische Hochschule Aachen, D-5100 Aachen

Delius, W., Doz. Dr. med., 1. Medizinische Klinik und Poliklinik r.d. Isar der TU München, Ismaninger Straße 22, D-8000 München 80

Dolder, M., Dr. med., Medizinische Klinik der Universität, Kardiologische Abteilung, Inselspital, CH-3008 Bern

Effert, S., Prof. Dr. med., Abteilung Innere Medizin 1 der Medizinischen Fakultät an der Rheinisch-Westfälischen Technischen Hochschule Aachen, Goethestraße 27/29, D-5100 Aachen

Fleischmann, D., Dr. med., Abteilung Innere Medizin 1 der Medizinischen Fakultät an der Rheinisch-Westfälischen Technischen Hochschule Aachen, Goethestraße 27/29, D-5100 Aachen

Gertsch, M., Dr. med., Medizinische Klinik der Universität, Kardiologische Abteilung, Inselspital, CH-3008 Bern

Guize, L., M. D., Hôpital Broussais, Clinique Cardiologique, 96, Rue Didot, F-75674 Paris Cedex 14

Gurtner, H. P., Prof. Dr. med., Medizinische Klinik der Universität, Kardiologische Abteilung, Inselspital, CH-3008 Bern

Jahrmärker, H., Prof. Dr. med., 1. Medizinische Klinik der Universität München, Ziemssenstraße 1, D-8000 München 2

Kahn, A. R., M. D., University of Minnesota, School of Medicine, Minneapolis, Minnesota 55418/USA

Krikler, D. M., M. D., F.R.C.P., Royal Postgraduate Medical School, Hammersmith Hospital, GB London W.12

Lammers, W. J. E. P., M. D., Medical Faculty Maastricht, Department of Physiology, Biomedical Center, Beeldsnijdersdreef 101, NL, Maastricht

Lang, K., Prof. Dr. med., 2. Medizinische Klinik der Universität, Langenbeckstraße 1, D-6500 Mainz

Lenzinger, H. R., Dr. med., Medizinische Klinik der Universität Inselspital, Kardiologische Abteilung, CH-3008 Bern

Lüderitz, B., Doz. Dr. med., Medizinische Klinik I der Universität München, Klinikum Großhadern, Marchioninistraße 15, D-8000 München 70

Narula, O. S., M. D., Division of Cardiology Department of Internal Medicine Mount Sinai Medical Center, Miami Beach, Florida/USA

Neuss, H., Dr. med., I. Medizinische Klinik, Klinikum Mannheim, der Universität Heidelberg, Postfach 23, D-6800 Mannheim 1

Pop, T., Dr. med., Abteilung Innere Medizin der Medizinischen Fakultät an der Rheinisch-Westfälischen Technischen Hochschule Aachen, Goethestraße 27/29, D-5100 Aachen

Puech, P., M. D., Prof., Cliniques Saint-Eloi, F-3400 Montpellier

Riecker, G. Prof. Dr. med., Medizinische Klinik I der Universität München, Klinikum Großhadern, Marchioninistraße 15, D-8000 München 70

Runge, M., Doz. Dr. med., Universitäts-Krankenhaus Eppendorf, 1. Medizinische Klinik, Martinistraße 52, D-2000 Hamburg 20

Schaumann, H.-J., Dr. med., I. Medizinische Klinik, Klinikum Mannheim, der Universität Heidelberg, Postfach 23, D-6800 Mannheim

Schlepper, M., Prof. Dr. med., Kerckhoff-Klinik, Benekestraße 6 – 8, D-6350 Bad Nauheim

Schopman, F. J. G., Department of Physiology University of Amsterdam, Eerste Constantijn Huygensstraat 20, NL Amsterdam

Seipel, L., Doz. Dr. med., I. Medizinische Klinik B der Universität Düsseldorf, Moorenstraße 5, D-4000 Düsseldorf 1

Stegaru, B., Dr. med., I. Medizinische Klinik, Klinikum Mannheim, der Universität Heidelberg, Postfach 23, D-6800 Mannheim 1

Spurrell, R. A. J., M. D., B. Sc., M.R.C.P., F.A.C.C., St. Bartholomew's Hospital, Department of Cardiology, West Smithfield, GB London EC 1 A 7 BE

Steinbeck, G., Dr. med., Medizinische Klinik I der Universität München, Klinikum Großhadern, Marchioninistraße 15, D-8000 München 70

Strauss, H. C., M. D., Departments of Medicine and Physiology and Pharmacology, Cardiovascular Division, Duke University, Medical Center Box 3845, Durham, N. C. 27710/USA

Theisen, K., Dr. med., 1. Medizinische Klinik der Universität München, Ziemssenstraße 1, D-8000 München 2

Wallace, A. G., M. D., Departments of Medicine and Physiology and Pharmacology, Duke University, Medical Center Box 3022, Durham, N. C. 27710/USA

Wellens, H. J. J., M. D. Prof., Department of Cardiology, University of Amsterdam, Wilhelmina Gasthuis, Eerste Helmersstraat 104, NL Amsterdam – Oud West

Wirtzfeld, A., Doz. Dr. med., 1. Medizinische Klinik und Poliklinik r. d. Isar der TU München, Ismaninger Straße 22, D-8000 München 80

Zacouto, F., M. D., Ph. D., Hôpital Boucicaut, 78, Rue de la Convention, F-75015 Paris 15[e]

Introduction

The history of electric cardiac stimulation is long and fascinating. The growing clinical importance has been recognized and renewed as Zoll in 1952 described a successful resusciation in cardiac standstill by external stimulation. Meanwhile, patients with disorders of cardiac rhythm have been treated all over the world for about 15 years. Recently the technical refinements of intracardiac stimulation in combination with a subtile analysis of endocavitary electrocardiograms improved the understanding of human intracardiac conduction. These new procedures include the possibility to study the initiation and termination of tachycardias. – The pertinent interest in these developments and the intention to learn more about the basic fundamentals of excitability and conduction under both normal and pathological circumstances were reasons to organize an international symposium on that topic. – The papers contained in this book were presented at this meeting on diagnostic and therapeutical tools of cardiac pacing, held at Munich on November 7 and 8, 1975, sponsored by the first Medical Clinic of the University of Munich and generously supported by Medtronic. Especially focused are the investigations on sinus node function, disturbances of av-conduction and electrophysiology of supraventricular and ventricular tachycardias. The content of the book that is emerging from the symposium were created by the authors. I wish to thank them for teaching us about the recent advances in cardiac tissue stimulation by electricity. Much credit is due Priv. Doz. Dr. B. Lüderitz, who organized the symposium and published these proceedings. I am sure that this meeting has contributed to the progress in understanding cardiac arrhythmias. I do hope that the advances in the field of diagnostic and therapeutic application of cardiac pacing will continue as rapid as before in order to give us further great help in taking care of the patient.

G. Riecker

I. Sinus Node

The Sinoatrial Node Function

F. I. M. Bonke

The impulse for the activation of the heart is generated normally in the sinoatrial node (SA node). This structure covers an area of only a few square millimeters. The cells have an irregular contour and are small (diameter less than 10 μ). Furthermore, they contain sparse myofilaments which are often not well organized. The intercellular junctions are different from normal myocardium since there are no intercalated discs, no real nexus, and only rare membrane junctions. The nodal cells often form clusters divided by connective tissue. One of the characteristic features of the SA nodal structure is the abundant innervation by autonomic fibers [15]. Since West [28] made the first impalement with a microelectrode in a fiber of a mammalian SA node, many researchers have studied the electrophysiologic characteristics of the node. Most of these studies were done with the rabbit heart. Although only little information about the human SA node is available, it seems reasonable to assume that there is no principal difference between man and rabbit in respect to the electrophysiology of the SA node.

Electrophysiology of the SA Node

The fibers of the SA node show a slow depolarization during diastole (phase 4 depolarization, prepotential) and, therefore, never have a real resting potential. Compared to atrial fibers, the maximal polarization of the membrane of the nodal fibers is less, the action potential has a lower amplitude and a longer duration, and depolarization is relatively slow.

However, the prepotential is not the same in all fibers of the node. In most of the fibers there is an abrupt transition from the prepotential into the depolarization phase of the action potential. It is clear that these fibers are brought to a discharge and are not generating a discharge themselves. If the prepotential was not interrupted these fibers would come to a spontaneous discharge. Therefore, they are called latent pacemaker fibers.

Any group of fibers in the SA node simultaneously coming to a spontaneous discharge, might act as the pacemaker of the heart. These fibers show a prominent prepotential (15 – 25 mV) and a smooth transition from prepotential to upstroke of the action potential. However, not all the fibers in the SA node in which these two conditions are fulfilled are dominant pacemaker fibers.

Only if the discharge of these fibers is conducted through the node to the atrium and serves as the impulse for the atrial activation, is it correct to call these fibers dominant pacemaker fibers. In the rabbit, therefore, the latency between the depolarization of such a fiber and the activation of atrial fibers just near the nodal region (crista terminalis) has to be at least 30 – 35 ms. Since impulse conduction is very slow in the SA node — 0.1 – 5 cm/s — it is possible that more groups of fibers come to a discharge more or less simultaneously without affecting each other. Only the group of which the impulse reaches the atrial border first will be the pacemaker. Normally this dominant pacemaker is located in the center of the SA node. The impulse is conducted through the node discharging the surrounding nodal fibers. The fibers that are located more at the periphery of the node will be discharged either by another group of spontaneously discharging fibers or by an impulse invading retrogradely the SA node from the crista terminalis.

The slow conduction velocity in the SA node is correlated with the relatively slow upstroke velocity of the action potential and the relatively bad electrotronic interactions [3]. The result is that the fibers in the SA node can work asynchronously. The advantage is that the function of pacemaker can be taken over by another group of fibers for a shorter or longer period. Therefore, the shape of the action potential is changeable and the pacemaker can shift through the node from place to place. This will, for instance, occur when the temperature in or surrounding the SA node is changed. A decrease in temperature is coupled with a lowering of the prepotential and consequently with a decrease in heart rate. The effect of a temperature change is more pronounced in fibers with a prominent prepotential than in typical latent pacemaker fibers. The prepotential in the dominant pacemaker fibers is more depressed than in other fibers and hence a shift of the pacemaker takes place [8]. When the vagal tone is increased, the slope of the prepotential is diminished and with further increase of the vagal tone, hyperpolarization might occur or even a complete arrest of impulse generation. In these cases a shift of the pacemaker is obvious as demonstrated by Toda and West [27] and Bouman et al. [7]. Hence, the acetylcholine, liberated at the ending of the vagal nerve, has a stronger effect on the dominant pacemaker fibers than on the latent fibers. One might assume that the pacemaker shift is caused by an unequal distribution of the acetylcholine through the node, but a pacemaker shift occurs also when acetylcholine is added to the fluid surrounding the SA node (e.g., isolated right atrium preparation).

On the other hand, stimulation of the sympathetic nerves or addition of adrenaline to the perfusion fluid in the isolated right atrium preparation is attended with an increase in heart rate based on a faster slope of the prepotential. The site of the pacemaker in the SA node is influenced by the above-mentioned maneuvers as demonstrated by Toda and Shimanoto [26] and Lu and Brooks [18]. Moderate changes in the sodium or potassium concentration of the extracellular fluid have little influence on the slope of the prepotential. However, changes in the calcium concentration have a striking effect. An increase in calcium concentration is attended with an increased slope of the prepotential and consequently an increased heart rate. [23]. Whether the extracellular calcium concentration has an influence on the site of the pacemaker has to be investigated.

As we have now seen, practically all factors influencing the SA nodal fibers influence both the rate of discharge of the pacemaker and the site of this pacemaker within the SA node.

A more basic problem in the electrophysiology of the SA node is the question of the mechanism that underlies the prepotential. Since the SA nodal fibers are difficult to impale with microelectrodes because of their small size and the close vicinity of the contracting atrial myocardium, most investigators used the Purkinje fiber preparation to study this problem. Besides, direct measurement of current flow in sinoatrial node cells is practically impossible because of the structural complexity of the nodal tissue. So far as I know only Irisawa [13] has tried to use a double sucrose gap technique for voltage clamping of SA nodal tissue of the rabbit. His results are, however, preliminary and many problems have to be solved. The Purkinje fiber preparation is of all cardiac preparations the most suitable for current analysis by means of the voltage clamp technique [14].

Customarily the same explanation for the formation of the action potential and for the development of the prepotential in both Purkinje fiber and sinoatrial node is used. It turns out, however, that this generalization is not absolutely valid since there are too many differences in behavior and in sensitivity to changes in the environment between both types of fibers. I will not go into more details here, but would refer the reader to the recent monograph of Brooks and Lu [9].

I would like to put forward here the following hypothesis about the sinoatrial nodal fiber:

The SA nodal fibers are in principle normal myocardial fibers the cell membrane of which has an abnormally high permeability for ions. Therefore, these nodal fibers will contain more sodium and less potassium than cardiac fibers normally do. The most leaky fibers will be the dominant pacemaker.

Because of the complex geometry of the SA node, chemical analysis of the ion contents of these cells is very difficult. Mazel and Holland [20] found that the sinus venosus fibers of frog and turtle contained obviously more sodium and less potassium than atrial and ventricular fibers. This is the only direct support for my hypothesis at this writing. However, the following observations can be explained with this hypothesis:

1. The nodal fibers are the least polarized cardiac fibers.
2. The ratio between potassium permeability and sodium permeability will be relatively low and the nodal fibers, therefore, are not very sensitive for changes in extracellular potassium concentration.
3. Since the nodal fibers are partly depolarized the sodium transport system will be more or less inactivated and in combination with the relatively small difference between the intra- and extracellular sodium concentration, this can explain the fact that sodium ions are far less important as current carriers during the upstroke of the action potential than is the case in other cardiac fibers. (Nodal fibers are TTX-insensitive, but can perhaps be made sensitive for this drug by hyperpolarization as assumed recently by Kreitner [16].)

4. If atrial fibers are partly depolarized artificially they start to show repetitive activity resembling very much the nodal action potentials [10].

5. The membrane of the nodal fibers — and especially of the fibers with a prominent prepotential — is polarized in a potential range in which in the working myocardial fibers a calcium transport system might be activated. Therefore, participation of a calcium inward current in the upstroke of the action potential as well as in the development of the prepotential in fibers of the SA node is very probable. This might explain the sensitivity of these fibers to manganese which is known to have a suppressive effect on the calcium permeability of the membrane. Furthermore, the positive chronotropic effect of adrenaline might be explained by an enhanced calcium inward current leading to a faster slope of the prepotential.

The Effect of Impulse Formation Outside the SA Node on the Behavior of the SA Nodal Fibers

Impulse formation – artificially induced or spontaneous – outside the SA node is called ectopic. Such an ectopic impulse can cause a premature beat. The dominant pacemaker, surrounded by slow-conducting nodal tissue, will be discharged by an ectopic impulse only if it is generated prematurely enough to reach the dominant pacemaker fibers before they discharge spontaneously. As long as the dominant pacemaker is not influenced by the ectopic impulse, the rhythm of the pacemaker is undisturbed and the atrium is activated subsequent to the premature beat with a slightly longer, but exactly compensatory, interval (late atrial premature beats).

If the ectopic impulse is generated earlier in the atrial cycle, the pacemaker in the SA node is discharged and another group of fibers will take over the function of pacemaker for one or a number of beats. The pacemaker shifts over a larger distance within the SA node as the premature impulse comes earlier in the atrial cycle. For a detailed analysis of the effects of atrial premature beats the reader is referred to the studies of Bonke et al. [5], Bonke et al. [6], and Miller and Strauss [21] on the isolated right atrium of the rabbit.

If an impulse from an ectopic pacemaker reaches the border of the SA node, it encounters fibers with a longer refractory period, the perinodal fibers [24], and this becomes more and more pronounced as the impulse penetrates deeper into the SA node. The impulse of very early atrial premature beats will therefore die out in the border of the SA node and only have electrotonic influence on the dominant pacemaker in the center of the SA node [6]. In these cases the rhythm of the dominant pacemaker is practically undisturbed and the atrial premature beat will be an interpolated beat between two spontaneous discharges of the dominant pacemaker in the SA node.

Since the impulse of the premature beat in this case is blocked in the border of the SA node, there is a sinoatrial node entrance block [4, 11, 25]. This conduction block protects the dominant pacemaker.

If ectopic impulse formation continues and a number of atrial premature beats appear, the situation is completely different. The pacemaker in the SA node has lost its dominance, nodal entrance block of varying degree might occur, and part of the SA node might be involved in a re-entry circuit [12]. Therefore, during a series of atrial premature beats or during atrial tachycardia, for instance, induced by a single premature beat [1, 2] or during artificial atrial pacing, the SA node no longer plays a dominant role and resembles the AV node. The effect of artificial drive on the pacemaker activity in the SA node has been investigated by Lange [17] in intact hearts and by Lu et al. [19] in isolated atrial preparations. It turned out that after a period of drive the pacemaker in the SA node did not immediately take over this function but was more or less suppressed. This postdrive suppression was stronger as the period of artificial drive was longer and also appeared to be dependent on the position of the driving electrode. The closer the stimulating electrode to the SA node, the more intensive the postdrive suppression. Lange [17] assumed that the postdrive suppression is — at least partly — due to the liberation of acetylcholine from the terminal vesicles in and around the SA node and the results of her pharmacologic studies on this phenomenon support this assumption. It is also in agreement with the findings of Lu et al. [19] who observed that during overdrive the fibers in the border of the SA node showed some hyperpolarization. In contrast, atrial fibers depolarize when the frequency of stimulation is increased [22].

Some investigators used the interval between the last driven beat and the first spontaneous discharge of the SA node as a measure of the amount of overdrive suppression (sinus node recovery time). However, a number of factors determine this "recovery time," namely the pacing rate, the duration of the pacing, the position of the stimulating electrode, the conduction velocity in the atrium and the SA node, the amount of transmittors — acetylcholine as well as (nor)adrenaline — that are liberated, and of course whether the SA node as a whole is following the stimulation rate or not. At least, it is possible that the first atrial activation after the cessation of the pacing is based on a reentrant beat from the SA node. Some of these factors can be controlled in case of an isolated atrium preparation, but for the human heart in vivo, it is very dangerous, in my opinion, to use the "recovery time" as an indicator of the sinus node function.

In conclusion, the relatively bad conduction properties and the long duration of the action potential of the SA node fibers, protect the SA node against high frequent impulses invading the node from the atrium. Although the blockade of the impulse might occur either at the border of the node or more to the center, it is called in general a sinoatrial entrance block. Once an impulse is generated in the SA node, it is conducted toward the atrium and will excite the atrial fibers. Only if the conduction is disturbed in the border of the node or in the atrium — for instance, because of an increased extracellular potassium concentration — will a sinoatrial exit block occur. In such a case there is a disturbance in conduction and not in impulse formation. In may opinion a lot of things have to happen before the sinus node loses its ability to generate impulses at a regular rate and becomes a sick sinus node.

Summary

As an introduction to clinical studies on the sinus node and the sick sinus syndrome, the electrophysiology of the impulse generation in fibers of the SA node is discussed briefly. In addition, attention is given to the following aspects of SA node function:

1. The conduction of the impulse from the group of fibers that acts as the pacemaker of the heart, via the surrounding nodal fibers, toward the atrial fibers (sinoatrial conduction and sinoatrial conduction time).
2. The effect of atrial premature beats; the difference between late atrial premature beats and early atrial premature beats.
3. The conduction of an impulse from the atrium into the SA node. Can the SA node play a role as part of a reentry circuit?
4. The effect of atrial tachycardia on the discharge pattern of the SA node; the effect of "overdrive suppression".

Acknowledgment

Most of the experiments in which I became familiar with the problems of the electrophysiology of the SA node were done together with Prof. Dr. L. N. Bouman (Department of Physiology of the University of Amsterdam) and some years ago we had long and fruitful discussions on this subject.

References

1. Allessie, M. A., Bonke, F. I. M., Schopman, F. J. G.: Circus movement in rabbit atrial muscle as a mechanism of tachycardia. Circulat. Res., **33**, 54 – 62 (1973)
2. Allessie, M. A., Bonke, F. I. M., Schopman, F. J. G., Lammers, W. J. E. P.: An in vitro model of circulating excitation in the absence of an anatomic obstacle. This volume, p. 175 – 184
3. Bonke, F. I. M.: Electrotonic spread in the sinoatrial node of the rabbit heart. Pflügers Arch. ges. Physiol. **339**, 17 – 23 (1973)
4. Bonke, F. I. M., Allessie, M. A., Bouman, L. N.: Reentry in the atrium. Bull. schweiz. Akad. med. Wiss. **31**, 33 – 44 (1974)
5. Bonke, F. I. M., Bouman, L. N., van Rijn, H. E.: Change of cardiac rhythm in the rabbit after an atrial premature beat. Circulat. Res. **24**, 533 – 544 (1969)
6. Bonke, F. I. M., Bouman, L. N., Schopman, F. J. G.: Effect of an early atrial premature beat on activity of the sionatrial node and atrial rhythm in the rabbit. Circulat. Res. **29**, 704 – 715 (1971)
7. Bouman, L. N., Gerlings, E. D., Biersteker, P. A., Bonke, F. I. M.: Pacemaker shift in the sino-atrial node during vagal stimulation. Pflügers Arch. ges. Physiol. **302**, 255 – 267 (1968)

8. Bouman, L. N., van der Westen, H. M.: Pacemaker shift in the sino atrial node induced by a change of temperature. Pflügers Arch. ges. Physiol. **318,** 262 (1970)
9. Brooks, C. McC., Lu, H. H.: The Sino-Atrial Pacemaker of the Heart. Springfield, Ill.: Charles C. Thomas, 1972
10. Brown, H. F., Noble, S. J.: Membrane currents underlying delayed rectification and pacemaker activity in frog atrial muscle. J. Physiol. **204,** 717 – 736 (1969)
11. Goldberger, B. N., Damato, A. N.: Sino-atrial-node entrance block. Circulation **44,** 789 – 802 (1971)
12. Han, J., Malozzi, A. M., Moe, G. K.: Sino-atrial reciprocation in the isolated rabbit heart. Circulat. Res. **22,** 355 – 362 (1968)
13. Irisawa, H.: Electrical activity of rabbit sino-atrial node. In: Symposium on the Electrical Field of the Heart. (Rylant, P., ed.), Brussels: Presses Académiques Européennes 1972
14. Johnson, E. A., Lieberman, M.: Heart: excitation and contraction. Ann. Rev. Physiol. **33,** 479 – 532 (1971)
15. Kawamura, K., James, T. N.: Comparative ultrastructure of cellular junctions in working myocardium and the conduction system under normal and pathologic conditions. J. Mol. Cell. Cardiol. **3,** 31 – 60 (1971)
16. Kreitner, D.: Evidence for the existence of a rapid sodium channel in the membrane of rabbit sino-atrial cells. J. Mol. Cell. Cardiol. **7,** 655 – 662 (1975)
17. Lange, G.: Action of driving stimuli from intrinsic and extrinsic sources on in situ cardiac pacemaker tissues. Cirulat. Res. **17,** 449 – 459 (1965)
18. Lu, H. H., Brooks, C. McC.: Intranodal shifts of pacemaker action. Circulation **40,** III – 136 (1969)
19. Lu, H. H., Lange, G., Brooks, C. McC.: Factors controlling pacemaker action in cells of the sino-atrial node. Circulat. Res. **17,** 460 – 471 (1965)
20. Mazel, P., Holland, W. C.: Acetylcholine and electrolyte metabolism in the various chambers of frog and turtle heart. Circulat. Res. **6,** 684 – 688 (1958)
21. Miller, H. C., Strauss, H. C.: Measurement of sinoatrial conduction time by premature atrial stimulation in the rabbit. Circulat. Res. **35,** 935 – 947 (1974)
22. Pasmooy, J. H., van Enst, G. C., Bouman, L. N., Allessie, M. A., Bonke, F. I. M.: The effect of heart rate on the membrane responsiveness of rabbit atrial muscle. Pflügers Arch. ges. Physiol. in press (1976)
23. Seifen, E., Schaer, H., Marshall, J. M.: Effect of calcium on the membrane potentials of single pacemaker fibers in isolated rabbit atria. Nature (Lond.) **202,** 1223 – 1224 (1964)
24. Strauss, H. C., Bigger, J. T.: Electrophysiological properties of the rabbit sinoatrial perinodal fiber. Circulat. Res. **31,** 490 – 506 (1972)
25. Strauss, H. C., Saroff, A. L., Bigger, J. T., Giardina, E. G.: Premature atrial stimulation as a key to the understanding of sino-atrial conduction in man. Circulation **47,** 86 – 93 (1973)
26. Toda, N., Shimamoto, K.: The influence of sympathetic stimulation on transmembrane potentials in the SA node. J. Pharmacol. exp. Ther. **159,** 298 – 305 (1968)
27. Toda, N., West, T. C.: Interactions of K, Na and vagal stimulation in the SA node of the rabbit. Amer. J. Physiol. **212,** 424 – 430 (1967)
28. West, T. C.: Ultramicroelectrode recording from the cardiac pacemaker. J. Pharmacol. exp. Ther. **115,** 283 – 290 (1955)

Clinical Aspects of the Sick Sinus Syndrome *

H. P. GURTNER, H. R. LENZINGER, and M. DOLDER

Introduction

The sick sinus syndrome (German, *Sinusknotensyndrom;* French, *maladie de l'oreillette*) encompasses a group of cardiac rhythm disturbances and their corresponding clinical manifestations which, in the last analysis, are a consequence of impaired formation and/or conduction of sinus node impulses [5, 9, 19]. This paper deals with clinical manifestations due to defective sinus node function as well as relevant problems in conjunction with pacemaker therapy. With respect to the latter, it appears reasonable and profitable to present our own findings on the clinical manifestations — which we believe attributable to disturbance of sinus node function — on a group of those of our patients whose illness could only be managed by pacemaker implantation (the mode of patient selection for this topic is presented in more detail under the heading "Discussion").

Material and Methods

During a 3-year 8-month period (January 1972 – September 1975) 259 pacemakers [1] were implanted as lasting therapy in patients presenting with bradycardiac rhythm disturbances at the Section of Cardiology and at the Department of Thoracic and Cardiovascular Surgery, both of the Bern University School of Medicine (see Table 1 for summary of indications).

Pacemakers were implanted in 133 of these patients because of complete atrioventricular (AV) block, but with normal atrial sinus rhythm (51%). A further 16 cases of total AV block were complicated by chronic atrial fibrillation or flutter (6%). Twenty-three cases presented with AV block II with complete right bundle branch block (RBBB) or left bundle branch block (LBBB). There were 12 digitalized cases of cardiac failure with bradycardiac sinus rhythm, atrial fibrillation, flutter, or AV block of second or even higher degree (4.6%), and 14 cases with intermittent or constant bilateral bundle branch block with syncope (5.4%). Finally, permanent pacemaker implantation was carried out in 61 patients (24%) due to chronic sinus bradycardia, episodic sinoatrial (SA) block or arrest, a combination of these disturbances with ectopic tachyventricular escape rhythms (bradycardia-tachycardia syndrome), or due to sinus arrest subsequent to cardioversion. It is this last series of 61 patients, who fulfill the criteria of the sick sinus syndrome, who are the subject of this paper (Table 2).

Patients have been excluded from this study who evidenced either transient sinus bradycardia subsequent to acute myocardial infarction or transient bradycardia-tachycardia syndrome following a surgical intervention in the region of the atria [6, 12], as in circumclusion of atrial septum defects (own observation), during which temporary pacing was utilized.

---

* With support of the Swiss National Fund for the Promotion of Scientific Research and the Swiss Foundation of Cardiology.

[1] Medtronic 5842 or 5944.

Table 1. Indications for pacemaker implantation

Indication	No. of patients
Total AV block (with sinus rhythm)	133
Total AV block (with atrial fibrillation or flutter)	16
AV block II with right or left bundle branch block	23
Sick sinus syndrome	61
Bilateral bundle branch block	14
Digitalized cardiac failure with prominent digitalis induced bradycardia	12
Total	259

Table 2. ECG criteria for diagnosis of sick sinus syndrome

Sinusbradycardia (pulse rate < 50/min)
SA block, sinus arrest
Bradycardia-tachycardia syndrome
Sinus arrest following cardioversion

Results

Patient Distribution According to Age and Sex. As illustrated in Figure 1, 91% of the patients receiving pacemakers were older than 60 years and 51% older than 70. Their average age was 69 (range: 47 – 93 years). The majority of patients were female in the ratio 2 : 1. Our data on age and sex correspond by and large with those in the literature devoted to the sick sinus syndrome even though our average for the age parameter is around 5 years higher [1, 2, 10, 13, 14, 16, 18, 19].

Etiology of the Disease. Allocation of factors causal for or implicated in the sick sinus syndrome into a formalized and meaningful etiologic classification system is indeed a difficult matter as anyone confronted with this task will readily attest. This difficulty was compounded in our own effort since we were required to identify the syndrome retrospectively.

With appropriate consideration and evaluation of anamnestic information and relevant clinical findings (blood pressure, presence and extent of generalized arteriosclerosis, quantity and quality of noxious environmental, i.e., risk factors) we propose that the following disease states observed in association with the syndrome are probably operational and even instrumental in its production (see Table 3 for summary):

1. Ischemic heart disease: 66% of patients, the disease observed most frequently;
2. Hypertension: 41% of patients;
3. Previous diphtheria: 10% of patients;

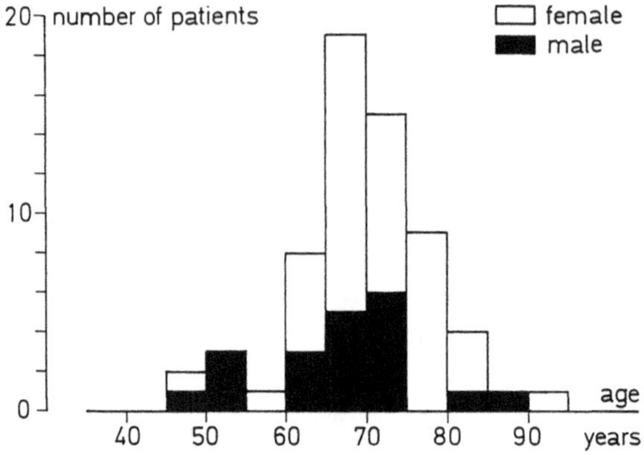

Fig. 1. Age of patients at pacemaker implantation. n=61

Table 3. Diseases associated with sick sinus snydrome

Disease	No. of patients =61 (%)
Coronary heart disease	40 (66)
Systemic hypertension	25 (41)
Diphtheria	6 (10)
Myocarditis	4 (7)
Rheumatic fever	4 (7)
No organic heart disease	2 (3)

4. Previous myocarditis of unknown origin: 7% of patients;
5. Rheumatic fever: 7% of patients, two with childhood rheumatic fever and two with valve lesions of rheumatic origin.

We were unable to implicate organic cardiovascular disease in only two patients (3%). This is a striking finding in comparison with corresponding data in the literature in which this category of the sick sinus patient assumes an important position occurring with a incidence ranging from 34% [10] to as high as 65% [1]. This discrepancy is most likely due to our broader interpretation of acceptable criteria constituting ischemic heart disease which not only include patients with angina pectoris and previous myocardial infarction but also older patients with generalized arteriosclerosis or cardiac failure even in the absence of hypertension, valvular lesion, or demonstrable myocardial lesion (we grant that we have no data — clinical or pathological — to buttress our diagnostic approach). In the literature, the incidence of coronary heart disease given as etiology for the syndrome varies from 14% [14] to 51% [10]. In our own material, we found diphtheria implicated in the sick sinus syndrome in 10% in our patients; other investigators report 6% [14] to 30% [1, 13]. Similar data divergence, with regard to the role of other disease states ultimately leading to myocardial ischemia, inflammation or degeneration, are reported in the literature (1 for review).

Symptoms [2] (Table 4). Syncope, encountered in 69% of our patients (45 – 71%), palpitations in 57% (15 – 59%), and dizziness (blackout) in 46% (7 – 67%) are the most frequently observed symptoms in the sick sinus syndrome. About two-thirds of our patients complained of increased tiredness and decreased performance of daily activities or other signs ascribable to cardiac failure such as dyspnea (at rest or effort) or dependent edema (10 – 70%). Recurrent or episodic attacks of angina pectoris occurred less frequently (20%) (14 – 26%). We observed apoplexy — manifested as transitory

Table 4. Symptoms encountered with sick sinus syndrome

Symptom	No. of patients =61 (%)
Syncope	42 (69)
Dizziness	28 (46)
Blackout, speech disturbance	11 (18)
Palpitations	35 (57)
Angina pectoris	12 (20)
Episodic dyspnea	13 (21)
Decrease in exercice tolerance	37 (61)
Heart failure (right and/or left)	30 (49)
Cerebrovascular insult	6 (10)

hemiplegia or temporary facial paresis — in six patients prior to pacemaker implantation (11 – 18%). None of our patients were asymptomatic. In the literature, the incidence of asymptomatic patients is related to the predominant rhythm disturbance and is highly variable (5 – 62%).

The appearance, development, and course of symptoms associated with the sick sinus syndrome are discussed below as they were observed in a 55-year-old male patient. This case analysis is presented to illustrate some of the varied clinical aspects of the sick sinus syndrome.

Case History (55-year-old white male).

Previous illness: Bouts of febrile tonsillitis in childhood. Purulent appendicitis at age 7. Mumps complicated with orchitis at 30. Cholecystectomy at age 53.

Sick sinus syndrome – related information: When the patient was 45 years old (1965) he first noticed irregularities in pulse rhythm. Four years later (1969) ventricular extrasystole was demonstrated electrocardiographically. During the 4-year interval 1969 – 1973, the patient experienced about 12 episodes of pain and discomfort in the chest which were independent of effort. These symptoms were transitory, lasting only a few minutes. We examined the patient in June,

[2] In the bracket is given the incidence range of individual symptoms as reported by other investigators for patients with the sick sinus syndrome [1, 2, 10, 13, 14, 16, 18, 19].

1973, and noted a sinus bradycardia (42/min.) in association with supraventricular extrasystoles. Following a course of treatment with digitalis and the beta-blocker practolol, the extrasystoles disappeared but the sinus bradycardia remained and alternated — both at rest and during effort — with a simple AV dissociation. After 60 steps in the one-step exercise test, the pulse rate increased from 42 to 85/min. On April 9, 1974, the patient evidenced transitory speech impediment and central facial paresis. The ECG taken during this period revealed supraventricular tachycardia (125/min) with rare ventricular extrasystoles and, later, alternating sinus bradycardia, atrial fibrillation and sinus rhythm.

Due to the above symptomatology, the patient received a permanent cardiac pacemaker on May 5, 1974. Subsequent to this implantation, he has received permanent daily medication — digoxin, 2×25 mg; practolol, 3×100 mg — and has remained essentially asymptomatic. The ECG under this regime first showed sinus rhythm, atrial fibrillation, and flutter, rarely occurring pacemaker escape, and occasional fusion beats, all alternating. A year later (May, 1975) an ECG showed atrial fibrillation with rarely occurring pacemaker escape and fusion beats; at this writing, the patient is doing well.

Analysis of our patient material has revealed the rather astonishing fact that only a small minority of patients were aware of any pulse irregularity or of palpitations prior to medical treatment. It is the exceptional patient, at least in Swiss society, who will palpate his own pulse upon perceiving palpitations, dizziness or clouding of consciousness and determine that it is irregular in rhythm or abnormal in frequency and thus seek professional advice. It is rather the direct perceptible expression of arrhythmia such as dizziness and syncope that arouses apprehension and induces an individual to seek medical help.

Incidence of Syncope Prior to Pacemaker Implantation. Nineteen patients (about 31%) experienced no syncope before receiving a pacemaker; 35 patients (better than 50%) had at least one and at most six attacks of syncope, and around 10% had seven or more before pacemaker implantation.

Incidence of Symptoms Prior to Pacemaker Implantation. More interesting and assertive than the above-mentioned frequency figures which, after all, depend on the subjective evaluation of syncope, is the relationship between the cumulative frequency of symptoms, especially of syncope, and the elapsed, latent period before pacemaker implantation. Figure 2 illustrates that:

1. General symptoms like dizziness, palpitation, dyspnea, and pain occur on the average 3 years before the first syncope.
2. Three years prior to pacemaker implantation 50% of the patients evidenced symptoms but only 10% initial syncope.
3. The history of general symptoms goes back more than 8 years in less than 10% of the patients and the history relating to syncope to more than 5 years in less than 5% of the patients.

Study of Figure 2 shows that the sick sinus syndrome is a chronic illness. As a rule, it persists for years, not months.

Our observations are in general agreement with those in the literature [1, 12–14, 16]. In a few cases, evidence of symptoms may reach back to two decades or even longer.

Arrhythmias in Relation to the Sick Sinus Syndrome. Tables 5 and 6 tabulate the diagnoses made electrocardiographically and prior to pacemaker implantation for our patient group of 61. Relevant diagnostic findings were not obtained with the facilities of either ECG telemetry or of continuously recording magnetic tape but via interpretation of ECGs taken with conventional equipment.

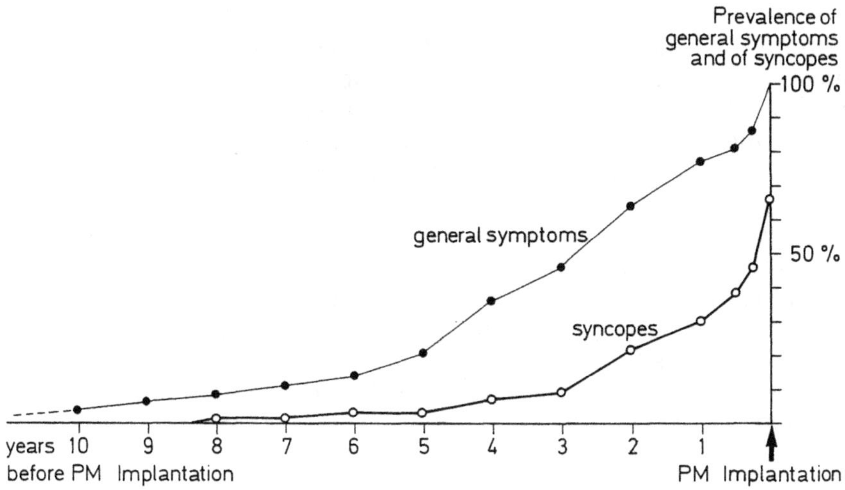

Fig. 2. Prevalence of general symptoms (filled in circles) and syncope (blank circles) in relation to time of appearence before pacemaker implantation

Table 5. Disturbances of impulse formation

Disturbance	No. of patients =61 (%)
Sinus bradycardia	48 (79)
SA block, sinus arrest	40 (66)
AV escape beat, AV escape rhythm	43 (71)
Atrial fibrillation and flutter Atrial tachycardia	44 (72)
Ventricular tachycardia	7 (12)

Table 6. Disturbances of impulse conduction

Disturbance	No. of patients =61 (%)
AV block I	15 (25)
AV block II	10 (16)
AV block III	8 (13)
Total left bundle branch block	6 (10)
Total right bundle branch block	1 (2)
Bilateral bundle branch block	8 (13)
Left anterior fascicular block	1 (2)

Disturbances of Impulse Formation. The frequency of diagnosed disturbances of impulse formation and sinoatrial conduction are given in Table 5. At one time or other before pacemaker installation, four-fifths of all patients evidenced sinus bradycardia and two-thirds sinoatrial block or arrest. AV escape beats and/or rhythms were observed in 71% of patients, ectopic supraventricular tachyarrhythmias in 72%, and episodic ventricular tachycardia in 12%.

Table 5 gives no information on the frequency and duration of the arrhythmic periods and, accordingly, no data on the predominance — related to time — of individual forms of arrhythmias. Since rhythm disturbances so far mentioned did not occur singly but in varying, multiple combinations in the majority of patients (see Table 7), the sums given in Table 5 exceed the extent of the stated absolute and percental values of the sample population (n=61=100%).

Table 7. Patient classification according to ECG criteria

Group, Disturbance	No. of patients =61(%)	AV block I, II, III
Group I		
Sinus bradycardia alone	9 (15)	3
Group II		
SA block or sinus arrest alone	7 (11)	2
Group I+II	17 (28)	5
Group III		
Bradycardia-tachycardia syndrome	28 (46)	12
Total	61 (100)	22

The incidence of additional electrocardiographically demonstrated atrioventricular and intraventricular *disturbances of impulse conduction* (related to patient number) before pacemaker implantation is given in Table 6. Twenty-five percent of these patients evidenced at one time or other an AV block I, 16% an AV block II, and 13% a total AV block. Furthermore, 13% of the patients had bilateral bundle branch block and 10% total left bundle branch block. One patient had total right bundle branch block and one left anterior fascicular block.

Disturbances of impulse formation and conduction viewed individually as isolated phenomena will not, of course, give the observer an integrated appreciation of the total rhythmologic spectrum of the sick sinus syndrome, i.e., individual stones do not constitute a mosaic. A more complete notion is obtained, accordingly, by simultaneous consideration of the varied and ever-fluctuating combinations of rhythm disturbances which are so characteristic of the syndrome. Drawing on the paper by Blömer et al., [1] we have categorized the arrhythmias found in our patient group (Table 7). As indicated in this table, 9 patients (15%) had sinus bradycardia alone and 7 (11%) only sinoatrial block or sinus arrest (with or without AV escape rhythms), i.e., a minority of the patient group. Combination of sinus bradycardia and sinoatrial block was observed twice as frequently (17 patients, 28%). Bradycardia-tachycardia syndrome, diagnosed via composite ECGs, was the most frequent anomaly; it was encountered in almost half of our patients (28 or 46%).

The association of sinus bradycardia and/or sinoatrial block with ectopic tachyarrhythmias was categorized under the bradycardia-tachycardia syndrome only when the ventricular rate at the time of tachycardiac episodes exceeded 100/min. This manner of classification explains the difference in frequency of patients with ectopic tachyarrhythmia (Table 5, n=44) and that of patients with bradycardia-tachycardia syndrome (Table 7, n=28).

Tachycardiac disturbances, usually supraventricular, were associated with sinus bradycardia in 12 patients (20%), with sinoatrial block in 6 (10%), and with combined sinus bradycardia and sinoatrial blockage in another 10 patients (17%).

Additional atrioventricular conduction disturbances are distributed rather uniformly in the groups listed in Table 7. Thus, about 30% of the patients in groups I, II and I+II had additional AV conduction disturbances, which were noted in 40% of patients with bradycardia-tachycardia syndrome. On the average, they were present in 36% of the patient population.

Clinical Course Following Pacemaker Implantation. Findings from follow-up examinations carried out for an average of 15 months on 55 of the 61-patient group are available for analysis (for reasons unknown, 6 patients did not appear for postoperative checkups). Results of pacemaker implantation for patient groups with sinus bradycardia and/or sinoatrial block as well as with bradycardia-tachycardia syndrome are listed separately in Table 8. Clinical response to pacemaker therapy was judged as "good" if syncope and dizziness disappeared, if cardiac failure (with or without glycoside therapy) improved noticeably, and if no further tachycardiac episodes were experi-

Table 8. Clinical success of pacemaker therapy

Group	Pacemaker implantation	No follow-up	Clinical success good	moderate to poor
Group I and or **II:** sinusbradycardia, SA block, sinus arrest	33	2	27	4
Group III: bradycardia-tachycardia syndrome	28	4	19	5
Total	61 (100%)	6 (10%)	46 (75%)	9 (15%)

enced. Response was evaluated as "moderate to poor" if dizziness or blackout were still encountered but no syncope (one exception), if further tachycardia was present despite adequate digitalization, and if no noteworthy improvement of cardiac failure was obtained.

It is concluded that pacemaker therapy is, in general, successful though to a different degree according to the disturbance (86% success with pure bradycardiac forms of sick sinus syndrome and 79% success with bradycardia-tachycardia syndrome). This difference in success is chiefly due to the fact that when digitalis was required along with pacemaker stimulation, only a part of the group III patients were free from tachyarrhythmias. We do not have reliable information or ECG data on patients still experiencing dizziness subsequent to pacemaker implantation which permits association of the symptom with any kind of rhythm disturbance.

Table 9. Sick sinus syndrome: Atrial rhythm after pacemaker implantation

Rhythm	No. of patients =61
Sinus rhythm	20
Sinusbradycardia	19
Atrial fibrillation and flutter	13
Retrograde atrial stimulation (with pacemaker rhythm)	9
Total	61

Atrial Rhythm Following Pacemaker Implantation. ECGs taken immediately after pacemaker insertion showed normal sinus rhythm in 20 patients, sinus bradycardia in 19, atrial fibrillation or flutter in 3, and retrograde atrial excitation in 9 patients (Table 9). The essential tendencies noted in the ECGs were as follows:

1. Ectopic atrial rhythms were only exceptionally encountered in group I and II patients but almost always for those in group III.
2. Conduction of impulses of supraventricular origin — partially as fusion beats — was frequently observed.

Discussion

Those topics will be discussed which are important to the title of this paper, "Clinical Aspects of the Sick Sinus Syndrome".

Diagnosis of the Sick Sinus Syndrome. We must initially point out that the sample population studied is not representative of parameters involved in the syndrome for two reasons.

First, our data arise uniquely from patients who received permanent pacemakers due to cardiac rhythmic disturbances associated with the sick sinus syndrome. This means that none of our findings include patients who were treated conservatively. This conservative group accounts for 15 – 78% of syndrome cases analyzed in the literature [1, 14, 16, 18, 19] and, in the only prospective study we are aware of, for 55% [14]. Second, we also included and evaluated patients who, in addition to suspected sick sinus syndrome, manifested atrioventricular and/or intraventricular conduction disturbances.

We are, to be sure, aware that disturbances in the lower conduction system are frequently observed with the syndrome as documented in numerous electrophysiologic studies [11, 15]. Nevertheless, our findings of 36% (16% for AV block II, and 13% for AV block III) are clearly higher than the percentage reported in the literature (AV block II, 0 – 5% with but a single exception, see [18, 19]; and 0% for AV block III, see [1, 2, 10, 13, 14, 16, 18]). Literature data on the incidence of AV block I and of intraventricular conduction disturbances are lower than ours in some reports [1, 2, 13, 14, 19] and higher in others [34].

It appears reasonable to assume that identification of the sick sinus syndrome in the presence of AV and/or IV conduction disturbances can only be reliable with the help of special investigative techniques. As of now, we have determined neither the sinus node recovery time, the sinoatrial conduction time nor AV conduction components by means of His-bundle electrocardiography. Exceptionally, we have conducted stress and other provocative tests which sometimes reveal impaired sinus function [1].

We wish to defuse any possible objection which may arise as to our inclusion of patients with AV conduction disturbances in whom impairment of sinus node function or sinoatrial conduction was not basic to the origin of the clinical symptomatology, with the following argument:

1. Patients without AV or IV conduction disturbances were included in our study when at least one of the criteria listed in Table 2 was fulfilled.
2. In the presence of AV or IV conduction disturbance, it was required that at least two of the criteria be met.

Future research is required to demonstrate whether or not the above two conditions are adequate and sufficient for identification of the sick sinus syndrome.

In this respect, consideration of the spectrum of indications which have been published by other centers using pacemakers may prove helpful. The fraction of patients with the sick sinus syndrome among those treated with pacemakers varies widely from country to country, e.g., France (Bordeaux) 8%, Germanspeaking regions of Europe, 12.5%, South Africa (Johannesburg) 20% [23]. In a prospective, 5-year Norwegian study [14], 98 patients with AV block and 51 with the sick sinus syndrome were observed, 23 of whom were given pacemakers, a relative frequency of 34%.

Symptoms and Course of the Sick Sinus Syndrome

There is no doubt that the clinical picture of the sick sinus syndrome is a manifestation chiefly of cerebral ischemia and, to a lesser extent, of primary cardiac disease which is partially etiologic. Mindful of the above, it is not surprising to encounter syncope, disorientation, blackout, dizziness, fleeting speech, and word association disturbances as the most obvious clinical expressions of the syndrome. Palpitation, even though signaling attendant arrhythmia immediately, is probably less prominent due to the variation of its awareness from patient to patient. To a variable extent, the clinical picture is supplemented with signs and symptoms of cardiac failure — on effort and at rest — as well as by angina pectoris. Episodes of dyspnea and pain at rest are no rarity. The underlying factor in these episodes (slowing of sinus bradycardia, SA block, or tachyarrhythmias) will vary from patient to patient. Cerebrovascular insult is not frequent but due to its gravity nevertheless important.

There is only a slight correlation between the symptoms and the pattern of the arrhythmia. There is consensus among investigators that syncope associated with the bradycardia-tachycardia syndrome (caused at the termination of a tachyarrhythmic attack by an extended interval until sinus activity or that of a substitute autonomous center sets in) is more frequent than with pure bradycardiac forms of the sick sinus syndrome [1, 16]; in our series, the percentages were 75 and 64%, respectively. In addition, rapid palpitation is limited to patients with the bradycardia tachycardia syndrome, of course. Otherwise, history and patient status do not help in differential diagnostic considerations. For a discussion of findings arising from the use of special techniques — for which we have no experience — see references [3, 21, and 22].

Prognosis of the Sick Sinus Syndrome

The sick sinus syndrome is predominantly an episodic disease and as such comparable to total heart block and to epilepsy. In common with these diseases, the syndrome is chronic and leads to momentary interruption of vital functions. Even in its milder (i.e., syncope-free) form, the sick sinus syndrome, like other paroxysmal arrhythmias, is at least disturbing to the patient [19]. Doubtless, the prognosis of the syndrome is better than that of total heart block [13, 14]. Nevertheless, grave and life-threatening complications do occur such as unexpected cumulative attacks of syncope in cases of long benign course, cerebrovascular insult, and, rarely, fatalities [19].

Little is known regarding the long-term progression of the disease for it has been recognized as an entity, but for a short time and mainly because numerous patients today are fitted with pacemakers. In some patients with the syndrome, repetitive His-bundle recordings have revealed progression of associated AV blockage [11].

Therapy of the Sick Sinus Syndrome

At first glance, it appears self-evident that predominantly bradycardiac forms of the syndrome should be treated with agents promoting an increase of heart rate. Experience — including our own — has shown, however, that except in very mild cases, neither belladona preparations nor, with few exceptions (e.g., 18), sympathicomimetic drugs are capable of accelerating the heart beat or of preventing episodes of cerebral ischemia [1, 8, 14, 16, 18, 24]. The treatment of the bradycardia-tachycardia syndrome with pharmacotherapy has proved especially difficult. This is true since although agents reducing heart rate can abort a tachycardiac episode, they also enhance the basic bradycardiac rhythm and, conversely, acceleration of a slow rhythm can trigger a tachyarrhythmia. Only the cardiac glycosides have been reported to be of occasional help in the prophylaxis of supraventricular tachyarrhythmias, a fact chiefly due to their action of shortening the recovery period of the sinus node without interfering with its inherent rhythmicity [4]. On the whole, however, conservative management of the sick sinus syndrome is unrewarding. It is, therefore, understandable that pacemaker implantation is resorted to more and more as the therapy of preference (survey: 1).

Pacemakers prevent bradycardia and asystole and, therefore, the occurrence of Adams-Stokes attacks. But only in some of the patients with bradycardia-tachycardia syndrome can tachycardiac rhythms be prevented with pacemaker therapy alone. However, in most cases, safe and effective pharmacotherapy along with pacemaker benefits will lead to successful management of the sick sinus syndrome.

Summary

During the last 45 months, 259 permanent pacemakers have been implanted in our hospital. Sixty-one patients (24%) suffered from sick sinus syndrome (SSS) with sinusbradycardia and/or sinoatrial block and/or supraventricular tachyarrhythmias alternating with episodes of bradycardia (bradycardia-tachycardia syndrome [BTS]). Half of the patients with SSS, in addition, had atrioventricular or intraventricular conduction defects. The mean age was 69 years. Females were found twice as often as males. Associated diseases were, in decreasing order, coronary heart disease, hypertension, diphtheria, myocarditis of unknown origin, and rheumatic fever. The clinical symptoms were mainly due to cerebral ischemia or to the associated heart lesion. The main symptoms were syncope, dizziness, blackout, and cerebral insult. Palpitation, angina pectoris, and manifestations of cardiac failure were less common. The clinical course of SSS is chronic, usually extending over years. Syncope was somewhat more frequent in patients with BTS than in patients with bradycardia alone. SSS is best treated with a cardiac pacemaker. Successful treatment with drugs alone is rare, but their use in combination with a pacemaker may prove helpful.

References

1. Blömer, H., Wirtzfeld, A., Delius, W., Sebening, H.: Das Sinusknoten-Syndrom. Z. Kardiol. **64,** 697 – 721 (1975)
2. Conde, C. A., Leppo, J., Lipski, J., Stimmel, B., Litwak, R., Donoso, E., Dack, S.: Effectiveness of pacemaker treatment in the bradycardia tachycardia syndrome. Amer. J. Cardiol. **32,** 209 – 214 (1973)
3. Delius, W., Wirtzfeld, A.: The significance of the sinus node recovery time in the sick sinus syndrome. This volume, p. 25 – 32
4. Engel, T. R., Schaal, S. F.: Digitalis in the sick sinus syndrome. The effects of digitalis on sinoatrial automaticity and atrioventricular conduction. Circulation **48,** 1201 – 1207 (1973)
5. Ferrer, I. M.: The sick sinus syndrome. Circulation **47,** 635 – 641 (1973)
6. Greenwood, R. D., Rosenthal, A., Stoss, L. J., La Corte, M., Nadas, A. S.: Sick sinus syndrome after surgery for congenital heart disease. Circulation **52,** 208 – 213 (1975)
7. Kaplan, B. M., Langendorf, R., Lev, M., Pick, A.: Tachycardia-bradycardia syndrome (so-called "sick sinus syndrome"). Amer. J. Cardiol. **31,** 497 – 508 (1973)
8. Kulbertus, H. E., De Leval-Rutten, F., Demoulin, J. C.: Sino-atrial disease: A report on 13 cases. J. Electrocardiol. **6,** 303 – 312 (1973)
9. Lown, B.: Electrical reversion of cardiac arrhythmias. Brit. Heart J. **29,** 469 – 489 (1967)
10. Moss, A. J., Davis, R. J.: Brady tachy syndrome. Progr. cardiovasc. Dis. **16,** 439 – 454 (1974)
11. Narula, O. S.: Atrioventricular conduction defects in patients with sinus bradycardia. Analysis by His bundle recordings. Circulation **44,** 1096 – 1110 (1971)
12. Niederhauser, H., Simonin, Ph., Friedli, B.: Sinus node function and conduction system after complete repair of tetralogy of Fallot. Circulation **52,** 214 – 220 (1975)
13. Rasmussen, K.: Chronic sinoatrial heart block. Amer. Heart J. **81,** 38 – 47 (1971)
14. Rokseth, R., Hatle, L.: Prospective study on the occurrence and management of chronic sinoatrial disease, with follow-up. Brit. Heart J. **36,** 582 – 587 (1974)
15. Rosen, K. M., Loeb, H. S., Sinno, M. Z., Rahmtoola, S. H., Gunnar, R. M.: Cardiac conduction in patients with symptomatic sinus node disease. Circulation **43,** 836 – 844 (1971)
16. Rubenstein, J. J., Schulman, C. L., Yurchak, P. M,. DeSanctis, R. W.: Clinical spectrum of the sick sinus syndrome. Circulation **46,** 5 – 13 (1972)
17. Seipel, L., Breithardt, G., Both, A., Loogen, F.: Diagnostische Probleme beim Sinusknotensyndrom. Z. Kardiol. **64,** 1 – 12 (1975)
18. Sigurd, B., Jensen, G., Meibom, J., Sandoe, E.: Adams-Stokes syndrome caused by sinoatrial block. Brit. Heart J. **35,** 1002 – 1008 (1973)
19. Slama, R., Waynberger, M., Motte, G., Bouvrain, Y.: La maladie rythmique auriculaire. Arch. Mal. Coeur **62,** 297 – 315 (1969)
20. Steinbeck, G., Koerber, H.-J., Lüderitz, B.: Die Bestimmung der sinuatrialen Leitungszeit beim Menschen durch gekoppelte atriale Einzelstimulation. Klin. Wschr. **52,** 1151 – 1157 (1974)
21. Steinbeck, G., Lüderitz, B.: Sinus node recovery time and sinoatrial conduction time. This volume, p. 45 – 57
22. Strauss, H. C., Wallace, A. G.: Premature atrial stimulation for evaluation of sinoatrial conduction in man. This volume, p. 33 – 44
23. Thalen, H. J. Th. (ed): Cardiac pacing. In: Proc. IV Internat. Symposium, Groningen. Assen: Van Gorcum, 1973
24. Wan, S. H., Lee, G. S., Toh, C. C. S.: The sick sinus syndrome. A study of 15 cases. Brit. Heart J. **34,** 942 – 952 (1972)

The Significance of the Sinus Node Recovery Time in the Sick Sinus Syndrome

W. Delius and A. Wirtzfeld

The phenomenon of the preautomatic interval after cessation of an artificially induced tachycardia has been known since the animal experiments of Gaskell in 1884 [8]. During the last 15 years numerous electrophysiologic experiments have contributed to our understanding of the transient suppression in sinus node automaticity induced by rapid atrial pacing [1, 11, 13]. The results suggest that the initially negative chronotropic effect on the normal sinus node is at least partly due to a release of acetylcholine by the electrostimulation but that in addition alterations of the extracellular potassium and sodium concentration as well as changes in membrane permeability may be involved.

Clinical cases of an impaired sinus nodal automaticity after termination of paroxysmal tachycardias were described in the past [12]. But the significance and high incidence of this phenomenon has only recently been appreciated, thanks to the modern methods of continuous ECG monitoring on magnetic tapes [3, 4, 7, 9, 10, 14, 18, 19, 20, 21, 26]. The longest preautomatic interval we were able to record on ECG tape was on a patient with spontaneously terminating atrial fibrillation, the interval amounting to 9.6 s. Prolonged preautomatic intervals or "sinus node recovery times" could also be demonstrated in patients with the sick sinus syndrome treated by cardiac pacing, if the pulse generator was inactivated by external chest wall stimulation.

Various test methods had been developed in order to differentiate between normal and disturbed sinus node function. Among these the determination of the sinus recovery time (SNRT) after atrial stimulation has gained wide acceptance. The SNRT is defined as the interval between the last artificially induced atrial systole and the first sinus beat after cessation of pacing. On discussing the significance of the SNRT one has to consider, however, that this definition can not be entirely satisfactory, as it includes the sinoatrial conduction time which might be normal or pathologically prolonged. Besides, the data of different centers regarding the incidence of a pathologically prolonged SNRT in patients with the clinical picture of the sick sinus syndrome are variable, varying from 35 – 93% of the cases [7, 10, 14, 16, 18, 19]. Accordingly, different views are taken confirming the clinical significance of the SNRT. In view of the different results published by various authors, an investigation of those factors that might influence the length of the recovery time appears necessary.

Methods and Patients

A unipolar pacing electrode was introduced into the right atrium under X-ray control and placed near the sinoatrial node or in the right atrial appendix. The stimulation was carried out with the double diastolic threshold with stimulating rates between 80 and 150 min, starting with the lowest frequency and increasing the stimulating rate by steps of 10 impulses per minute. On each step, pacing was performed for 30 s and then the stimulation was stopped for another period of 30 s. Besides the absolute SNRT (upper limit 1400 ms) and the corrected recovery time (difference between absolute recovery time minus average P – P interval prior to stimulation, upper limit 525 ms [16]), the total interval following cessation of pacing until the prepacing sinus rate had been reestablished was determined; this interval was called the "entire SNRT". In seven patients, the arterial pressure was monitored during the procedure with an indwelling catheter in the brachial artery. Atrial stimulation, starting again with the lowest rate, was subsequently repeated after i.v. injection of 1.0 mg of atropine. Digitalis as well as antiarrhythmic drugs were discontinued at least 5 days prior to the examination.

Twenty-one patients (13 females and 8 males between the ages of 19 and 80) were admitted to our study, all of whom fulfilled the diagnostic criteria for the sick sinus syndrome as established by Ferrer [7]. The various arrhythmias observed in our patients were recorded on routine ECG registrations or during ECG magnetic tape recording. Of 21 patients, 19, i.e., 90% of the cases, turned out to have a SNRT over 1400 ms and in 80% of the patients the corrected SNRT was longer than 525 ms. Only in two cases was the SNRT normal at every pacing rate although the symptomatology and the underlying cardiac arrhythmias of these patients did not differ from those who showed prolonged SNRT. The reproductibility of the test results proved to be good. According to Seipel et al. [19], the absolute deviations on repeated pacing are longer in patients with long recovery intervals but the relative changes in comparison to the length of the recovery interval are small. Normalization of a pathologically prolonged interval on repeating the test was never observed. The duration of pacing does not significantly influence the SNRT [14, 15], but in general, a stimulation time of at least 30 s is used; an SNRT of several seconds duration may be observed after only a few seconds of pacing or of spontaneously occurring and terminating atrial tachyarrhythmias.

Of greater significance for the SNRT is the pacing rate. Whereas in normals a variation in stimulating rate does not significantly influence the recovery time, most authors found an increase of the SNRT on increasing the pacing rate in patients with disturbed sinus node function [7, 9, 14, 16, 19]. It has also been described that the SNRT increases with higher pacing rates, reaching its maximum at the frequency of 120 – 130/min and decreasing thereafter. In our experience, however, it is not sufficient to pace only at the higher rates, as there is no way to predict in an individual case at which rate the longest preautomatic interval is to be expected. In 14 out of 21 patients we found the maximal interval at pacing rates below 120/min. On confining the stimulation test to rates above 100/min only, there would have been quite a few patients in whom no pathologic prolongation of the SNRT would have been demonstrated. The diagnostic significance, especially of the low stimulating rates, may be documented in the following examples:

In the case of a 75-year-old male with the typical symptomatology of the sick sinus syndrome, a stimulating rate of 80/min was sufficient to suppress sinus nodal automaticity for 4 s. At the highest stimulating rate of 90/min, the sinus node recovery interval could not be determined because prolonged asystole developed and the external pacemaker had to be switched on after 7 s in order to avoid a syncopal attack. This example suggests an extreme sensitivity to low-frequency stimulation of an apparently severely damaged sinus node and it demonstrates how much the patient might be endangered by spontaneously occurring ectopic atrial activity.

In another patient, a 39-year-old woman with symptomless bradycardia, an SNRT of 3.2 s was seen following atrial pacing at rates between 65 and 80/min. On increasing frequency, the SNRT shortened progressively and at a rate of 130 and above the absolute as well as the corrected recovery times were normal.

In this case, besides a progressive shortening of the recovery time on increasing stimulating rates, another remarkable phenomenon could be observed: the depressive effect on the sinus node was more pronounced in the 2nd and 3rd P – P intervals following cessation of pacing so that these intervals turned out to be longer than the actual SNRT. After the administration of atropine, the recovery intervals were almost normal. Therefore, there seems to be an increased sensitivity to vagal influences of the sinus node automaticity or the conducting tissue at the sinoatrial junction. It is conceivable that the release of acetylcholine from parasympathetic nerve endings by atrial stimulation may be operative and that this parasympathetic effect is neutralized by atropine. The possibility must be recognized, however, that the observed shortening of the SNRT upon increasing stimulating rates may not be real but rather an expression of a sinus node entrance block occurring at higher rates.

SNRT Following Atropine Administration

The effect of atropine on the length of the SNRT was evident in most patients (Fig. 1). In 16 out of 19 cases there was a more or less pronounced shortening of the absolute as well as the corrected SNRT. In two of the seven cases showing normal intervals following atropine administration, however, the SNRT was below 1400 ms prior to administration of the drug. It was impressive that in the remaining five patients with normalized SNRT following atropine administration, the longest pretreatment intervals had been found at relatively low stimulating rates. In one case, for

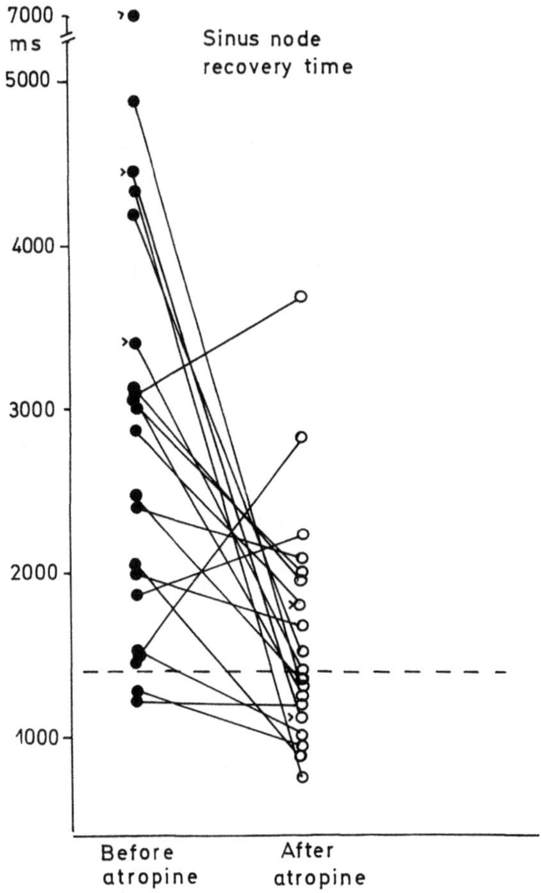

Fig. 1. Maximal SNRT prior to and following administration of atropine. Circles marked by > signify appearance of junctional escape beats after cessation of pacing so that a longer interval than the one depicted must be assumed. Dashed line marks upper limit of normal (1400 ms).

instance, atrial pacing at the rate of 80/min was followed by an interval of 3000 ms, in another case by an interval of 4880 ms; following atropine the recovery times amounted to 1200 and 1320 ms, respectively. In two cases the recovery times could not be determined because of AV nodal escape systoles occurring before the sinus node had taken over. Finally, there were three patients who showed a paradoxical prolongation of the SNRT following atropine, a phenomenon which has also been described by other groups in a few cases [2, 10, 19, 22]. This might be explained on the assumption that atropine had improved the retrograde sinoatrial conduction, thereby permitting the sinus node to be depolarized by higher stimulating rates [10, 19, 20].

The Significance of the "Entire SNRT"

Not only the SNRT proper but the total interval following cessation of pacing until the prepacing sinus rate has been reestablished, seems to be important. Even in cases with a normal sinus node function the depressive effect of the overdrive stimulation appears not to be restricted exclusively to the first P – P interval following stimulation but it can be demonstrated also to be operative following the next spontaneous beats. In our control group this effect lasted for 3.8 s on the average. This interval, "the entire SNRT", was determined in 17 patients with a sick sinus syndrome and amounted to 6000 ± 3800 ms at the rate of 90/min and reached its mean maximum of 8300 ± 7450 ms at the rate of 120/min. As compared to the controls, these intervals were significantly prolonged. As a matter of fact this "entire SNRT" includes sinoatrial conduction as well and will be prolonged if SA conduction is impaired.

An additional and — in our experience — a very characteristic phenomenon on the poststimulating period in patients with the sick sinus syndrome is the appearance of AV nodal escape systoles. In our patients, junctional beats were seen in one-third of the cases prior to and in over two-thirds following the administration of atropine. Apparently the positive bathmotropic effect of atropine cannot affect a damaged sinus node to its normal extent but is able to accelerate the AV node. As is demonstrated in Figure 2, the SNRT may be normal or only slightly prolonged despite the second P – P interval being markedly longer. The relatively short interval between the last artificially stimulated atrial systole and the first sinus beat has been explained on the basis of a sinus node reentry phenomenon or as evidence of the retrograde sinus nodal entrance block explained before [22]. In any event, the measured interval, i.e., the interval between the last stimulated P wave and the first spontaneous atrial depolarization would not represent the true SNRT.

Finally, there might be an additional mechanism influencing the length of the P – P intervals after overdrive pacing. The marked alterations in arterial pressure occurring after cessation of pacing which are dependent upon the cycle length of the preceding diastoles (Fig. 2), will activate baroreflex mechanisms which might subsequently influence the automaticity of the sinus node as well as the conducting properties at the SA junction. In this context some results of former investigations performed by our group in Uppsala, Sweden, measuring sympathetic activity in peripheral nerves should be considered. These studies demonstrated a close baroreflex-mediated relation between sympathetic activity and changes in arterial pressure [5, 6, 23, 24, 25]. Depending on the heart rate, an acute rise in arterial pressure may influence the next or the following interval as the time required for reflex conduction from the baroreceptors to the heart only takes about 475 ms [5, 17]. Such a mechanism may be operative in those cases that show a normal or only slightly prolonged SNRT but a much longer 2nd P – P interval. In the example shown in Figure 2 the inhibitory effect of the rise in blood pressure apparently primarily influences the sino-

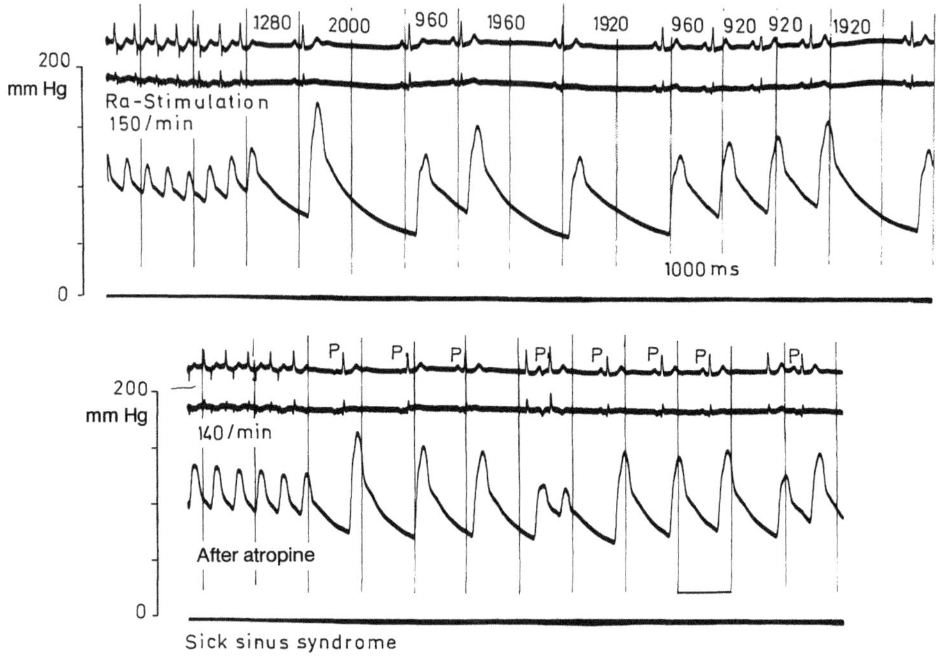

Fig. 2. Apparent influence of arterial pressure (dependent upon cycle length of preceding diastole) on length of P – P intervals following cessation of pacing. Ever acute rise in blood pressure obviously produces a (baroreflex-mediated?) 2 : 1 sinoatrial exit block (*upper tracing*). After atropine the inhibitory effect of blood pressure is no longer present (*lower tracing*).

atrial conduction because it provokes a 2 : 1 sinus nodal exit block. Following the drop in pressure, on the other hand, sympathetic activity decreases and the inhibitory effect on SA conduction is abolished, as evidenced by the shorter P – P-cycle length. This hypothesis is supported by the observation, that following atropine administration the P – P interval is much less dependent on the arterial pressure.

Conclusions

In summarizing our experiences on the SNRT in patients with the sick sinus syndrome, the following conclusions may be drawn:

An SNRT over 1400 ms is suggestive of the diagnosis of the sick sinus syndrome; in some cases this might imply a reduction in the sinus node automaticity whereas in other cases there may be a primary disturbance in sinoatrial conduction. The diagnosis may be further confirmed by the additional finding of a pathologic prolongation of the SNRT following atropine administration. Besides, the consideration of the "entire SNRT," i.e., the total poststimulation period until return of the prestimulation sinus rate, may be important. The frequent occurrence of junctional escape beats and escape rhythms, especially after atropine administration, is a further sign of an impaired sinus node function. The clinical significance of an SNRT which is prolonged prior to Atropine but normalizes after atropine administration is less certain. But even in cases with a typical sick sinus syndrome, an enhanced sensitivity of the SA node to parasympathetic influences which may be mediated by baroreflex mechanisms induced by abrupt changes secondary to alterations in heart rate appears to be operative. Our observations suggest that this inhibitory effect preferentially influences sinoatrial conduction rather than the automaticity of the SA node.

Summary

The sinus node recovery time (SNRT) prior to and following administration of atropine has been investigated in 30 patients with the clinical diagnosis of sick sinus syndrome and the results are extensively discussed and compared with those of other groups. From our study the following conclusions may be drawn: An SNRT over 1400 ms strongly suggests the diagnosis of a sick sinus syndrome; normal values are unusual in this syndrome. Characteristically the SNRT remains prolonged even after administration of atropine. Further information concerning a disturbed sinus node function may be obtained by assessing the total poststimulation period, i.e., the interval until the return of the patient's original rate and rhythm. This interval tends to be markedly prolonged in patients with the sick sinus syndrome; in addition AV escape beats and rhythms may be observed, particularly after atropine administration. The clinical significance of a pathologic SNRT which normalizes after atropine is less well known. An enhanced sensitivity of the sinus node to vagal stimuli may play an important part in these cases.

References

1. Amory, D. W., West, T. C.: Chronotropic response following direct electrical stimulation of the isolated sinoatrial node: A pharmacologic evaluation. J. Pharmacol. exp. Ther. **137**, 14 – 23 (1962)
2. Bashour, T., Hemb, R., Wickramesekaran, R., Strauss, H. C., Bigger, J. T.: An unusual effect of atropine on overdrive suppression. Circulation **48**, 911 – 912 (1973)
3. Bleifeld, W., Rupp, M., Fleischmann, D., Effert, S.: Syndrom des kranken Sinusknotens. Dtsch. med. Wschr. **99**, 795 – 802 (1974)
4. Blömer, H., Wirtzfeld, A., Delius, W., Sebening, H.: Das Sinusknoten-Syndrom. Z. Kardiol. **64**, 697 – 721 (1975)
5. Delius, W., Hagbarth, K.-E., Hongell, A., Wallin, B. G.: General characteristics of sympathetic activity in human muscle nerves. Acta physiol. scand. **84**, 65 – 81 (1972)
6. Delius, W., Wallin, G., Hallén, A., Sundlöf, G.: Registrierung sympathischer Nervenaktivität beim Menschen während elektrischer Stimulation der Carotissinusnerven. Verh. dtsch. Ges. Kreisl.-Forsch. **39**, 240 – 243 (1973)
7. Ferrer, I.: The sick sinus syndrome. Circulation **47**, 635 – 641 (1973)
8. Gaskell, W. H.: On the innervation of the heart with especial reference to the heart of the tortoise. J. Physiol. **4**, 43 (1884)

9. Grohmann, H. W., Theisen, K., Halbritter, R., Jahrmärker, H.: Zum Verhalten des Sinusknotens bei der Vorhofstimulation. Verh. dtsch. Ges. inn. Med. **78**, 1091 – 1093 (1972)
10. Gupta, P. K., Lichstein, E., Chadda, K. D., Badui, E.: Appraisal of sinus nodal recovery time in patients with sick sinus syndrome. Amer. J. Cardiol. **34**, 265 – 260 (1974)
11. Lange, G.: Action of driving stimuli from intrinsic and extrinsic sources on in situ cardiac pacemaker tissues. Circulat. Res. **17**, 449 – 459 (1965)
12. Levine, S. A.: Observations on sino-auricular heart block. Arch. int. Med. **17**, 153 – 175 (1916)
13. Lu, H. H., Lange, G., Brooks, Ch.: Factors controlling pacemaker action in cells of the sinoatrial node. Circulat. Res. **17**, 460 – 471 (1965)
14. Mandel, W. J., Hayakawa, H., Allen, H. N., Danzig, R., Kermaier, A. I.: Assesment of sinus node function in patients with the sicksinus syndrome. Circulation **46**, 761 – 769 (1972)
15. Moss, A. J., Davis, R. J.: Brady-tachy syndrome. Progr. cardiovasc. Dis. **16**, 439 – 454 (1974)
16. Narula, O. S., Samet, P., Javier, R. P.: Significance of the sinusnode recovery time. Circulation **45**, 140 – 158 (1972)
17. Pickering, T. G., Davies, J.: Estimation of the conduction time of the baroreceptor – cardiac reflex in man. Cardiovasc. Res. **7**, 213 – 219 (1973)
18. Rosen, K. M., Loeb, H. S., Sinno, M. Z., Rahimtoola, S. H., Gunnar, R. M.: Cardiac conduction in patients with symptomatic sinus node disease. Circulation **43**, 836 – 844 (1971)
19. Seipel, L., Breithardt, G., Both, A., Loogen, F.: Diagnostische Probleme beim Sinusknotensyndrom. Z. Kardiol. **64**, 1 – 12 (1975)
20. Steinbeck, G., Körber, H. J., Lüderitz, B.: Die Bestimmung der sinuatrialen Leitungszeit beim Menschen durch gekoppelte atriale Einzelstimulation. Klin. Wschr. **52**, 1151 – 1157 (1974)
21. Strauss, H. C., Saroff, A. L., Bigger, J. T., Giardina, E. G. V.: Premature atrial stimulation as a key to the understanding of sinoatrial conduction in man. Circulation **47**, 86 – 93 (1973)
22. Ticzon, A. R., Strauss, H. C., Gallagher, J. G., Wallace, A. G.: Sinus nodal function in the intact dog heart evaluated by premature atrial stimulation and atrial pacing. Amer. J. Cardiol. **35**, 492 – 503 (1975)
23. Wallin, G., Delius, W., Hagbarth, K.-E.: Comparison of sympathetic nerve activity in normotensive and hypertensive subjects. Circulat. Res. **33**, 9 – 21 (1973)
24. Wallin, B. G., Delius, W., Sundlöf, G.: Human muscle nerve sympathetic activity in cardiac arrhythmias. Scand. J. clin. Lab. Invest. **34**, 293 – 300 (1974)
25. Wallin, G., Delius, W.: Neue Aspekte zur sympathischen Kontrolle der Haut- und Muskelgefäße beim wachen Menschen. Klin. Wschr. **52**, 457 – 465 (1974)
26. Wirtzfeld, A., Sebening, H.: Das Sinusknotensyndrom. Dtsch. med. Wschr. **98**, 1 – 7 (1973)

Premature Atrial Stimulation for Evaluation of Sinoatrial Conduction in Man

H. C. STRAUSS and A. G. WALLACE

Recent interest in the pathophysiology of sinus node dysfunction has stimulated the development of techniques that would provide a means of quantitating disturbances of sinoatrial conduction and sinus node automaticity in this group of patients [3, 6, 7, 8, 10, 11, 14, 15, 18, 20, 23, 25, 28, 30]. Such information might be useful not only in the understanding of the underlying pathophysiology but might also provide some insight into the mechanism(s) by which cardioactive agents depress sinus node function. A lack of such knowledge undoubtedly contributes to our empiricism in the selection of safe pharmacologic agents for use in these patients. One such example is the effects of digitalis in patients with sick sinus syndrome. Greenwood and Finkelstein in a review of the literature stated that 22% of all reported instances of sinoatrial (SA) block were due to digitalis excess [9]. It would not be unreasonable to assume that digitalis would cause SA block in a large number of patients with sinus node dysfunction, yet, except for the occasional patient with sinus node dysfunction [16], most of these patients tolerate digitalis remarkably well [6]. Another such example relates to the effects of quinidine and procainamide in patients with the brady-cardia-tachycardia syndrome. Short reported on the markedly depressant effect of these drugs in his patients [24]. Yet we have since come to realize that not all patients with the brady-tachy syndrome experience a marked depression of sinus node function during therapy with procainamide or quinidine. Thus, the electrocardiographic descriptors seem to be incapable of predicting which patients will tolerate the effects of different pharmacologic agents and which patients will not. Variation in response to a given pharmacologic agent could therefore reflect different degrees of depression of sinus node automaticity and/or sinoatrial conduction in these patients. For these reasons documentation of the disturbances of sinus node automaticity and/or sinoatrial conduction in patients with sinus node dysfunction may be of therapeutic benefit to these patients.

It is the purpose of the present communication to discuss sinoatrial conduction disturbances in patients with sinus node dysfunction. An understanding of the pathophysiology of sinoatrial conduction disturbances is facilitated by our consideration of the results of in vitro experiments performed on isolated rabbit right atrial preparations [19, 22, 26]. Impulses formed within the sinus node propagate through the zone of perinodal fibers to the crista terminalis where they then spread to activate the rest of

Supported in part by U.S. Public Health Service Grants HL-15190, HL-08845, HL-05736, the Walker P. Inman Fund, and a N. C. Heart Association Grant-In-Aid, and by RR-30 from the General Clinical Research Centers Program of the Division of Research Resources, NIH.

the atrium. Failure of impulse propagation could therefore occur either in the sinus node proper or in the zone of perinodal fibers. In either case the disturbance would result in the absence of a P wave and this could be diagnosed as second degree SA block. A less or more severe disturbance of sinoatrial conduction (1st or 3rd degree SA block) cannot be detected using conventional electrocardiographic recording techniques.

In 1906, Wenckebach postulated that an atrial premature depolarization (APD or A_2) could gain access to the sinus node, reset it, and the resulting atrial return cycle (A_2A_3) would therefore be determined by the retrograde conduction time between the atrium and the sinus node, the sinus node return cycle, and the antegrade conduction time between the sinus node and atrium [32]. Langendorf et al. [13], in an analysis of the electrocardiographic records of a patient with atrial parasystole, stated that the atrial response to the variably coupled APDs was determined in part by the sinoatrial conduction times. With this background we began to investigate the atrial responses to APDs in patients with sinus node dysfunction. Using routine electrophysiologic stimulation and recording techniques, programmed stimuli were delivered through two poles of an atrial electrode catheter so that APDs were elicited following every eighth spontaneous sinus cycle (A_1A_1). The A_1A_2 interval was varied so that APDs were elicited at different coupling intervals throughout diastole. The last undisturbed sinus cycle (A_1A_1), the cycle terminated by an APD (A_1A_2), the return cycle (A_2A_3), and the postreturn cycle (A_3A_4) were measured. The A_1A_2, A_2A_3, and A_3A_4 intervals were normalized by dividing each by the A_1A_1 cycle. The normalized A_2A_3 and A_3A_4 cycles were plotted as a function of the normalized A_1A_2 cycle as shown in Figure 1. Late APDs (long A_1A_2 intervals) were invariably followed by compensatory return cycles (A_2A_3); as the A_1A_2 coupling interval decreased, the A_2A_3 cycles became less than compensatory.

We reasoned that A_2A_3 cycles were compensatory ($A_1A_2 + A_2A_3 = 2\,A_1A_1$) and fell about the compensatory line in Figure 1 a and b because the APDs failed to gain access to the sinus node and collisions between the emerging sinus node impulse and the retrogradely conducting A_2 were occurring somewhere between the sinus node and the crista terminalis [26, 30]. Atrial premature depolarizations followed by such compensatory A_2A_3 cycles were said to be elicited during zone I of the spontaneous sinus cycle. As A_1A_2 decreased, A_2A_3 cycles became less than compensatory, but constant in duration and formed a plateau in the graph depicted in Figure 1 a. The duration of the A_2A_3 response in the plateau was determined by the sum of the $A_2SAN_2 + SAN_2SAN_3 + SAN_3A_3$ intervals. If sinus node automaticity was undisturbed by A_2 then it would seem likely that SAN_1SAN_1 or A_1A_1 would equal SAN_2SAN_3 and $A_2A_3 - A_1A_1$ would therefore equal $A_2SAN_2 + SAN_3A_3$. This value derived by subtracting the A_1A_1 cycle from the A_2A_3 cycle should correspond to a value that is double the sinoatrial conduction time. It also follows that changes in either the A_2SAN_2 or the SAN_2SAN_3 or the SAN_3A_3 intervals would be reflected in a change in the estimated "sinoatrial conduction time" (SACT). Early APDs were shown to

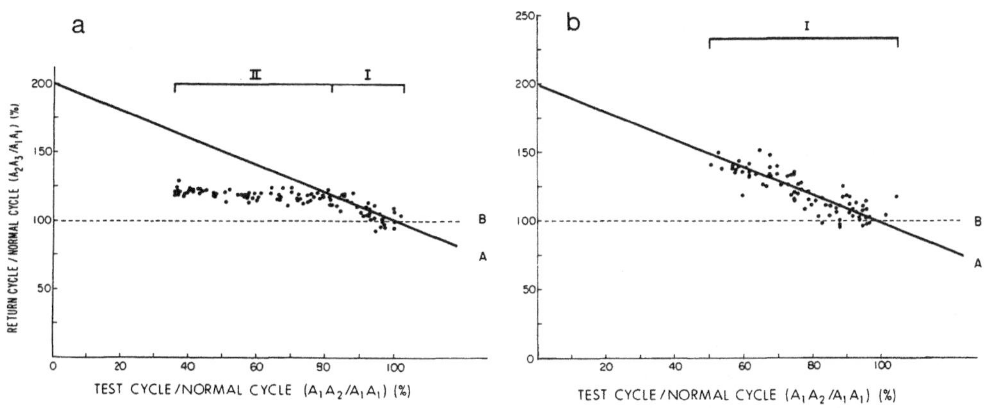

Fig. 1 a and b. Return cycles are plotted as a function of test cycles for two patients [30]. The return (A_2A_3) and premature (A_1A_2) cycles are normalized by dividing them by the last undisturbed spontaneous sinus cycle (A_1A_1). The compensatory line *A* is shown in both panels. Line *B* represents value of one A_1A_1 cycle. The mean value for the A_1A_1 cycle for all data points depicted in panel (a) is 1176 ms. In panel (a), late in diastole, atrial premature depolarizations (APDs-A_2) are followed by compensatory A_2A_3 cycles, which fall about the compensatory line (zone I). As A_1A_2 decreases, A_2A_3 cycles become less than compensatory, fall below line *A*, and form a plateau in zone II. Points in the last third of the plateau in zone II (65 – 80% of the A_1A_1 cycle) are selected for further analysis. The mean values of the A_1A_1 and A_2A_3 cycles were 1179 ± 50 ms (M ± SD) and 117.1 ± 3.26%. The slope of the line through these points is – 0.036. The estimated SACT is 202 ms. In panel (b), zone I is markedly prolonged. Since the mean value for the A_1A_1 cycle is 949 ms at an A_1A_2 coupling interval of 48.9%, compensatory responses are still present and estimated $SACT_{A+R}$ has to exceed 464 ms. (Reproduced by permission of Circulation)

depress sinus node automaticity and to encounter refractoriness in the sinus node and perinodal fibers so that retrograde conduction to the sinus node (A_2SAN_2) was prolonged [1, 12, 26]. To minimize such complications, we believe that only the A_2A_3 cycles falling in the last third of zone II (adjacent to zone I) should be used in the calculation of the estimated SACT.

Using such an approach, the plateau in zone II is identified in a graph, divided into thirds, and the A_1A_1, A_2A_3, and A_3A_4 cycles falling in the last third are selected for analysis and their mean values determined. In addition, we perform a regression analysis on the values of the normalized A_2A_3 and A_1A_2 cycles. The number of APDs that should be introduced and therefore the number of cycles that should be analyzed in the calculation of the estimated SACT is determined by the range of spontaneous sinus cycle length. If marked sinus arrhythmia is present, marked scatter in data point distribution occurs and prevents the estimation of SACT. To estimate SACT when sinus arrhythmia is moderate, a greater number of APDs would have to be elicited than when sinus arrhythmia is absent. Differences in the number of APDs required to estimate SACT would be due to: 1. variation of sinoatrial conduction time with sinus arrhythmia; 2. cyclic variation in sinus cycle length, so that when A_1A_1 is progressively decreasing in value, an A_2 elicited at an A_1A_2 coupling interval will be followed by shorter SAN_2SAN_3 and A_2A_3 cycles than an A_2 elicited at an identical coupling interval when A_1A_1 is progressively increasing in value; and 3. variation in autonomic nervous system tone. Thus, in patients with sinus arrhythmia the number of cycles that should be analyzed will depend on the magnitude of the variation in spontaneous sinus cycle length. Finally, in patients with spontaneous second degree SA block, the prolonged A_2A_3 cycles resulting from blockade of the sinus node impulse following A_2 may reflect either its spontaneous occurrence or an unmasking of SA block. Hence, determination of whether a prolonged A_2A_3 cycle compatible with second degree SA block is due to its spontaneous occurrence or to its being unmasked by an APD will depend on the frequency with which spontaneous SA block occurs.

According to the Wenkebach hypothesis, to derive a value for the estimated SACT, it should not matter whether the transition between zones I or II or the A_2A_3 cycles falling in the last third of zone II are used. However, in almost all of the animal studies and many of the human studies, the A_1A_2 interval at which A_2A_3 becomes less than compensatory and the A_1A_2 interval at which A_2A_3 becomes constant and forms a plateau in the graph do not closely agree [27].

Studies designed to evaluate the accuracy of the premature atrial stimulation technique in the estimation of the sinoatrial conduction time also demonstrated why deviation from the compensatory line did not coincide with sinus node capture and reset by the APD [17]. In such studies performed on isolated rabbit right atrial preparations, recordings of transmembrane action potentials from the sinus node and bipolar electrogram recordings from the crista terminalis showed that late APDs failed to capture the sinus node and were followed by compensatory A_2A_3 cycles [17]. As the A_1A_2 coupling interval decreased the sinus node action potentials, sinus node and atrial return cycles began to shorten. The shortening of the A_2A_3 cycle prior to sinus node capture indicated that deviation from the compensatory line did not coincide with sinus node reset. The shortening of the sinus node action potential, sinus node, and atrial return cycles following A_2 indicated that the use of the premature atrial stimulation technique in measuring SACT will result in an underestimation of the real value. If the retrograde and antegrade sinoatrial conduction time ($SACT_{R+A}$) equals 200 ms and the error corresponds to the range of shortening of sinus node action potentials seen in our in vitro study (6 – 54 ms), then the error of the estimated $SACT_{R+A}$ will range from –3 to –27% [17]. These findings would also serve to explain the gradual transition from the compensatory response to the plateau response, seen in the feline, lapine, canine, and some of the human studies [2, 5, 17, 27 – 29, 31]. Thus, the findings of our in vitro study would seem to be relevant to the clinical studies in those instances where there is a gradual transition from the compensatory response to the plateau response. If deviation from the compensatory line does not coincide with sinus node capture, should the value of the A_2A_3 cycle on deviation from the compensatory line, or in the plateau, be used to calculate the SACT? The experimental data depicted in Figure 2 a and b provides the answer to this question. In this experiment, APDs were elicited at different coupling intervals and the normalized A_2A_3, A_3A_4, and SAN_2SAN_3 cycles were plotted as a function of the normalized A_1A_2 cycles. As the antegrade SACT was 140 ms, reset only occurred with APDs elicited at A_1A_2 coupling intervals less than 45% of the spontaneous sinus cycle, and yet deviation from the compensatory line occurred at an A_1A_2 coupling interval 75% of A_1A_1.

That the deviation from the compensatory line should not closely agree with sinus node capture, even when the sinoatrial conduction time is long, is not surprising. The sinoatrial conduction time is determined not only by the distance of the sinus node from the crista terminalis but also by factors that determine conduction velocity, such as membrane capacitance, the radius of the fibers, intercellular resistance, the values of the ionic conductances, the ionic driving forces that occur during depolarization, and the length constant. The shortening of the sinus node action potential, which is due to electrotonic interactions between cells during a change in activation sequence of cells around the sinus node, should be determined by the

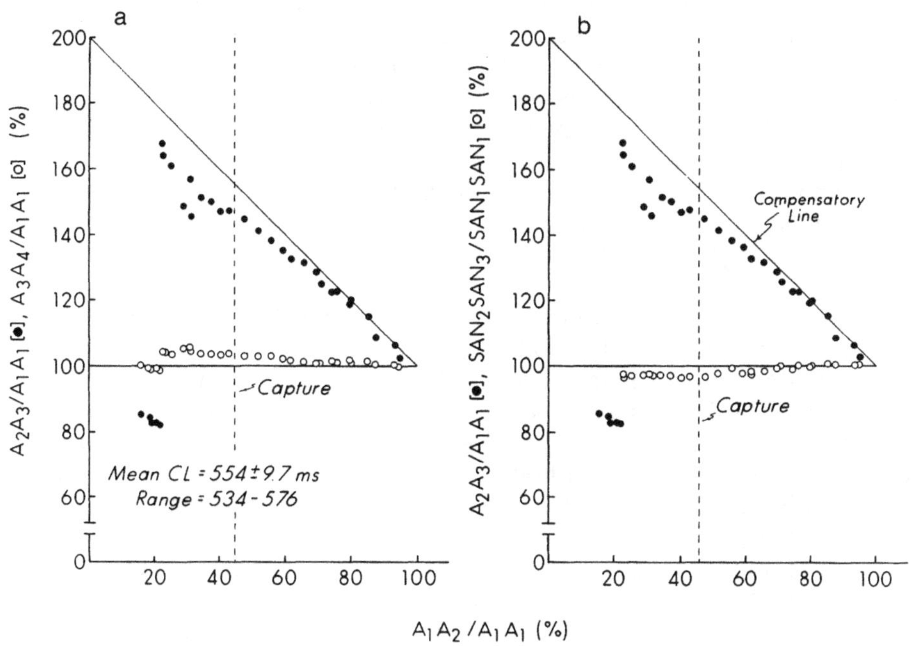

Fig. 2 a and b. Return and postreturn cycles plotted as a function of premature cycle, from a rabbit study. In left-hand panel (a), normalized atrial return (A_2A_3/A_1A_1) and postreturn (A_3A_4/A_1A_1) cycles are plotted as a function of normalized atrial premature cycle (A_1A_2/A_1A_1). In right-hand panel (b) atrial return (A_2A_3/A_1A_1) and sinus node return (SAN_2SAN_3/SAN_1SAN_1) cycles are plotted as a function of test cycle (A_1A_2/A_1A_1). Since the antegrade sinoatrial conduction time was 140 ms, capture of sinus node did not occur until an A_1A_2 interval of 45% was reached; yet deviation from the compensatory line occurred at A_1A_2 interval of 75%. Note A_2A_3 cycles less than 100% indicate incompletely interpolated A_2A_3 cycles.

length constant, the propagation velocity of the electronic potential, values of the conductances, and ionic driving forces that occur during repolarization, and action potential duration. Since the sinoatrial conduction time is dependent on many more factors than distance, and since the point at which A_2A_3 becomes less than compensatory would most likely be principally determined by the action potential duration in cells of the sinus node and the distance of the site of block from the sinus node, then it is not surprising that there is a discrepancy between the value of A_2A_3 cycle on deviation from the compensatory line, and in the plateau. Preparations where action potential duration in cells of the sinus node is long would be expected to have a greater discrepancy in A_1A_2 values between onset of sinus node shortening and sinus node capture than preparations where action potential duration in cells of the sinus node is short. Since we are interested in obtaining a value that approximates the sinoatrial conduction time, we believe that SACT should be derived from the mean value of the A_2A_3 cycle during the last third of the plateau in zone II.

While we have dwelled on the shortening of sinus node action potential and its anticipated effects on the estimation of sinoatrial conduction time, using the premature atrial stimulation technique, other variables also affect the accuracy of the estimation of the SACT. The A_2A_3 cycle is determined by the conduction time between the site of stimulation in the atrium and the sinus node, the SAN_2SAN_3 cycle, and the SAN_3A_3 interval. The intra-atrial conduction time may become a significant factor in the presence of diseased atrial tissue, and may result in a relatively large value for the estimated SACT when, in fact, the conduction time between the crista terminalis and sinus node may be within normal limits. More importantly, changes in estimated SACT that occur following administration of a given pharmacologic agent may result, in part, from changes in intra-atrial conduction [4].

Changes in sinus node automaticity following APDs have been recognized in studies on isolated rabbit atrial preparations [1, 2, 12, 17]. In our studies, the depression of sinus node automaticity was usually not marked (Fig. 3 a – c) [17]. If, as a result of depression of sinus node automaticity, the SAN_2SAN_3 cycle exceeded the SAN_1SAN_1 cycle, this could cause an underestimation of SACT. Although we previously stated that the A_3A_4 cycle could be used to monitor changes in sinus node automaticity [31], we now know that, in most instances, a prolongation of the A_3A_4 cycle reflects a shift of pacemaker following A_2, so that SAN_3A_3 is shorter than SAN_1A_1 [1, 27]. Since SAN_4A_4 returns to control values, this results in an A_3A_4 cycle that is longer than the SAN_3SAN_4 cycle [1, 27]. This difference between the SAN_3SAN_4 and A_3A_4 cycles indicates that, in most instances, we would be unable to use the A_3A_4 cycle to monitor different degrees of depression of SAN automaticity following A_2.

As the A_1A_2 interval decreases, the retrograde conduction time into the sinus node increases, prolonging the A_2SAN_2 interval and causing a lengthening of the A_2A_3 cycle (Fig. 3 a – c). This effect is most marked at short A_1A_2 coupling intervals. Thus, either a prolongation of the retrograde

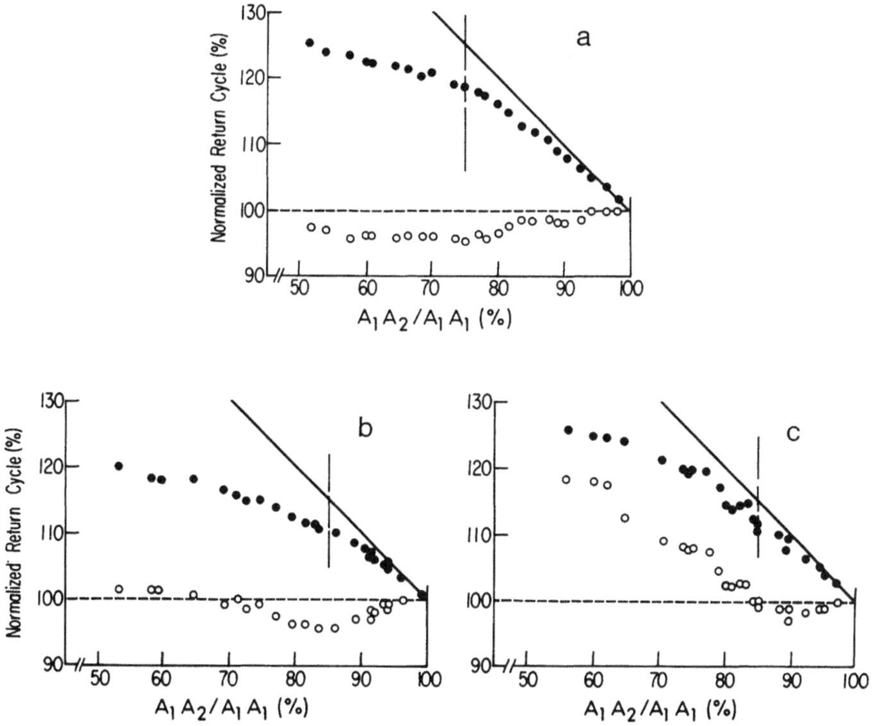

Fig. 3 a – c. The normalized atrial (*solid circles*) and sinus node return (*empty circles*) cycles are plotted as a function of the normalized atrial premature (A_1A_2) cycles in experiments on three different isolated rabbit right atrial preparations [17]. Although values of atrial return cycles are similar, sinus node return cycles differ. As A_1A_2 decreases, sinus node return cycles remain short (panel a), return to control values (panel b), or lengthen (panel c). The marked lengthening of sinus node return cycle depicted in panel c was an unusual response in this series of experiments [25]. (Reproduced by permission of Circulat. Res.)

sinoatrial conduction time or a depression of sinus node automaticity can result in a lengthening of the A_2A_3 cycle, as shown in Figure 3 a – c. Differentiation between an increase in A_2SAN_2 or SAN_2SAN_3 as a cause of a lengthening of the A_2A_3 cycle is presently impossible. Finally, the accuracy of the technique in certain respects is cycle length – dependent. For example, at a cycle length of 600 ms, a 2.5% error in determination of cycle length would result in an error of 15 ms. If $SACT_{A+R}$ were 100 ms, this would result in a 15% error. If the cycle length was 1200 ms, a 2.5% error in determination of cycle length would result in an error of 30 ms, or a 30% error in the estimated value ($SACT_{A+R} = 100$ ms).

The technique has been used in the evaluation of sinus node function in many patients and the following patterns of response which have been found would indicate less than ideal behavior. In two patients, late APDs that fell in zone I were followed by greater than compensatory A_2A_3 cycles [28]. Further, the A_3A_4 cycles in zone I were similarly prolonged, when in all of our other patients, the A_3A_4 cycles equaled the A_1A_1 cycles in zone I. How then, can we explain the prolongation of the A_2A_3 and A_3A_4 cycles in zone I, a zone in which APDs fail to gain access to the sinus node and should therefore be followed by a compensatory response? The most likely explanation would seem to lie in the fact that, in some humans, either the stimulus itself, or the APD, is capable of releasing acetylcholine from nerve terminals, thereby depressing sinus node automaticity and prolonging the A_2A_3 and A_3A_4 cycles. Using these prolonged A_2A_3 cycles for analysis of SACT would provide for an artificially high value for the conduction time. It is for this reason that, when the A_2A_3 cycle is prolonged in zone I, subtraction of the A_3A_4 cycle from the A_2A_3 cycle is indicated to derive a corrected value for the estimated sinoatrial conduction time.

In one patient, late APDs that ordinarily fall in zone I were followed by less than compensatory A_2A_3 cycles (Fig. 4 a and b). In this patient, these observations occurred following administration of digoxin 0.02 mg/kg i.v. in divided doses over 24 hours [16]. Under control conditions, traditional compensatory responses were observed; however, following administration of digoxin in this patient, the compensatory responses following late APDs were never observed (Fig. 4 a and b). This would indicate that these late APDs caused the sinus node return cycle or the SAN_3A_3 interval to shorten, thereby causing the A_2A_3 cycle to be less than compensatory. Whether a similar augmentation of shortening of the sinus node return cycle occurred during zone II is unknown, but if it did, it would mean that the estimated SACT deviates from the true value even more markedly than it did under control conditions.

Although we have talked extensively about the use of the A_2A_3 cycle in the plateau for the calculation of the SACT, we have not commented on the slope of the line drawn through the data points (A_2A_3 vs. A_1A_2) in the last third of zone II. In 23 patients with sinus node dysfunction, the slope of the lines through the data points falling in the last third of zone II ranged between +0.239 and –0.756 [28, 29]. In only 6 of 23 patients did the slope range between –0.1and +0.1. The slope ranged between –0.1 and –0.3 in 3 of 23, between –0.3 and –0.5 in 9 of 23, was more negative than –0.5 in 2 of 23, and more positive than 0.1 in 3 of 23 patients. Thus, in 14 of 23 patients, the A_2A_3 cycles in zone II increased progressively in value as A_1A_2 shortened. Three factors could account for this negative slope: 1. an increase in A_2SAN_2 conduction time because of a prolonged refractory period; 2. a depression of sinus node automaticity; 3. or a prolongation of the SAN_3A_3 conduction time. The latter possibility has not been observed in our laboratory [17] or in the data reported by Bonke et al. [2]. The first two possibilities occurred in all previously published studies on sinus node function in isolated rabbit atria and is exemplified in Figure 3 a – c; differentiation between the two possibilities is impossible at present [1, 2, 12, 17]. Thus, whether the retrograde SACT is truly prolonged in these patients (due to a prolongation of refractoriness) is a matter of speculation. Further, the reported changes in estimated SACT following a given pharmacologic

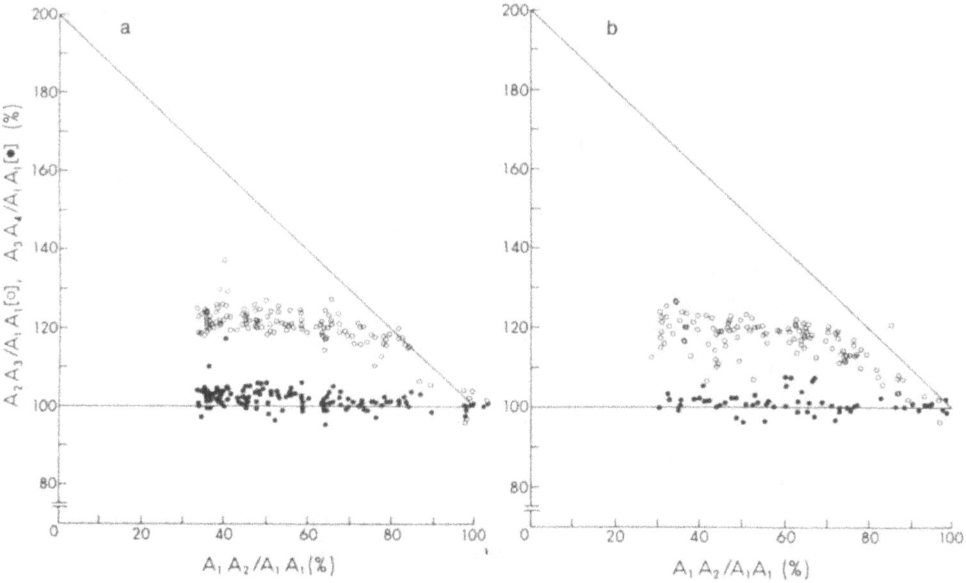

Fig. 4 a and b. Effects of digoxin on return and postreturn cycles. Normalized A_2A_3 (*unfilled circles*) and A_3A_4 (*filled circles*) are plotted as previously described. In left-hand panel (a), deviation from compensatory line occurs at A_1A_2 coupling interval of 84.6%. After 1.125 mg of digoxin over 24 h, late APDs fall below compensatory line, indicating shortening of A_2A_3 cycle at a time when APDs were followed by compensatory A_2A_3 cycles under control conditions. (Reproduced by permission of Circulation)

intervention such as digitalis, ouabain, or propranolol can either reflect a real change in sinoatrial conduction time or a depression of sinus node automaticity [4, 29].

With these additional reservations in mind, let us examine the $SACT_{A+R}$ in 24 patients with sinus node dysfunction. If a value of 215 ms can be considered to represent the upper limits of normal [28], then the $SACT_{A+R}$ in 7 of 23 (30%) patients was found to exceed this value.

The majority of patients (13/23) had an estimated $SACT_{A+R}$ that ranged between 100 and 215 ms. In three patients the estimated $SACT_{A+R}$ was less than 100 ms [28]. Yet, these three patients also had sinus node dysfunction. How can these results be interpreted? One may conclude that those patients had only a depression of sinus node automaticity and that sinoatrial conduction was normal. A second interpretation would be that the value of the estimated SACT was markedly less than the real value. A third interpretation is that, due to extensive sinus node damage, third degree SA block had appeared and the functioning pacemaker had shifted closer to the crista terminalis, resulting in shorter than anticipated sinoatrial conduction times, as occurs in patients with short AV conduction times that are in atrial or in AV junctional rhythms. Such a shift in pacemaker site might produce only a subtle change in P wave morphology and go undetected, save for the relatively short SACT. Thus, not all patients with sick sinus syndrome may have prolonged sinoatrial conduction times.

Although the accuracy of the premature atrial stimulation technique has been questioned, what about its sensitivity? Can this detect abnormal conduction in those patients in whom SA conduction defects would be anticipated, i.e., those patients with intermittent second degree SA block? At present, we have too few patients to answer this question. Second, can this technique predict which patients will respond poorly to cardioactive agents? Third, can this technique help to quantitate the disturbances of sinus node function in patients with sick sinus syndrome? These questions have yet to be answered. Some of these problems can only be settled by examining the SACT in normal patients. The control population should be matched for heart rate, since one clinical study has indicated that the estimated SACT is cycle length – dependent [21]. In our rabbit studies, over a range of cycle lengths, 400 – 635 ms, no significant correlation between $SACT_A$ and cycle length could be detected [17]. Whether such data are relevant to the clinical studies is uncertain, but may indicate that even when the heart rate variable is controlled, the range of normal sinoatrial conduction times will be quite wide.

In summary, we have shown that there are a lot of uncertainties about the premature atrial stimulation technique. Its role in the evaluation of patients with sinus node function and its ability to predict which patients will not tolerate a given cardioactive agent remain to be determined in future clinical studies.

Summary

Recent interest in the pathophysiology of sinus node dysfunction has stimulated the development of techniques that would provide a means of quantitating disturbances of sinoatrial conduction and sinus node automaticity in patients. Since electrical activity in the sinus node can only be recorded using intracellular recording techniques, evaluation of sinoatrial conduction time must be indirect. Premature atrial stimulation was introduced in an attempt to provide an indirect determination of sinoatrial conduction time. In essence, atrial premature depolarizations (APDs) are elicited following every eighth spontaneous cycle, so that the atrial return cycles (A_2A_3) following APDs elicited at the different coupling intervals can be determined. Late APDs are followed by compensatory return cycles; as the coupling interval of the APD is decreased, a transition to a less than compensatory atrial return cycle occurs. The duration of the less than compensatory atrial return cycle is determined by the retrograde sinoatrial conduction time A_2SAN_2, the sinus node return cycle (SAN_2SAN_3) and the antegrade sinoatrial conduction time (SAN_3A_3). The original Wenckebach hypothesis, seemingly confirmed in our early clinical studies, suggested that the sinoatrial conduction time $= \frac{1}{2}(A_2A_3) - (A_1A_1) = \frac{1}{2}(A_2SAN_2 + SAN_2SAN_3 + SAN_3A_3) = \frac{1}{2}(A_2SAN_2 + SAN_3A_3)$.

Inherent in this derivation are the assumptions that $A_1A_1 = SAN_2SAN_3$; and that the sinoatrial conduction times in either direction are not markedly different.

Studies in cats, rabbits, dogs, and in some clinical studies have shown that the transition to a constant less than compensatory response does not occur at a discrete point in diastole. Microelectrode studies have shown that late APDs shorten the sinus node action potential and the sinus node return cycle. The shortening of the sinus node return cycle causes the premature atrial stimulation technique to imprecisely estimate the sinoatrial conduction time. Other factors decreasing the accuracy of the premature atrial stimulation technique include the intraatrial conduction time; variable degree of depression of sinus node automaticity following an APD that cannot be readily identified; pacemaker shifts that follow early APDs (that reset the sinus node) so that the SAN_3A_3 intervals are shortened and the A_3A_4 cycles are prolonged; encroachment of late APDs on the relative refractory period of the sinoatrial junction. Nonetheless, despite these limitations, the technique is adequate to estimate prolonged sinoatrial conduction times. In our recent evaluation of patients with sinus node dysfunction, 30% of 23 patients were found to have an estimated sinoatrial conduction time that exceeded 210 ms. The sinoatrial conduction time in patients with sinus pauses and spontaneous sinoatrial block will be discussed.

Acknowledgment

We gratefully acknowledge the valuable assistance of Ms. Joy Bonar in the preparation of this manuscript.

References

1. Bonke, F. I. M., Bouman, L. N., Schopman, F. J. G.: Effect of an early atrial premature beat on activity of the sinoatrial node and atrial rhythm in the rabbit. Circulat. Res. **29,** 704 (1971)
2. Bonke, F. I. M., Bouman, L. N., Van Rijn, H. E.: Change of cardiac rhythm in the rabbit after an atrial premature beat. Circulat. Res. **24,** 533 (1969)
3. Dighton, D. H.: Sinus bradycardia: Autonomic influences and clinical assessment. Brit. Heart J. **36,** 791 (1974)
4. Dhingra, R. C., Amat-Y-Leon, F., Wyndham, C., Wu, D., Denes, P., Rosen, K. M.: The electrophysiological effects of ouabain on sinus node and atrium in man. J. clin. Invest. **56,** 555 (1975)
5. Eccles, H. C., Hoff, H. E.: The rhythm of the heart beat. II. Disturbance of rhythm produced by late premature beats. Proc. roy. Soc. B **115,** 327 (1934)
6. Engel, T. R., Schaal, S. F.: Digitalis in the sick sinus syndrome: The effects on sinoatrial automaticity and atrioventricular conduction. Circulation **48,** 1201 (1973)
7. Ferrer, M. I.: The sick sinus syndrome. Circulation **47,** 635 (1973)
8. Goldreyer, B. N., Damato, A. N.: Sinoatrial node entrance block. Circulation **44,** 789 (1971)
9. Greenwood, R. J., Finkelstein, D.: Sinoatrial Heart Block. Springfield, Ill.: Charles C. Thomas, 1964, p. 37

10. Gupta, P. K., Lichstein, E., Chadda, K. D., Badui, E.: Appraisal of sinus nodal recovery time in patients with sick sinus syndrome. Amer. J. Cardiol. **34,** 265 (1974)
11. Kaplan, B. M., Langendorf, R., Lev, M., Pick, A.: Tachycardia-bradycardia syndrome (so-called "Sick Sinus Syndrome"). Amer. J. Cardiol. **31,** 497 (1973)
12. Klein, H., Singer, D. H., Hoffman, B. F.: Effects of atrial premature systoles on sinus rhythm in the rabbit. Circulat. Res. **32,** 480 (1973)
13. Langendorf, R., Lesser, M. E., Plotkin, P., Levin, B. D.: Atrial parasystole with interpolation. Observations on prolonged sinoatrial conduction. Amer. Heart J. **63,** 649 (1962)
14. Mandel, W., Hayakawa, H., Danzig, R., Marcus, H. S.: Evaluation of sinoatrial node function in man by overdrive suppression. Circulation **44,** 59 (1971)
15. Mandel, W. J., Hayakawa, H., Hirokazu, A., Allen, H. N., Danzig, R., Kermaier, A. I.: Assessment of sinus node function in patients with the sick sinus syndrome. Circulation **46,** 761 (1972)
16. Margolis, J. R., Strauss, H. C., Miller, H. C., Gilbert, M., Wallace, A. G.: Digitalis and the sick sinus syndrome. Circulation **52,** 162 (1975)
17. Miller, H. C., Strauss, H. C.: Measurement of sinoatrial conduction time by premature atrial stimulation in the rabbit. Circulat. Res. **35,** 935 (1974)
18. Narula, O. S., Samet, P., Javier, R. P.: Significance of the sinus node recovery time. Circulation **45,** 140 (1972)
19. Paes de Carvalho, A., de Mello, W. C., Hoffman, B. F.: Electrophysiological evidence for specialized fiber types in rabbit atrium. Amer. J. Physiol. **196,** 483 (1959)
20. Rosen, K. M., Loeb, H. S., Sinno, M. Z., Rahimtoola, S. H., Gunnar, R. M.: Cardiac conduction in patients with symptomatic sinus node disease. Circulation **43,** 836 (1971)
21. Reiffel, J. A., Bigger, J. T., Jr., Konstam, M. A.: The relationship between sinoatrial conduction time and sinus cycle length during spontaneous sinus arrhythmia in adults. Circulation **50,** 924 (1974)
22. Sano, T., Yamagishi, S.: Spread of excitation from the sinus node. Circulat. Res. **16,** 423 (1965)
23. Seipel, L., Breithardt, A., Both, A., Loogen, F.: Messung der sinu-atrialen Leitungszeit mittels vorzeitiger Vorhofstimulation beim Menschen. Dtsch. med. Wschr. **99,** 1895 (1974)
24. Short, D. S.: The syndrome of alternating bradycardia and tachycardia. Brit. Heart J. **16,** 208 (1954)
25. Sims, B. A.: Pathogenesis of atrial arrhythmias. Brit. Heart J. **34,** 336 (1972)
26. Strauss, H. C., Bigger, J. T., Jr.: The electrophysiological properties of the rabbit sinoatrial perinodal fibers. Circulat. Res. **31,** 490 (1972)
27. Strauss, H. C., Wallace, A. G.: Direct and indirect techniques in the evaluation of sinus node functions. In: The Conduction System of the Heart. Structure, Function, and Clinical Implications, Wellens, H. J. J., Lie, K. I., Janse, M. J. (ed.). Leiden, H. E. Stenfert Kroese B. V. 1976, p. 227
28. Strauss, H. C., Bigger, J. T., Jr., Saroff, A. L., Giardina, E. G. V.: Electrophysiologic evaluation of sinus node function in patients with sinus node dysfunction. Circulation **53,** 763 (1976)
29. Strauss, H. C., Gilbert, M., Svenson, R. H., Miller, H. C., Wallace, A. G.: Electrophysiological effects of propranolol on sinus node function in patients with sinus node dysfunction. Submitted for publication
30. Strauss, H. C., Saroff, A. L., Bigger, J. T., Jr., Giardina, E. G. V.: Premature atrial stimulation as a key to the understanding of sinoatrial conduction in man. Circulation **47,** 86 (1973)
31. Ticzon, A. R., Strauss, H. C., Gallagher, J. J., Wallace, A. G.: Sinus node function in the intact dog heart evaluated by premature atrial stimulation and atrial pacing. Amer. J. Cardiol. **35,** 492 (1975)
32. Wenckebach, K. F.: Über die Dauer der compensatorischen Pause nach Reizung der Vorkammer des Säugetierherzens. Arch. Anat. Physiol. (Physiol. Abt.) **57,** 1903

Sinus Node Recovery Time and Sinoatrial Conduction Time *

G. STEINBECK and B. LÜDERITZ

Recently, disorders of sinus node function gained clinical importance. Impaired sinus node function in sinoatrial disease, which includes sinus bradycardia, sinus arrest, sinoatrial block, and the bradycardia-tachycardia syndrome [8, 11, 14, 19], cannot easily be assessed, as the recording of electrical activity of sinus node pacemaker cells is not available in man. The analysis of atrial activity in the surface electrogram permits only an overall estimation of sinus node function. This involves the ability to act as an impulse generator and includes the conduction of the impulse from the pacemaker site to the atrium.

Therefore, methods of provocative atrial stimulation have been developed which are thought to allow the indirect estimation of sinus node automaticity and sinoatrial conduction in man [15, 20, 22, 33]. In this paper the results of rapid atrial stimulation as well as premature atrial stimulation are presented in a total of 28 patients, 18 of whom had electrocardiographic evidence of sinoatrial disease.

Methods

No patient received cardioactive drugs unless stated otherwise. After informed consent had been obtained, a quadripolar electrode catheter was inserted via the basilic vein and the tip placed at the lateral wall of the right atrium. The distal pair of electrodes was used for stimulation; from the proximal pair of electrodes a high right atrial electrogram was recorded together with the standard leads. The stimulation procedure is described in detail elsewhere [29, 30]. Using premature atrial stimulation, the postextrasystolic cycle (A_3A_4) was determined after single beats with increasing prematurity (A_2A_3).

A_3A_4 was plotted in a diagram as a function of A_2A_3 ; both were related to the preceding spontaneous atrial interval A_1A_2 . For indirect calculation of the sinoatrial conduction time (SACT), we used a transitional postextrasystolic atrial cycle that was on the borderline between a compensatory and a noncompensatory pause.

Sinus node recovery time (SNRT) is defined as the time interval between the last paced atrial activation of rapid stimulation and the first spontaneous atrial activity of sinus origin after cessation of pacing. Each pacing period lasted 1 min. Sinus node recovery time was measured first with rates slightly above sinus rate; thereafter, pacing rate was increased by increments of 10 or 20 impulses/min. The maximum sinus node recovery time (max. SNRT) is the longest time interval seen at any of the pacing rates.

Results and Discussion

The results of provocative atrial stimulation are listed in Tables 1 and 2.

* Supported by Deutsche Forschungsgemeinschaft.

Table 1. Results of atrial stimulation studies in 10 controls

No.	Sex and Age	Sinus-rate/min	Max. SNRT/ms	SACT/ms	Atropine 1 mg		
					Sinus-rate/min	Max. SNRT/ms	SACT/ms
1	M, 32	65	1280	–	–	–	–
2	F, 66	85	–	70	–	–	–
3	F, 27	96	1050	60	120	600	25
4	M, 50	96	–	40	–	–	–
5	M, 51	65	1205	50	95	895	35
6	F, 33	64	–	60	–	–	–
7	M, 16	83	–	70	–	–	–
8	F, 19	80	1000	–	–	–	–
9	M, 71	91	1145	50	97	815	45
10	M, 72	97	930	110	–	–	–
		82 ± 13	1101 ± 131	63 ± 21	104 ± 13	770 ± 152	35 ± 10

Table 2. Results of atrial stimulation studies in 18 patients with sinoatrial disease

No.	Sex and Age	Sinus-rate/min	Max. SNRT/ms	SACT/ms	Atropine 1 mg		
					Sinus-rate/min	Max. SNRT/ms	SACT/ms
1	M, 57	62	1330	145	83	1070	55
2	F, 50	69	1275	[a]	83	900	45
3	F, 69	60	3215	150	–	–	–
4	F, 61	57	3880	105; 2° SA block	86	–	2° SA block
5	M, 69	47	2540	–	48	4420	–
6	M, 65	77	1230	–	102	800	–
7	M, 76	50	1600	–	80	–	–
8	F, 66	66	1405	–	88	1100	–
9	M, 53	63	2395	60; 2° SA block	70	2160	65; 2° SA block
10	M, 64	76	–	70	–	–	–
11	M, 47	59	1290	[a]	84	800	35
12	M, 61	76	1845	135	86	1440	135
13	F, 57	67	1340	70	88	945	40
14	F, 60	63	1690	[a]	91	990	50
15	M, 69	61	1475	70	75	1035	40
16	M, 62	61	1370	65	74	1090	40
17	M, 68	59	1270	[a]	87	850	35
18	F, 68	47	1675	2° SA block	65	4115	35
		62 ± 8	1813 ± 763	96 ± 37	80 ± 12	1551 ± 1203	57 ± 30

[a] Exact calculation of SACT was not possible because of severe sinus arrhythmia.

1. Controls

In patients without sinus node dysfunction max. SNRT was 1101 ms and SACT 63 ms. Included in this group is, however, patient No. 10, suffering from a hypersensitive carotid sinus, who exhibited a markedly prolonged SACT of 110 ms. If this by all means pathologic finding is excluded, our normal values range between 40 and 70 ms, which is understood as half the conduction time into and out of the sinus node. In respect to SNRT we obtained results similar to other authors [9, 13, 20]. Different values, however, were reported by Seipel et al. [26] and Dhingra et al. [7]: concerning SACT, these authors could observe a constancy of the postextrasystolic cycle throughout the zone of the noncompensatory pause. A similar finding was reported by Strauss et al. in their early clinical studies in 1973. However, it was subsequently noted that in 17 out of 23 patients with sinus node dysfunction the slope of the line drawn through the data points falling in the last third of the noncompensatory pause (adjacent to the zone of compensatory pause) was not zero [35]. Out of a series of 22 patients 15 of whom were restudied after atropine 1 mg i.v. (see Tables 1 and 2), we observed in 18 cases a continuous prolongation by various degrees of the postextrasystolic cycle within the noncompensatory pause with increasing prematurity of stimulation, whereas only four cases demonstrated a plateau phase. These results are in accordance with experimental evidence that either sinus node automaticity or sinoatrial conduction or both are not constant following premature atrial beats falling in the zone of noncompensatory pause [2, 3, 12]. To avoid the possibility of sinus node depression by the premature beat challenging indirect calculation of SACT, we, therefore, decided to take the postextrasystolic cycle at the borderline between the compensatory and the noncompensatory pause for SACT determination.

In order to test whether sinoatrial conduction time might be derived indirectly from the length of the postextrasystolic atrial cycle after single premature atrial beats, recordings of transmembrane potentials of single pacemaker cells within the sinoatrial node, and bipolar electrograms from the crista terminalis were obtained in the isolated, spontaneously beating right atrium of the rabbit [18]. In this study it was observed that atrial premature depolarizations, elicited late in atrial diastole, caused a noncompensatory postextrasystolic cycle, although the premature beat did not reach the impaled cell within the pacemaker area. This phenomenon was attributed to a shortening of the sinus node action potential due to electrotonic interaction between the sinoatrial node and adjacent cells, which had been passively discharged by the premature beat, during repolarization. The authors conclude therefrom that calculation of SACT by the use of transition from compensatory to less than compensatory postextrasystolic atrial cycles consistently underestimates "true sinoatrial conduction time".

On the other hand it can be speculated whether such a definite true sinoatrial conduction time exists at all. Measurements of the electrotonic spread in the sinoatrial node of the rabbit heart demonstrated a relatively small value of the space constant amounting to $465 \pm 55\ \mu$ [4]. Conduction velocity within the sinoatrial node is slow [23]. As a consequence, a premature beat coming from the right atrium will not discharge the whole of the sinoatrial node, and if the original pacemaker is reached, another group of fibers can take over pacemaker function [4]. It is therefore questionable whether the latency between activation of the pacemaker cell impaled by the microelectrode and activation of the crista terminalis truly reflects sinoatrial conduction properties, as the time interval depends on the location of the electrode within the sinoatrial node recording the pacemaker potential, and this latency is expected to change when a transmembrane potential from another group of pacemaker fibers is recorded. Transition from the compensatory to the noncompensatory atrial cycle could signify the following events:

1. Influence of the dominant pacemaker fiber, which thereafter reaches threshold first and continues to activate the atrium.
2. Influence of the dominant pacemaker cell; however, a spontaneous impulse from a latent pacemaker fiber which had been excited earlier gains access to the atrium first after the premature beat and controls the heart rate for one or several beats.

In the former event, the difference between the postextrasystolic cycle at transition from compensatory to noncompensatory pause and spontaneous atrial cycle will represent indirect estimation of retrograde and antegrade conduction properties between the atrium and the dominant pacemaker.

In the latter case, this difference will account for the sum of conduction time between the atrium and the latent pacemaker if the basic rhythm of the latent pacemaker is not significantly different from that of the dominant one. The slower the rate of spontaneous depolarization of the cell to which the actual pacemaker function has shifted, the more will the calculated sinoatrial conduction time be overestimated. However, for practical purposes it may be said that the calculated value is a maximal one, which despite the limitations mentioned does permit differentiation from prolonged sinoatrial conduction times. In any case, it might be preferable to estimate functional sinoatrial conduction properties using the transition from the compensatory to the noncompensatory pause rather than the noncompensatory pause itself, where the gradual increase of postextrasystolic cycle may be caused by depression of sinus node automaticity, prolongation of retrograde sinoatrial conduction, or a combination of both so that differentiation is impossible.

Further uncertainties of SACT calculation are the inherent assumption of identical conduction times in both directions, and the unknown amount of intra-atrial conduction time contributing to SACT. In order to minimize the latter possibility of error, we positioned the electrodes, used for recording a bipolar electrogram, at the junction of the superior vena cava and the right atrium. Stimulation was performed via a distal pair of electrodes at the tip of the catheter which was placed at the lateral wall of the right atrium, in order to avoid a stimulation-induced release of transmitters from nerve terminals influencing the response of the sinus node to provocative atrial stimulation.

Besides the different methods of SACT calculation, such differences may in part account for the different values of SACT reported in the literature.

Despite the limitations of indirect SACT calculation mentioned, our results are similar to experimental data derived from transmembrane action potential measurements in a spontaneously beating preparation of the isolated right atrium of the rabbit [2, 10, 23, 32, 36].

2. Sinoatrial Disease

In patients with electrocardiographic evidence of sinoatrial disease, mean values of max. SNRT and SACT are both increased; however, this is not true for every case (see Table 2). In three patients some premature beats were followed by markedly prolonged postextrasystolic cycles exceeding the other intervals by one basic cycle. As an explanation it is therefore tempting to assume an intermittent sinoatrial node exit block after stimulation [28].

Our results of SNRT agree with those of other authors [6, 16, 20, 25].

Using a method of SACT-determination similar to ours, Masini et al. [17] reported a mean value of 126,5 ms in seven patients with sinoatrial block. When, however, the noncompensatory pause is taken for SACT estimation, much larger values have been reported [5, 35].

3. Atropine

It is obvious from Table 2 that SACT may be prolonged in the presence of a normal SNRT and vice versa. If sinus node recovery time is to provide a valid indicator of sinus node automaticity, every paced beat during rapid atrial stimulation should be conducted in retrograde direction to the sinus node, and, after termination of pacing, antegrade sinoatrial conduction should be equally unaffected [34]. We were interested in studying how an impaired sinoatrial conduction may influence the apparent recovery interval of the sinus node. For this reason, we repeated the stimulation studies in patients with and without SA conduction disturbances after administration of atropine which is able to improve SA conduction (Tables 1 and 2). In three controls, atropine 1 mg induces an increase in sinus rate and a decrease of both SNRT and SACT.

In patients with sinoatrial disease, max. SNRT was shortened to a different degree in 12 of 14 cases. It was, however, increased in two. SACT values were nearly unchanged in two patients, and reduced in the others. An example of an unexpected effect of atropine on max. SNRT is depicted in Figure 1. These data are taken from a 68-year-old patient in whom a phenomenon, which we interpret as a sinus node exit block, was elicited by premature atrial beats. This behavior could, however, no longer be observed after atropine. The max. SNRT amounted to 1675 ms. It increased extensively after drug administration, rising to 4115 ms despite an increase in spontaneous sinus rate. As an explanation for this finding we think it reasonable to assume that an impaired retrograde sinoatrial conduction prevented the sinus node from being depolarized by every paced beat, thus giving shorter recovery intervals than would be expected in the presence of an adequate SA conduction. Since atropine improves sinoatrial conduction, the real extent of impairment of sinus node automaticity is disclosed after drug administration. Similar, apparently paradoxical atropine effects have been reported by others [1, 20, 21].

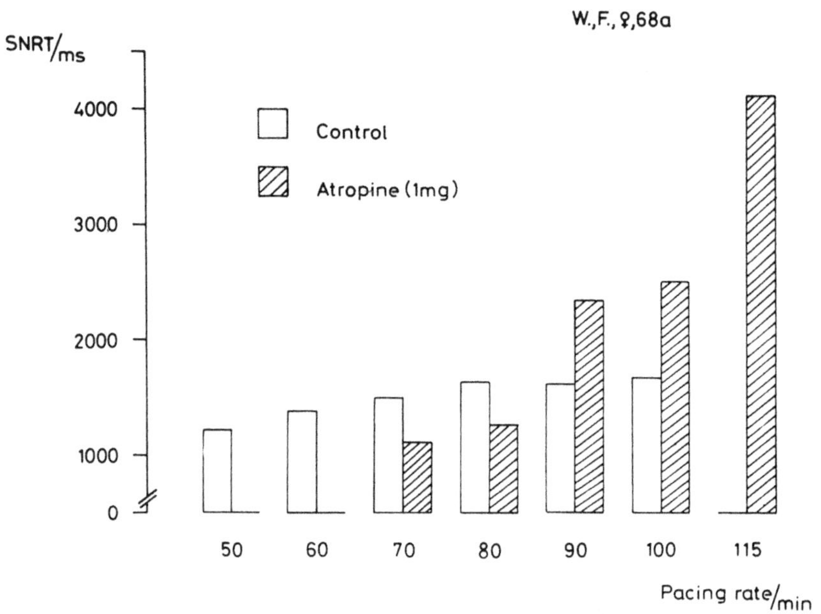

Fig. 1. Rapid atrial pacing in 68-year-old female before (*white columns*) and after atropine administration (*hatched columns*). On the ordinate the sinus node recovery time is given in ms, on the abscissa the pacing rates chosen. Spontaneous sinus rate was 47/min and after drug administration 65/min. Stimulation with 115/min was not performed before atropine because of onset of angina.

An impairment of sinoatrial conduction may significantly influence the sinus node recovery interval: a sinus node entrance block during rapid atrial stimulation leads to a shortening of SNRT, whereas an apparent sinus node exit block after cessation of rapid atrial pacing could be demonstrated to result in a marked prolongation of SNRT [30].

In four patients the zone of compensatory and noncompensatory pause could not be discriminated because of a wide scattering of the A_3A_4 cycles due to a sinus arrhythmia. Such an example is shown in Figure 2 (top diagram). No further information can be obtained by observation of the post-postextrasystolic cycle A_4A_5 (second diagram). Atropine not only increased spontaneous sinus rate but also reduced standard deviation of the

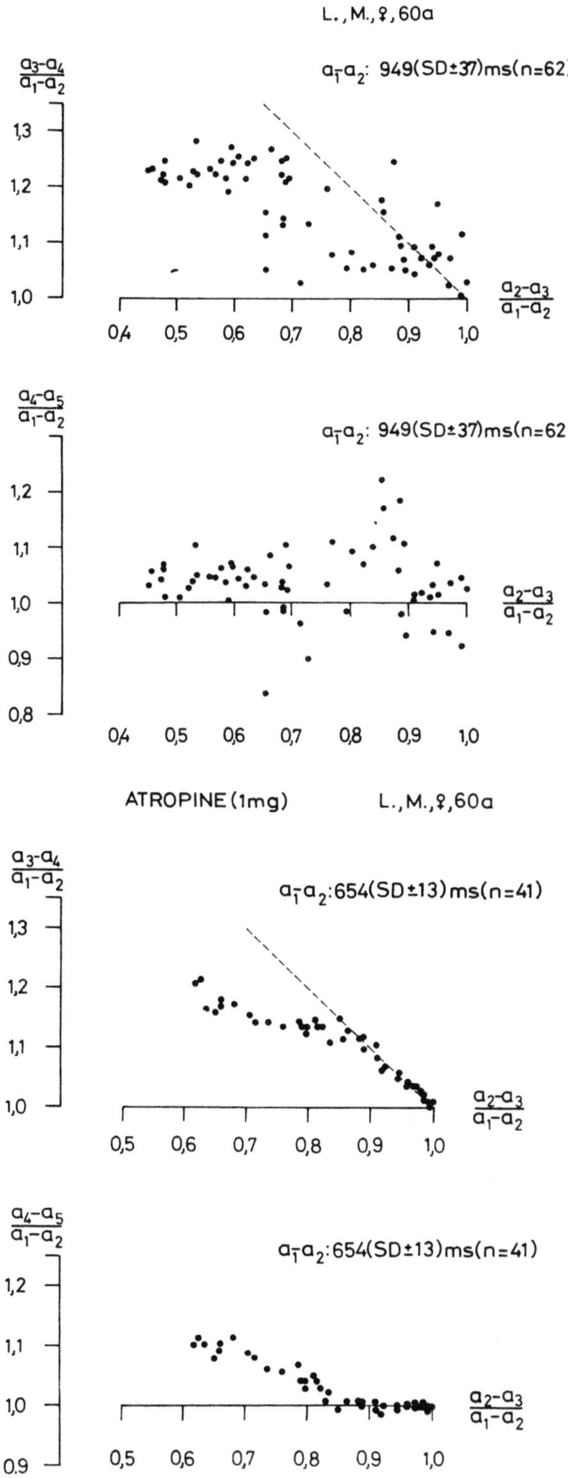

Fig. 2. Results of premature atrial stimulation in 60-year-old female with sinus arrhythmia before (*above*) and after (*below*) administration of atropine. *Top:* Postextrasystolic cycle A_3A_4 as a function of curtailed cycle A_2A_3; both values are related to spontaneous A_1A_2 interval. *Bottom:* Post-post-extrasystolic cycle A_4A_5 as function of A_2A_3.

mean spontaneous atrial cycle A_1A_2. As a consequence, the compensatory and noncompensatory pause can clearly be identified (third diagram). The borderline between these two zones coincides with a change in atrial rate after stimulation, which is indicated by a continuous lengthening of the A_4A_5 interval within the noncompensatory pause with increasing prematurity of stimulation (bottom diagram), from which a SACT of 50 ms could be calculated.

As Figures 1 and 2 demonstrate, repetition of both pacing techniques after administration of atropine is of appreciable additional value in assessing sinus node function in sinoatrial disease.

4. Mechanism of Sinoatrial Block

In five patients a clear prolongation of SACT was measured by use of the premature atrial stimulation technique (see Tables 1 and 2). Thus, a first degree of sinoatrial block exists in our opinion with its possible progression to a higher degree of sinoatrial block. This event may constitute one of the pathophysiologic mechanisms underlying sinoatrial disease. However, one should be aware of the fact that an exact anatomical localization of the site of conduction impairment is not possible with the techniques used until now. Such a delay of conduction may be confined to the area of pacemaker fibers, to the junction between the sinus node and the atria, as supposed by Strauss and Bigger [32], as well as to the atrium itself, which was suggested by Sano et al. [24].

When some intervals between spontaneous atrial activations from the sinus node are more or less approximate multiples of the normal period, this behavior has been widely accepted as indirect evidence of an intermittent, complete conduction block between the sinus node and the atria. However, the simplicity of this conclusion does not provide evidence for the presence of this conduction disturbance [27]. We had the opportunity to observe a similar behaviour of atrial cycle lengths in an animal experiment (Fig. 3).

In the top panel on the left, the right atrium is driven electrically at a rate of 293/min. Every paced beat is conducted retrogradely to the pacemaker cell. Following the cessation of pacing, sinus node recovery time lasts for 940 ms. In the middle panel, stimulation rate is increased to 333/min. Again, every impulse is conducted retrogradely. The recovery interval, however, is markedly prolonged with 1870 ms, thereafter being nearly normal. If only the length of the atrial intervals were observed, one might suppose that within the prolonged period of 1870 ms the sinus node pacemaker discharges spontaneously, but does not activate the atrium, which means a sinoatrial exit block. However, this tracing clearly demonstrates that at least the pacemaker cell under observation does not spontaneously discharge at all. Instead, only a subthreshold wave is observed of a period similar to the control interval.

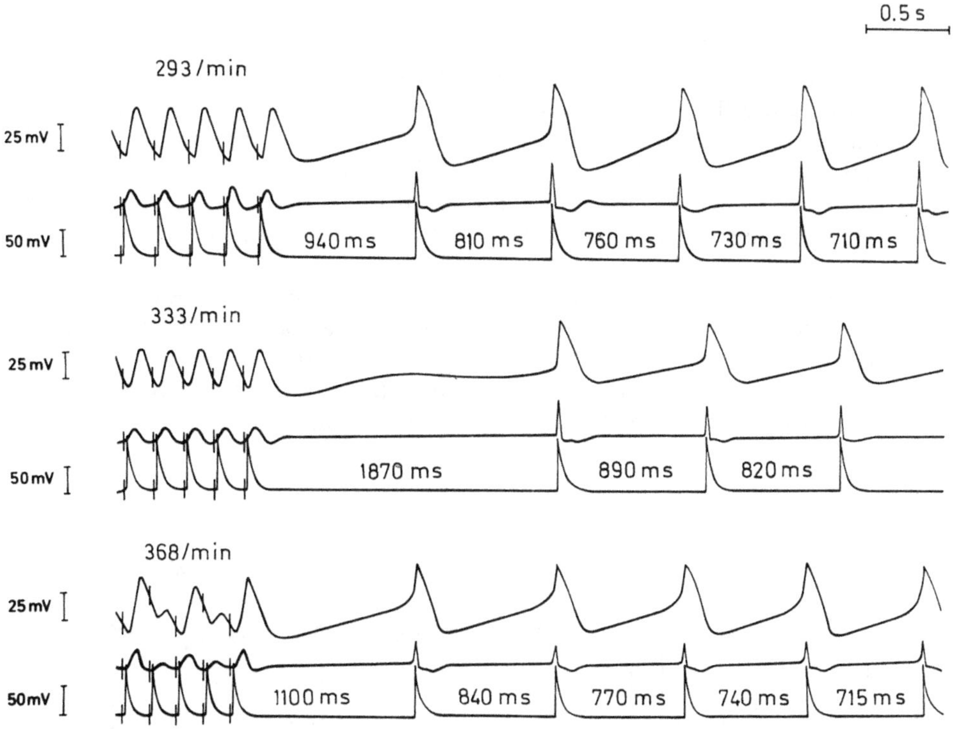

Fig. 3. Tracings of transmembrance potentials by use of standard microelectrode technique, taken from spontaneously beating right atrium of rabbit in vitro. In all three panels the transmembrane voltage change is recorded from the same latent pacemaker cell, showing slow diastolic depolarization and smooth transition to upstroke of action potential (*above*), the differentiated signal (*middle*), and an action potential recorded from crista terminalis (*bottom*).

In the bottom panel, pacing rate is further increased. Only one-half of the beats elicited in the right atrium is conducted retrogradely; every second activation influences the pacemaker cell only electrotonically. As a consequence of this 2 : 1 sinoatrial entrance block, the sinus node recovery interval decreases.

Similar, spontaneously occurring subthreshold waves were observed under various experimental conditions [37]. West noted that the peak-to-peak period of such oscillations was almost identical with the frequency of spontaneous discharge of the same cell. Whether such disturbances of automaticity may occur spontaneously or following rapid as well as premature atrial stimulation in humans mimicing sinoatrial conduction block, cannot be proved. However, we think that the phenomenon of periodically dropped atrial beats resulting in multiples of the preceeding cycle length should be no longer taken as unequivocal evidence for a sinoatrial conduction block.

5. Pacemaker Shift

In four patients we observed a phenomenon which we ascribed to a premature beat-followed shift of the dominant pacemaker of the heart. Such an example is shown in Figure 4 a and b. In panel a, a premature beat elicited late in atrial diastole is followed by a compensatory pause. The pattern of the following atrial activations in the bipolar atrial electrogram (AE) is unchanged when compared with the prepacing atrial configurations.

In panel b the curtailed cycle is shortened. After this premature beat interval, a sudden change in configuration of the atrial activation terminating the postextrasystolic pause can be observed in the high right atrial electrogram. This change in activation pattern persists for two beats, thereafter returning to the prepacing atrial configuration.

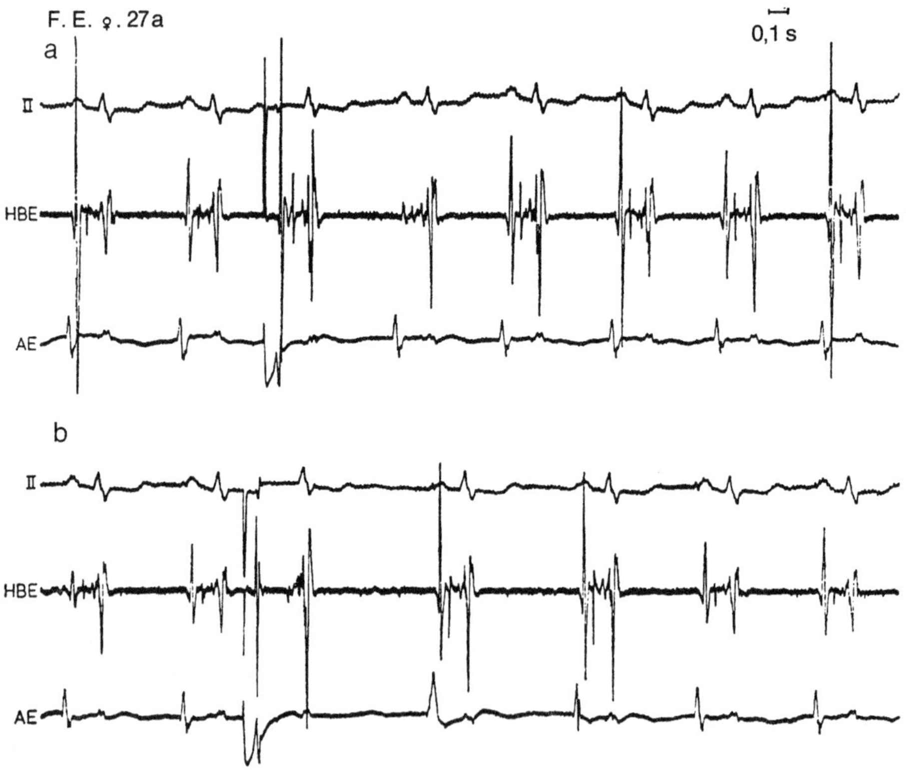

Fig. 4 a and b. Recording of lead II, a His bundle electrogram (HBE) and a high right atrial bipolar electrogram (AE) from a 27-year-old female patient without sinus node dysfunction (case No. 3, Table 1). After the second atrial activation of sinus origin a premature beat is elicited late in atrial diastole in panel a.
In panel (b), prematurity of stimulus-induced atrial activation is increased.
For further explanation see text.

In all four patients the occurrence of a premature beat-followed change of atrial activation contour was associated with a sudden change of atrial rate which was abruptly slowed (not graphically shown). The simultaneous occurrence of both phenomena indicates a passive discharge of the sinoatrial node, thus helping to clearly identify the zone of compensatory and noncompensatory pause. Following experimental observations of a stimulation-induced pacemaker shift [2], we therefore assume that during the zone of noncompensatory pause the premature beat is conducted retrogradely to the sinus node and does discharge the pacemaker fibers. After discharge, however, another cell takes over pacemaker function. To explain our findings, two assumptions have to be made: first, the dominant pacemaker has to shift over such a wide area (within the sinus node or out of it) that impulse propagation from the new pacemaker cell is changed, thus causing the altered activation pattern in our bipolar electrograms, and second, the rate of the new pacemaker cell has to be slower than the original one, which is reflected by the prolonged A_4A_5 intervals following a noncompensatory pause. It is stressed that the standard leads in all cases were not able to truly reflect the change in atrial activation contour seen in the high right atrial electrogram.

Until now such a pacemaker shift could clearly be identified in four patients, two of whom had sinoatrial disease. This phenomenon was seen after rapid atrial stimulation too, and in all patients it persisted after atropine administration [31]. Whereas the practical relevance of these findings remains to be clarified, the observation of a pacemaker shift helps to clearly discriminate between compensatory and noncompensatory atrial cycles. Thus, the phenomenon serves as further evidence that the borderline between these two zones rather than the zone of noncompensatory pause itself should be used for the indirect estimation of sinoatrial conduction properties in man.

Summary

Atrial stimulation studies were performed in a total of 28 patients, 18 of whom had electrocardiographic evidence of sinoatrial disease. In the latter group, "maximum sinus node recovery time" (max. SNRT) ranged between 1230 and 3880 ms. "Sinoatrial conduction time" (SACT) was normal in 3/14 patients, and prolonged in 4/14 patients. In three cases a probable exit block of the next spontaneous sinus impulse was observed after premature atrial stimulation. In the same patients, variation of the spontaneous atrial cycle by nearly one basic interval occurred from one beat to another after cessation of rapid atrial pacing. In four patients, at a critical premature beat interval, an altered configuration of the postextrasystolic atrial activation and a change of the successive cycle lengths were observed. The simultaneous occurrence of both phenomena suggests a pacemaker shift as the underlying mechanism, following those premature atrial depolarizations which discharged the sinus node. Thus, this observation served for clear discrimination between compensatory and noncompensatory pauses allowing a more accurate calculation of SACT. We conclude from our results that at least a differentiation is possible between normal and abnormal sinoatrial conduction properties using premature atrial stimulation. Our determinations of SNRT in patients with sinoatrial disease before and after an atropine-induced reduction of SACT indicate that sinoatrial conduction properties may significantly influence SNRT. On the contrary, sinus arrhythmia may challenge indirect estimation of SACT. Because of the dependence of SNRT on sinoatrial conduction properties on one hand, and of the validity of SACT calculation on sinus node automaticity on the other — both of which may be marked —, the two stimulation methods shoud be applied when sinus node function is studied in man. Repetition of both pacing techniques after administration of atropine is of appreciable additional value in assessing sinus node function in sinoatrial disease.

References

1. Bashour, T., Hemb, R., Wickramesekaran, R.: An unusual effect of atropine on overdrive suppression. Circulation **48,** 911 (1973)
2. Bonke, F. I. M., Bouman, L. N., van Rijn, H. E.: Change of cardiac rhythm in the rabbit after an atrial premature beat. Circulat. Res. **24,** 533 – 544 (1969)
3. Bonke, F. I. M., Bouman, L. N., Schopman, F. J. Cr.: Effect of an early atrial premature beat on activity of the sinoatrial node and atrial rhythm in the rabbit. Circulat. Res. **29,** 704 – 715 (1971)
4. Bonke, F. I. M.: Electrotonic spread in the sinoatrial node of the rabbit heart. Pflügers Arch. ges. Physiol. **339,** 17 – 23 (1973)
5. Breithardt, G., Seipel, L.: The influence of drugs on sinoatrial conduction time in man. This volume, p. 58 – 72
6. Delius, W., Wirtzfeld, A.: Significance of the sinus node recovery time. This volume, p. 25 – 32
7. Dhingra, R. C., Wyndham, C., Amat-Y-Leon, F., Denes, P., Wu, D., Rosen, K. M.: Sinus nodal responses to atrial extrastimuli in patients without apparent sinus node disease. Amer. J. Cardiol. **36,** 445 – 452 (1975)
8. Ferrer, M. I.: The sick sinus syndrome in atrial disease. J. Amer. med. Ass. **206,** 645 – 646 (1968)
9. Gupta, P. K., Lichstein, E., Chadda, K. D., Badui, E.: Appraisal of sinus nodal recovery time in patients with sick sinus syndrome. Amer. J. Cardiol. **34,** 265 – 270 (1974)
10. Hoffman, B. F., Cranefield, P. F.: Electrophysiology of the Heart. New York: McGraw-Hill, 1960
11. Kaplan, B. M., Langendorf, R., Lev, M., Pick, A.: Tachycardia-bradycardia syndrome (so-called "sick sinus syndrome"). Amer. J. Cardiol. **31,** 497 – 508 (1973)
12. Klein, H. O., Singer, D. H., Hoffman, B. F.: Effects of atrial premature systoles on sinus rhythm in the rabbit. Circulat. Res. **32,** 480 – 491 (1973)
13. Kulbertus, H. E., De Leval-Rutten, F., Mary, L., Casters, P.: Sinus node recovery time in the elderly. Brit. Heart J. **37,** 420 – 425 (1975)
14. Lown, B.: Electrical reversion of cardiac arrhythmias. Brit. Heart J. **29,** 469 – 489 (1967)
15. Mandel, W. J., Hayakawa, H., Danzig, R., Marcus, H. S.: Evaluation of sino-atrial node function in man by overdrive suppression. Circulation **44,** 59 – 66 (1971)
16. Mandel, W. J., Hayakawa, H., Allen, H. N., Danzig, R., Kermaier, A. I.: Assessment of sinus node function in patients with the sick sinus syndrome. Circulation **46,** 761 – 769 (1972)
17. Masini, G., Dianda, R., Graziina, A.: Analysis of sino-atrial conduction in man using premature atrial stimulation. Cardiovasc. Res. **9,** 498 – 508 (1975)

18. Miller, H. C., Strauss, H. C.: Measurement of sinoatrial conduction time by premature atrial stimulation in the rabbit. Circulat. Res. **35**, 935 – 947 (1974)
19. Moss, A. J., Davis, R. J.: Brady-tachy syndrome. Progr. cardiovasc. Dis. **16**, 439 – 454 (1974)
20. Narula O. S., Samet, P., Javier, R. P.: Significance of the sinus-node redovery time. Circulation **45**, 140 – 158 (1972)
21. Reiffel, J. A., Bigger, J. T., Giardina, E. G. V.: "Paradoxical" prolongation of sinus nodal recovery time after atropine in the sick sinus syndrome. Amer. J. Cardiol. **36**, 98 – 104 (1975)
22. Rosen, K. M., Loeb, H. S., Sinno, M. Z., Rahimtoola, S. H., Gunnar, R. M.: Cardiac conduction in patients with symptomatic sinus node disease. Circulation **43**, 836 – 844 (1971)
23. Sano, T., Yamagishi, S.: Spread of excitation from the sinus node. Circulat. Res. **16**, 423 – 430 (1965)
24. Sano, T., Iida, Y., Yamagishi, S.: Sites of conduction block in the atria in excess potassium and a doubt on the existence of the sino-atrial block. Proc. Jap. Acad. **42**, 1197 – 1201 (1966)
25. Seipel, L., Breithardt, G., Both, A., Loogen, F.: Diagnostische Probleme beim Sinusknotensyndrom. Z. Kardiol. **64**, 1 – 12 (1975)
26. Seipel, L., Breithardt, A., Both, A., Loogen, F.: Messung der sinu-atrialen Leitungszeit mittels vorzeitiger Vorhofstimulation beim Menschen. Dtsch. med. Wschr. **99**, 1895 – 1900 (1974)
27. Sherf, D.: The mechanism of sinoatrial block. Amer. J. Cardiol. **23**, 769 – 770 (1969)
28. Steinbeck, G., Körber, H.-J., Lüderitz, B.: Untersuchungen zur Sinusknotenfunktion beim Bradykardie-Tachykardie-Syndrom. Verh. dtsch. Ges. inn. Med. **80**, 1126 – 1129 (1974 a)
29. Steinbeck, G., Körber, H.-J., Lüderitz, B.: Die Bestimmung der sinuatrialen Leitungszeit beim Menschen durch gekoppelte atriale Einzelstimulation. Klin. Wschr. **52**, 1151 – 1157 (1974 b)
30. Steinbeck, G., Lüderitz, B.: Comparative study of sinoatrial conduction time and sinus node recovery time. Brit. Heart J. **37**, 956 – 962 (1975)
31. Steinbeck, G., Lüderitz, B.: Right atrial pacemaker shift following atrial stimulation in man. Submitted for publication (1976)
32. Strauss, H. C., Bigger, Jr., J. T.: Electrophysiological properties of the rabbit sinoatrial perinodal fibers. Circulat. Res. **31**, 490 – 506 (1972)
33. Strauss, H. C., Saroff, A. L., Bigger, J. T., Giardina, E. G. V.: Premature atrial stimulation as a key to the understanding of sinoatrial conduction in man. Ciruculation **47**, 88 – 93 (1973)
34. Strauss, H. C., and Bigger, J. T. Jr.: The authors reply. An unusual effect of atropine on overdrive suppression. Circulation **48**, 911 – 913 (1973)
35. Strauss, H. C., Wallace, A. G.: Premature atrial stimulation for evaluation of sinoatrial conduction in man. This volume, p. 33 – 44
36. West, T. C.: Ultramicroelectrode recording from the cardiac pacemaker. J. Pharmacol. exp. Ther. **115**, 283 – 290 (1955)
37. West, T. C.: Electrophysiology of the sinoatrial node. In: Electrical Phenomena in the Heart. de Mello, W.C. (ed.), New York and London: Academic Press, 1972, pp. 191 – 217

The Influence of Drugs on Sinoatrial Conduction Time in Man

G. Breithardt and L. Seipel

In contrast to the growing knowledge of the effect of drugs on atrioventricular and intraventricular conduction in man, the effects on sinus node function are less well known. Sinus node automaticity can be evaluated by high rate atrial stimulation and estimation of sinus node recovery time [25, 26, 32]. This parameter has been used for evaluation of the effect of drugs on sinus node function [3, 15, 17, 45, 46]. However, the properties of sinoatrial conduction have not yet been clearly established, because sinus node potentials cannot be accurately recorded in man.

Recently, Strauss et al. [47] proposed to calculate sinoatrial conduction time (SACT) from the length of the postextrasystolic pause and the spontaneous cycle using premature atrial stimulation. In the meanwhile, this approach has been adopted by several investigators [9, 27, 39, 44, 49]. The effect of drugs on calculated SACT has only been studied in a few instances [5, 9, 10, 11, 40, 48]. Therefore we systematically studied the effect of some known or new drugs on calculated SACT in 77 patients.

Methods

A detailed description of the method has been given elsewhere [9, 27, 41, 44, 47, 49]. In short, premature atrial stimuli are introduced during spontaneous sinus rhythm with increasing prematurity until the effective refractory period of the atrium is reached. The following intervals are measured from a high right atrial electrogram:

1. A_1A_1, the spontaneous cycle length preceding the premature stimulus
2. A_1A_2, the coupling interval or the test interval between the last spontaneous beat and the premature stimulus
3. A_2A_3, the return cycle length or the postextrasystolic pause.
4. A_3A_4, the postreturn cycle, i.e., the spontaneous cycle following the return cycle.

Additionally, intra-artrial conduction time (P-A interval, i.e., the interval between the onset of the P wave and the low right atrial electrogram in the His bundle electrogram) was measured. Paper speed was 50 or 100 mm/s.

SACT is calculated from the length of the return cycle (A_2A_3) and the spontaneous cycle (A_1A_1) during reset responses of the sinus node according to the following equation:

$$SACT = \frac{(\overline{A_2A_3}) - (\overline{A_1A_1})}{2} \qquad [9, 44, 47]$$

Sinus node recovery time (SRT) was measured as the interval between the last stimulus-induced atrial beat and the first beat of sinus origin after abrupt cessation of high rate atrial stimulation [25, 26, 32]. The rate of stimulation was increased stepwise at increments of 10 – 20 beats/min starting just above the spontaneous rate. Duration of stimulation was at least 30 s.

The following protocol was adopted for testing the effects of drugs on sinus node function: Patients having given informed consent were studied in the nonsedative, postabsorptive state. After introduction of the catheters for His bundle electrography and high rate atrial stimulation, control registrations were done during a 10-min period. Then, high rate stimulation (for estimation of SRT) and single premature stimulation (for estimation of SACT) were performed. The drugs to be tested were injected i.v. within 3 – 5 min. After drug injection two different protocols were followed. Either the sequence was "high rate, premature, and high rate atrial stimulation" or "premature atrial, high rate atrial, and premature atrial stimulation." The maximum deviation from the control value of each parameter was used for further evaluation.

The effect of the following drugs was studied (number of patients and dose in parenthesis):

1. Atropine (1 mg or 0.02 mg/kg i.v., n = 18)
2. Proprafenone (1 mg/kg i.v., n = 10) (Helopharm, Berlin)
3. Verapamil (0.1 mg/kg i.v., n = 11)
4. Disopyramide (1.5 – 2.0 mg/kg i.v., n = 8) (Hoechst AG, Werk Albert)
5. Diphenylhydantoin (5.0 mg/kg i.v., n = 3)
6. 564-A-1 (1.0 mg/kg i.v., n = 12) (Knoll AG, Ludwigshafen)
7. Mexiletine (3.0 mg/kg i.v., n = 3) (Boehringer, Ingelheim)
8. R 818 (1.0 – 1.5 mg/kg i.v., n = 9) (Kettelhack Riker, Borken)
9. CI 661 (0.5 mg/kg i.v., n = 3) (Parke-Davis, Munich)

Statistical evaluation was done by use of student's t test for paired data. Results are given as mean ± standard deviation ($\bar{x} \pm s_x$).

Results

A total of 77 patients was studied before and after application of the different drugs. The results will be discussed for each drug seperately.

Atropine was tested in 18 patients, 5 of whom exhibited persistent or transient bradycardia. Seven patients showed the typical signs of the sick sinus syndrome [16]. Two typical examples of the effect of atropine on calculated SACT are shown in Figure 1.

Spontaneous cycle length in 15 patients with a typical biphasic pattern of the return cycles decreased from 1075.4 ± 265.0 ms to 785.2 ± 174.9 ms ($\bar{x} \pm s_x$; $P < 0.01$). Before atropine calculated SACT was 123.8 ± 46.4 ms, decreasing to 74.4 ± 24.0 ms ($P < 0.001$) after atropine. In 3 patients with a chaotic pattern of the return cycles (in whom SACT cannot be calculated due to methodologic reasons [9, 44]) a typical biphasic pattern of the return cycles appeared after atropine (Fig. 1).

The percentage of decrease of the spontaneous cycle length in patients without sinus node dysfunction was – 19.7%, in patients with sinus node dysfunction (sinus bradycardia and sick sinus syndrome) – 26.1%, and in the 3 patients with a chaotic pattern of the return cycles – 32.2%. The control values of the spontaneous cycle length were 894.8 ± 100.6 ms, 1122.8 ± 216.1 ms, and 1294.7 ± 452.5 ms, respectively. The effect of atropine on calculated SACT was not different in patients without and with sinus node dysfunction (– 41.0 and – 39.5%, respectively). In 6 patients the stimulation procedure was performed twice after drug application in order to establish the duration of action on calculated SACT. This was relatively short with a maximal effect usually during the first minutes. After more than 5 – 10 min, the effect decreased progressively (Fig. 1).

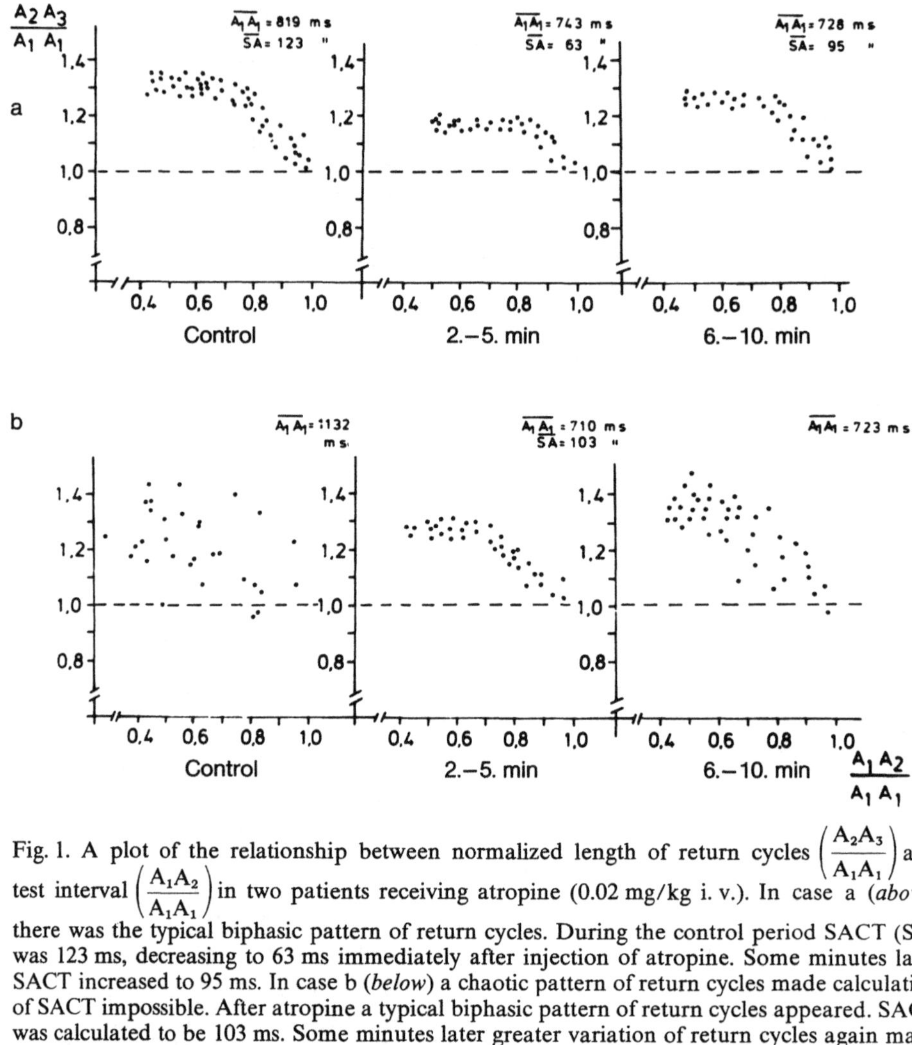

Fig. 1. A plot of the relationship between normalized length of return cycles $\left(\frac{A_2A_3}{A_1A_1}\right)$ and test interval $\left(\frac{A_1A_2}{A_1A_1}\right)$ in two patients receiving atropine (0.02 mg/kg i. v.). In case a (*above*) there was the typical biphasic pattern of return cycles. During the control period SACT (SA) was 123 ms, decreasing to 63 ms immediately after injection of atropine. Some minutes later SACT increased to 95 ms. In case b (*below*) a chaotic pattern of return cycles made calculation of SACT impossible. After atropine a typical biphasic pattern of return cycles appeared. SACT was calculated to be 103 ms. Some minutes later greater variation of return cycles again made calculation of SACT impossible.

The effect of *Propafenone*, a new antiarrhythmic drug which has just been introduced into clinical trials [1, 2, 43], was studied in 10 patients. Two patients exhibited sinus bradycardia and one patient a sick sinus syndrome. In 8 patients premature atrial stimulation was performed twice.

Spontaneous cycle length increased from 867.9 ± 231.9 ms to 928.8 ± 200.0 ms during the first period after drug application ($P < 0.025$). During the second period it lengthened further to 977.3 ± 210.7 ms ($P < 0.0025$). Calculated SACT increased from a control value of 104.7 ± 27.0 ms to 126.2 ± 35.5 ms and 122.2 ± 27.4 ms ($P < 0.01$). Using the longest value of SACT during one of both periods, maximal prolongation was 26.5% ($P < 0.0025$).

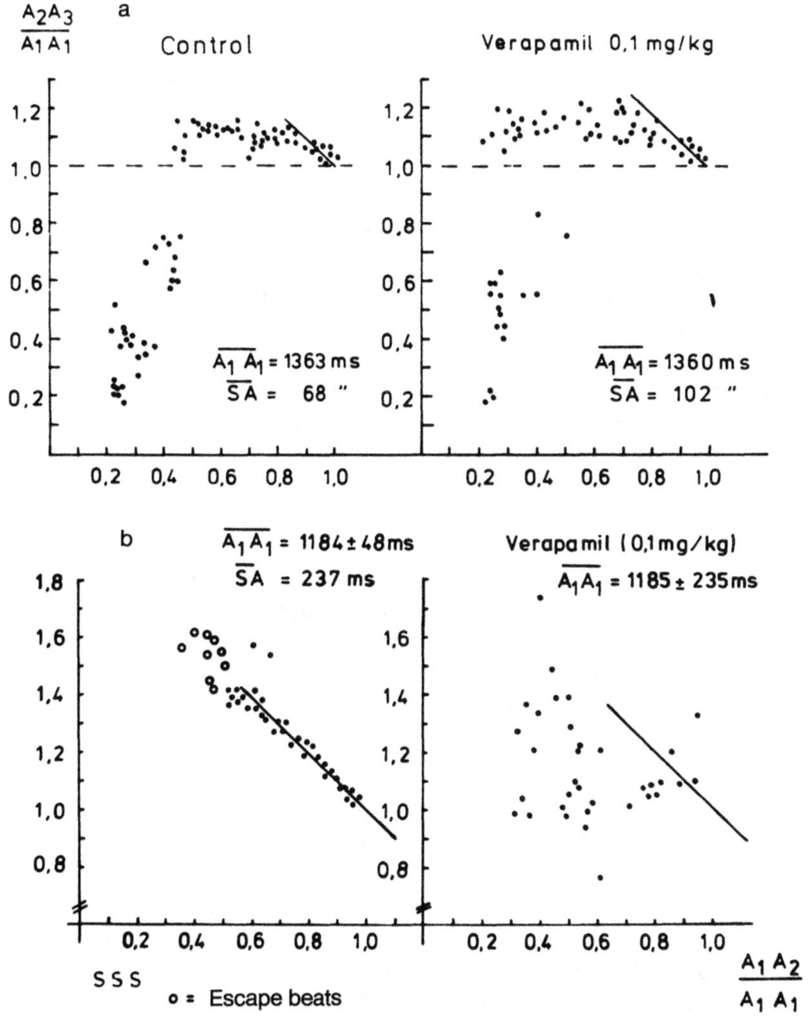

Fig. 2. A plot similar to Fig. 1. In case a (*above*) there was the typical biphasic pattern of the return cycles. Calculated SACT was 68 ms. At early coupling intervals very short return cycles occurred probably due to sinoatrial entrance block [18] and sinus node reentry [30, 36, 37]. After injection of verapamil SACT increased to 102 ms without a change of spontaneous cycle length (A_1A_1). The return cycles showed greater variation than before. There was still a small zone of very short return cycles. In case b (*below*) SACT was 237 ms. At test cycles less than 50% of spontaneous cycle length His bundle escape beats occurred (*open circles*). After verapamil there was an atypical chaotic pattern of the return cycles signifying great impairment of sinoatrial conduction.

There was no difference between patients with (n = 3) and without sinus node dysfunction.

Verapamil was tested in 13 patients, 5 with a sick sinus syndrome. One of the latter patients had an ectopic atrial rhythm during the study as judged from the P wave configuration in lead I – III.

The response of spontaneous sinus cycle length to verapamil was different. In 8 patients spontaneous cycle length decreased by an average of 78.0 ms, whereas in 4 patients it increased by an average of 138.0 ms. However, within the whole group verapamil caused no significant change of the spontaneous cycle length, which increased slightly from an average of 963.9 ± 249.0 ms to 965.2 ± 224.9 ms.

During the control study calculated SACT was 104.5 ± 53.7 ms. After verapamil it increased by an average of 47.5 ± 32.2 ms in 6 patients. A typical example is shown in Figure 2. In 2 patients calculated SACT remained essentially unchanged. It decreased in 2 further patients by −31 and −65 ms. In one patient with a sick sinus syndrome and a very long SACT of 237 ms, a chaotic pattern of the return cycles was observed after application of verapamil (Fig. 2), which makes calculation of SACT impossible. In the aforementioned patient with an atrial ectopic rhythm during the study, the calculated conduction time (probably representing conduction time in and out of the ectopic focus) was not influenced by verapamil. Spontaneous cycle length remained unchanged, too. In one patient a progressive increase in the return cycle length occurred during the control study. There was no plateau zone. This pattern suggests nonreset of the sinus node [47]. After verapamil, in spite of an increase in spontaneous cycle length from 695 to 751 ms, this pattern remained unchanged.

In those 2 patients who demonstrated a decrease of calculated SACT, maximal sinus node recovery time decreased, too (1050 − 700 ms, and 4080 − 2880 ms). This was in contrast to the prolongation of sinus node recovery time in the remaining patients.

The effect of *564-A-1,* a new antiarrhythmic drug, which is not yet in clinical use, was studied in 12 patients, one presenting with a sick sinus syndrome. Spontaneous cycle length during the control study was 937.3 ± 123.9 ms, increasing to 960.3 ± 143.1 ms after the drug was injected (N.S.). Calculated SACT before 564-A-1 was 115.6 ± 30.8 ms. In 5 patients there was a marked increase of calculated SACT of about + 32.3 ± 9.7 ms. In the remaining patients this effect was smaller (+ 2.8 ± 7.6 ms). Mean calculated SACT after drug injection was 130.4 ± 33.5 ms ($P < 0.025$). In no patients did an atypical pattern of the return cycles or sinoatrial exit block occur. The effect in one patient with a sick sinus syndrome was similar to the effects in other patients.

The effect of *Diphenylhydantoin (DPH)* in three patients will be reported on a preliminary basis. In 2 patients spontaneous cycle length was not affected by DPH, increasing only slightly from 936 to 956 ms. Calculated SACT during the control study was 70 and 118 ms, respectively. After DPH, calculated SACT increased to 110 and 145 ms.

One 17-year-old patient was studied during digitalis intoxication due to suicidal ingestion of the drug. Serum digoxin level at the time of study was 6.3 ng/ml (we are indebted to Dr. Risler, 1st Medical Clinic A, for serum digoxin estimation). During the study she was in regular sinus rhythm with a spontaneous cycle length of 1086 ms. Calculated SACT was 120 ms

(Fig. 3). After injection of DPH, heart rate remained unchanged. Calculated SACT increased to 144 ms. Five days later, serum digoxin was 0.3 ng/ml and calculated SACT had declined to 66 ms at a spontaneous cycle length of 875 ms.

CI 661 is a further new drug, which was tested in 3 patients on a preliminary basis, too. Mean spontaneous cycle length decreased from 944.3 ±22.5 ms to 913.3 ± 142.5 ms (N.S.). This difference did not reach statistical significance due to the limited number of patients.

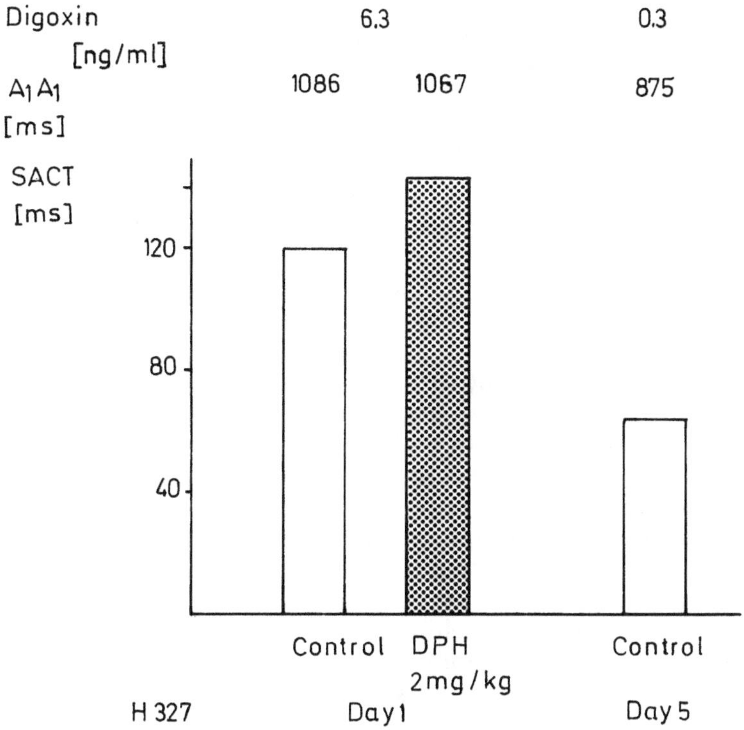

Fig. 3. SACT in a case of digoxin intoxication. At a serum level of 6.3 ng/ml digoxin, SACT was 120 ms. After injection of diphenylhydantoin (2 mg/kg i. v.) SACT increased to 144 ms without change of spontaneous cycle length. Five days later SACT was 62 ms at a serum digoxin level of 0.3 ng/ml.

R 818, which is in preclinical evaluation as well, was tested in 9 patients. Two patients were studied because of sinus bradycardia. Spontaneous cycle length decreased from 928.0 ± 222.4 ms to 902.9 ± 206.5 ms (N.S.). During the control study calculated SACT was 87.2 ± 28.5 ms. It increased slightly during the first stimulation period after drug application (93.3 ± 35.9 ms, n = 9), but it decreased to 79.8 ± 14.0 ms in seven patients in whom the stimulation procedure was repeated. These changes were not significant. There was no difference between the reaction of patients without and with sinus node dysfunction.

Disopyramide (B 712) has been in clinical use for some time [3, 8, 38]. It was tested in eight patients. Mean spontaneous cycle length before injection of the drug was 861.0±133.8 ms. Mean calculated SACT was 111.1±32.4 ms. After drug application there was neither a significant change of the mean spontaneous cycle length (858.0±128.1 ms and 884.8 ±81.0 ms, respectively) nor of the calculated SACT (108.2±36.4 and 111.4 ±39.3 ms, respectively). Nevertheless, there were marked changes of calculated SACT in individual patients. In four patients calculated SACT was prolonged by disopyramide between 7.9 to 23.6% (range; mean prolongation +16.3±6.9%) whereas in the remaining four patients, it decreased between 15.5 and 27.0% (range; mean decrease −20.7±5.7%).

The effect of *Mexiletine (Kö 1173)* was studied in 3 patients. It decreased the spontaneous cycle length from an average of 609.3±16.0 ms to 567.0±18.7 ms. The decreases in the individual cases were 23, 23, and 71 ms, respectively. Calculated SACT decreased by 5,4, and 17 ms.

In 5 patients atropine was tested for its effect after prior administration of either R 818, disopyramide, or 564-A-1. In 3 cases these drugs caused a reduction of calculated SACT, whereas in the remaining 2 cases, SACT increased. After atropine, calculated SACT decreased significantly ($P < 0.01$) in all cases by an average of 45.1 ms during a 20−30 min period after administration of one of these drugs.

In 67 patients the influence of the drugs tested on the relationship between calculated SACT and sinus node recovery time was studied. In each patient, in whom both parameters were evaluated, the stimulation rate with maximal overdrive suppression of the sinus node and the calculated SACT were defined both before and after drug administration. The results are shown in Figure 4 in which the absolute changes of stimulation rate and calculated SACT are plotted. The drugs were treated as a whole because there was no difference between the individual drugs.

Figure 4 shows an inverse relationship between the change of stimulation rate with maximal sinus node suppression and the change of calculated SACT. After application of drugs that caused a prolongation of calculated SACT, the stimulation rate with maximal sinus node depression decreased in many cases, above all in those who had abnormally long values of calculated SACT during the control period. The opposite effect occurred when calculated SACT decreased, e.g., by the action of atropine, mexiletine, and in some cases disopyramide. However, in 15 patients no change of the stimulation rate with maximal sinus node depression occurred in spite of marked changes of calculated SACT. This was the case mainly in patients with normal or only slightly prolonged values of calculated SACT.

Since changes of intra-atrial conduction time and of sinus node automaticity after drug application may influence the length of the return cycles (and thus the value of calculated SACT), the P-A intervals and the length of the postreturn cycles were evaluated. Intra-atrial conduction time (P-A interval) was prolonged only to a small degree by the following drugs:
Verapamil: +2.6 ms;
Propafenone: +6 ms;

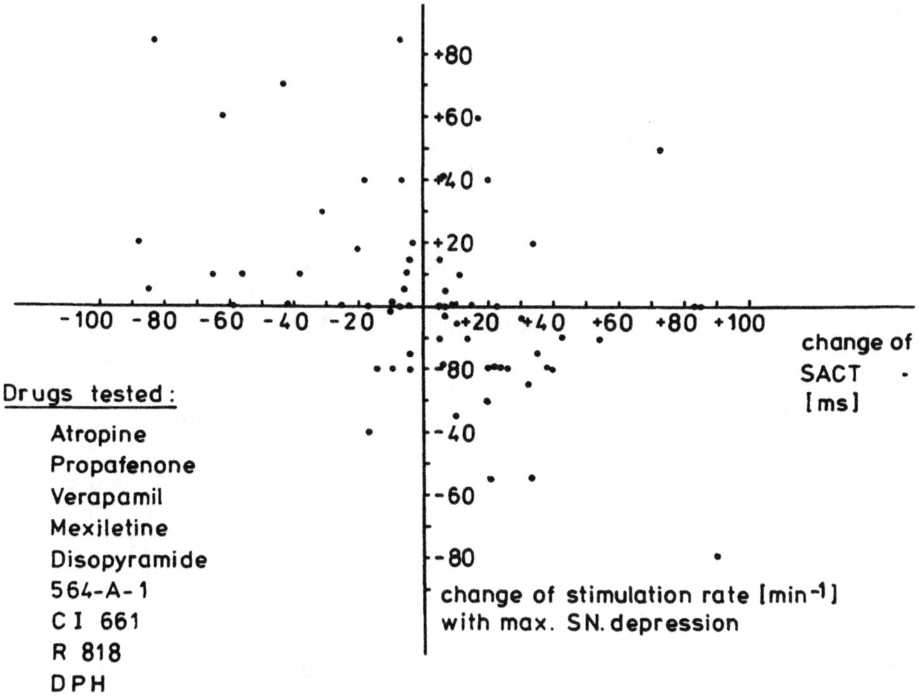

Fig. 4. A plot of changes of SACT vs. changes of stimulation rate at which maximal sinus node depression after drug administration occurred. (See text for further explanation.)

Disopyramide: +0.4 ms;
564-A-1: +2.1 ms;
R 818: +3.6 ms;
Atropine: −2.5 ms.

These changes were not significant in any of the groups. Similar results were obtained with the remaining three drugs which were only tested in a few patients. Additionally, the lengths of the postreturn cycles (A_3A_4) were compared to the spontaneous cycle length (A_1A_1) before and after drug administration. Mean (A_3A_4 minus A_1A_1) did not change significantly in any group after drug administration. The following mean values of (A_3A_4 minus A_1A_1) were found before and after drug administration:

	Before	After
Verapamil:	19.3 ± 20.9 ms	10.5 ± 24.3 ms
Propafenone:	7.4 ± 28.4 ms	18.9 ± 40.3 ms
Disopyramide:	28.6 ± 13.1 ms	7.9 ± 32.6 ms
564-A-1:	41.2 ± 32.7 ms	22.3 ± 47.4 ms
R 818:	12.3 ± 22.5 ms	14.3 ± 25.8 ms
Atropine:	27.2 ± 26.5 ms	24.2 ± 22.5 ms

Discussion

The intention of the present study was to evaluate the effects of different drugs on calculated SACT in man. The methodologic approach and the limitations of this method for indirect estimation of sinoatrial conduction properties has been widely discussed elsewhere [9, 28, 39, 41, 44, 47, 49].

Several well-known drugs such as atropine, verapamil, and diphenylhydantoin were studied [13, 17, 20, 23, 45]. Additionally, we tested some new antiarrhythmic drugs such as propafenone, CI 661, 564-A-1, R 818, disopyramide (B 712), and mexiletine (Kö 1173). Propafenone [2], disopyramide (B 712), [8, 34, 38], and mexiletine (Kö 1173) [51] have been used in some clinical trials, whereas CI 661 [43, 45], R 818, and 564-A-1 are new antiarrhythmic drugs about which only electrophysiologic data exist in man (unpublished data). Propafenone, CI 661, and R 818 slow conduction velocity in all compartments of the heart to nearly the same degree as revealed by His bundle electrography. They have a slightly more pronounced effect on conduction velocity in the His-Purkinje system (H-V time) [1, 42, 43, 45, unpublished data]. On the other side, mexiletine (Kö 1173) 564-A-1, and disopyramide have either no effect on intracardiac conduction or exert only small effects on the His-Purkinje system [3, 21, 24, 42, 50, unpublished data].

SACT is calculated from the length of the return cycle and the spontaneous cycle after reset of the sinus node [9, 27, 44, 47]. The following three components constitute the length of the return cycle: they may change independently after drug application:

1. The time for antegrade and retrograde conduction in the sinoatrial node and the perinodal region (true sinoatrial conduction time).
2. The sinus nodal cycle length during the return cycle.
3. The time for conduction of the impulse between the site of stimulation and the sinoatrial node [9, 31, 41].

Since only the first component reflects true sinoatrial conduction time, changes of the other two components should be excluded when studying the effect of drugs on SACT. In our study, no drug caused a significant change of either intra-atrial conduction time or of the difference between the length of the postreturn cycle and the spontaneous cycle length. A change of the postreturn cycle relative to the spontaneous cycle length may indicate a change of sinus node automaticity after premature discharge of the sinus node [6, 7, 41]. Though in most cases some sinus node depression occurred, this was not different after drug administration compared to the control period. Therefore, we conclude that the changes of calculated SACT that we observed reflect true changes of sinoatrial conduction.

The effects of the drugs tested in this study on calculated SACT were different (Table 1). Propafenone, 564-A-1, verapamil, DPH, and CI 661 prolonged calculated SACT between 12 and 30%, on an average. R 818 and disopyramide had no effect on calculated SACT, whereas atropine and probably also mexiletine (Kö 1173) shortened SACT. These differences were

Table 1. A summary of the effects of different drugs on spontaneous cycle length (A_1A_1) and calculated SACT

Drug	A_1A_1	SACT
1. Propafenone n=10	**↑** +13%	**↑** +27%
2. Verapamil n=10	→ 0%	↑ +18%
3. DPH n=3	→ + 2%	↑ +30%
4. CI 661 n=3	→ − 3%	↑ +17%
5. 564-A-1 n=12	→ + 2%	**↑** +12%
6. R 818 n=9	→ − 3%	↑ +7%
7. Disopyramide n=8	→ + 3%	→ − 3%
8. Atropine n=15	**↓** −24%	**↓** −27%
9. Mexilentine n=3	↓ −7%	↓ − 9%

↑ = nonsignificant changes
↑ = significant changes ($P < 0.025$)
↑ = prolongation
→ = no effect
↓ = shortening

significant only in case of propafenone (P <0.01), 564-A-1 (P <0.025), and atropine (P <0.001). Due to the limited number of cases receiving DPH, CI 661, and mexiletine, these results have to be regarded as preliminary. Verapamil caused marked changes of SACT in most patients. However, since a decrease of SACT and sinus node recovery time occurred in two patients, the results were not significant within the whole group.

Verapamil is a potent antiarrhythmic drug which has been in clinical use for many years [4, 23]. It is the main representative of a group of drugs which inhibit slow-channel conduction [12, 22] by their calcium-antagonistic action [12, 22]. Experimental studies have shown that the action potentials of the sinus node and the AV node are slow-channel – dependent [52], in contrast to the action potentials of most other tissues which depend on rapid sodium channels. This may explain why the site of action of verapamil is in the AV node as demonstrated by His bundle electrography [17, 20, 33, 45]. Atrial, His-Purkinje and intraventricular conduction is not affected by verapamil [17, 20, 33, 45].

The effect of verapamil on the SA node in man still needs further elucidation. In patients with normal sinus node function, verapamil caused no or only minor changes of sinus node recovery time [17, 20, 33, 45, 46]. Some clinical observations suggest that verapamil may have deleterious effects on sinus node function [19, 29, 35]. SACT has not yet been studied after verapamil. In this study, verapamil caused marked prolongation of SACT in 8 of 10 patients. This is consonant with the aforementioned experimental studies which have demonstrated that the SA node is calcium-dependent. The opposite reaction of SACT (and SRT) in two patients in whom shortening of both parameters occurred remains unexplained. Verapamil has no effect on the atrial myocardium because the P-A intervals remained constant. This is further substantiated by the findings in one patient with an ectopic atrial rhythm both before and after verapamil. In this case neither spontaneous cycle length nor conduction time between the site of stimulation and the ectopic focus was changed by verapamil.

Atropine, by its vagolytic actions, exerted marked effects on spontaneous sinus node discharge and on calculated SACT. The effect on heart rate was more marked in patients with sinus node dysfunction, whereas the effect on SACT in patients with and without sinus node dysfunction was the same. The effect of atropine on both heart rate and calculated SACT was short, decreasing in some cases already during the second period after drug injection.

Disopyramide, though demonstrating no significant effect on calculated SACT in the whole group, caused opposite changes in individual patients. These opposite effects may be due to two different properties of the drug that have been elucidated in animal studies [14, 53]. On the one hand, it has a vagolytic action. On the other, it depresses conductivity within the AV node. It may be speculated whether disopyramide exerts a similar twofold action on the SA node. The net effect would then depend on the actual state of vegetative innervation.

The effect of diphenylhydantoin in a case of digitalis intoxication deserves notice because it prolonged SACT. This was also the case in two additional patients. This may indicate that DPH in the case of digitalis intoxication is not able to antagonize the negative dromotropic effects of digitalis.

In a few cases we observed a chaotic pattern of the return cycles. The electrophysiologic mechanism is hitherto unexplained [9, 44]. Atropine was able to restore a typical biphasic pattern of the return cycles, probably by enhancing sinoatrial conduction. The opposite reaction was observed in a case with maximally prolonged calculated SACT. In this case, a chaotic pattern of the return cycles appeared after injection of verapamil, which has been shown to slow sinoatrial conduction in most patients. It may be concluded that the chaotic pattern of the return cycles is due to greatly impaired sinoatrial conduction. Additionally, disturbances of sinus node automaticity may play an important part because spontaneous cycle lengths varied to a greater extent than during a regular biphasic pattern of the return cycles.

Reiffel et al. [39] found an inverse relationship between spontaneous cycle length and calculated SACT in patients with sinus arrhythmia. They concluded that "in order to interpret the effect of a medication on the SACT, one must know the direction and degree of change in SACT to be expected simply from a change in sinoatrial cycle length induced by the drug." In view of these findings, drugs which prolong spontaneous cycle length such as propafenon should lead to a decrease of calculated SACT or, vice versa, drugs which shorten spontaneous cycle length, such as atropine, should prolong SACT. The opposite effect was observed in our study. Therefore we conclude that the effects of the drugs tested on SACT are independent of their effects on heart rate. We doubt whether the approach of Reiffel et al. [39] is correct because their mode of calculation still assumes that the sinus cycle length during the A_1A_1 and the A_2A_3 intervals are identical, which was certainly not the case in view of the spontaneous sinus arrhythmia in their patients. Furthermore, we were unable to find any relationship between sinus cycle length and calculated SACT in 64 patients [41].

In case of adverse effects of a drug on sinus node function, it seems important to know whether it may be overcome by an antagonistic drug. Therefore, we tested the effect of atropine on SACT after prior administration of an antiarrhythmic drug. These preliminary results showed a reduction of SACT in all five cases, suggesting atropine as a possible antidote in case of adverse side-effects.

We were able to establish an inverse relationship between changes of the atrial stimulation rate leading to maximal sinus node depression and calculated SACT after drug application. This was most apparent in patients with abnormally long values of SACT during the control period. This inverse relationship after pharmacologic intervention probably is due to either impairment or improvement of sinoatrial conduction.

In addition to His bundle electrography, estimation of SACT gives a further characterization of the effects of antiarrhythmic drugs in man. The practical conclusions which may be drawn from the results of the present study may be that some of the drugs will be useful in terminating tachycardias due to sinus node reentry [30, 36, 37]. This point deserves further evaluation. Furthermore, they may be used for provocative tests to detect latent disturbances of sinoatrial function.

Summary

Seventy-seven patients were studied by high rate and programmed premature atrial stimulation for estimation of sinus node recovery time and sinoatrial conduction time (SACT) before and after administration of nine different drugs. The drugs tested were: atropine, propafenone, disopyramide, mexiletine, verapamil, diphenylhydantoin, and four new antiarrhythmic drugs which are not yet in clinical use. Three different reactions of calculated SACT after drug administration occurred: a prolongation of calculated SACT (propafenone, verapamil, diphenylhydantoin, CI 661, 564-A-1), no change of calculated SACT (R 818, disopyramide), and a reduction of calculated SACT (atropine, mexiletine). Atropine was shown to have an antidotal effect after prior administration of some of these drugs. A comparison of the changes of the stimulation rate with maximal sinus node depression and of calculated SACT revealed an inverse relationship between both parameters after drug administration. This indicates that the properties of sinoatrial conduction may be important to achieve maximal sinus node depression by high rate atrial stimulation.

References

1. Beck, O. A., Witt, E., Hochrein, H.: Der Einfluß des Antiarrhythmikums Propafenon auf die intrakardiale Erregungsleitung. Klinische Untersuchungen mit Hilfe der His-Bündel-Elektrographie. Z. Kardiol. **64,** 179 (1975)
2. Beck, O. A., Krämer, K.-D., Wolf, R., Müller, A., Hochrein, H.: Propafenon, ein neues Antiarrhythmikum zur Therapie tachykarder und extrasystolischer Herzrhythmusstörungen. Med. Klin. **70,** 95 (1975)
3. Befeler, B., Castellanos, Jr., A., Wells, D. E., Vagueiro, M. C.,Yeh, B. K.: Electrophysiologic effects of the antiarrhythmic agent disopyramide phosphate. Amer. J. Cardiol. **35,** 282 (1975)
4. Belz, G. G., Bender, F.: Therapie der Herzrhythmusstörungen mit Verapamil, Stuttgart: G. Fischer 1974
5. Bond, R. C., Engel, T. R., Schaal, S. F.: The effect of digitalis on sinoatrial conduction in man. Circulation suppl. **4,** 147 (1973)
6. Bonke, F. I. M., Bouman, L. N., van Rijn, H. E.: Change of cardiac rhythm in the rabbit after an atrial premature beat. Circulat. Res. **24,** 533 (1969)
7. Bouman, L. N., Gerlings, E. D., Biersteker, P. A., Bonke, F. I. M.: Pacemaker shift in the sino-atrial node during vagal stimulation. Pflügers Arch. ges. Physiol. **302,** 255 (1968)
8. Bouvrain, Y.: Le disopyramide, Ann. Cardiol. Angeiol. **19,** 352 (1970)
9. Breithardt, G., Seipel, L., Both, A.: Die Messung der „sinu-atrialen Leitungszeit" beim Menschen. In: Symposium His-Bündel-Elektrographie (Seipel, L., ed.), Stuttgart: Schattauer, 1975
10. Breithardt, G., Seipel, L., Both, A., Loogen, F.: The effect of atropine on sino-atrial conduction time in man. Europ. J. Cardiol. In press
11. Breithardt, G., Seipel, L., Höhfeld, E., Both, A., Loogen, F.: Pharmakologische Beeinflussung der „sinu-atrialen Leitungszeit" und der Sinusknotenautomatie beim Menschen. Z. Kardiol. **64,** 895 (1975)
12. Cranefield, P. F., Aronson, R. S., Wit, A. L.: Effect of verapamil on the normal action potential and on a calcium dependent slow response of canine cardiac Purkinje fibers. Circulat. Res. **34,** 204 (1974)
13. Damato, A. N., Berkowitz, W. D., Patton, R. D., Lau, S. H.: The effect of diphenylhydantoin on atrioventricular and intraventricular conduction in man. Amer. Heart J. **79,** 51 (1970)
14. Dean, R. R., Ferguson, D. M.: Effects of disopyramide on the A-V conduction system. Arch. int. Pharmacodyn. **190,** 183 (1971)

15. Engel, T. R., Schaal, S. F.: Digitalis in the sick sinus syndrome. The effects of digitalis on sinoatrial automaticity and atrioventricular conduction. Circulation **48,** 1201 (1973)
16. Ferrer, M. I.: The sick sinus syndrome. Circulation **47,** 635 (1973)
17. Gleichmann, U., Seipel, L., Loogen, F.: Der Einfluß von Antiarrhythmika auf die intrakardiale Erregungsleitung (His-Bündel-Elektrographie) und Sinusknotenautomatie beim Menschen. Dtsch. med. Wschr. **98,** 1487 (1973)
18. Goldreyer, B. N., Damato, A. N.: Sinoatrial-node entrance block, Circulation **44,** 789 (1971)
19. Heck, J., Heim, R. R., Elbers, C.: Letaler Ausgang nach intravenöser Behandlung mit Isoptin. Z. Kreisl.-Forsch. **61,** 621 (1972)
20. Husaini, M. H., Kvasnicka, J., Rydén, L., Holmberg, S.: Action of verapamil on sinus node, atrioventricular and intraventricular conduction. Brit. Heart J. **35,** 734 (1973)
21. Josephson, M. E., Caracta, A. R., Lau, S. H., Gallagher, J. J., Damato, A. N.: Electrophysiological evaluation of disopyramide in man. Amer. Heart J. **86,** 771 (1973)
22. Kohlhardt, M., Bauer, B., Krause, H., Fleckenstein, A.: Differentiation of the transmembrane Na and Ca channels in mammalian cardiac fibers by the use of specific inhibitors. Pflügers Arch. ges. Physiol. **335,** 309 (1972)
23. Krikler, D.: Verapamil in cardiology. Europ. J. Cardiol. **2,** 3 (1974)
24. Lang, K. F., Just, H., Limbourg, P.: Untersuchungen über die Einwirkungen von Mexiletin (Kö 1173) auf die A-V Überleitungszeit und Sinusimpulsautomatie bei Herzgesunden und Patienten mit Erkrankung des Reizleitungssystems. Z. Kardiol. In press
25. Lange, G.: Action of driving stimuli from intrinsic and extrinsic sources on in situ cardiac pacemaker tissues. Circulat. Res. **17,** 449 (1965)
26. Mandel, W., Hayakawa, H., Danzig, R., Marcus, H. S.: Evaluation of sino-atrial node function in man by overdrive suppression. Circulation **46,** 59 (1971)
27. Masini, G., Dianda, R., Graziina, A.: Analysis of sino-atrial conduction in man using premature atrial stimulation. Cardiovasc. Res. **9,** 498 (1975)
28. Miller, H. C., Strauss, H. C.: Measurement of sinoatrial conduction time by premature atrial stimulation in the rabbit. Circulat. Res. **35,** 935 (1974)
29. Motté, G., Bellanger, P., Vogel, M., Behausen, B., Welti, J. J.: Asystole suive de choc cardiogénique aprés intraveneuse de vérapamil. Ann. Cardiol. Angéiol. **24,** 157 (1975)
30. Narula, O. S.: Sinus node reentry. A mechanism for supraventricular tachycardia. Circulation **50,** 1114 (1974)
31. Narula, O. S.: Disorders of sinus node function: Electrophysiological evaluation. In: His Bundle electrography and Clinical Electrophysiology, Narula, O. S. (ed.). Philadelphia: F. A. Davis, 1975
32. Narula, O. S., Samet, P., Javier, R. P.: Significance of the sinus-node recovery time. Circulation **45,** 140 (1972)
33. Neuß, H., Schlepper, M.: Der Einfluß von Verapamil auf die atrioventrikuläre Überleitung. Lokalisation des Wirkungsortes mit His-Bündel-Elektrogrammen. Verh. dtsch. Ges. Kreisl.-Forsch. **37,** 433 (1971)
34. Olbermann, M., Just, H., Guckenbiehl, H., Lang, K. F.: Antiarrhythmische Wirkung von Disopyramid. Verh. dtsch. Ges. inn. Med. 1975, in press
35. own observations
36. Paulay, K. L., Damato, A. N.: Effect of digoxin on sinus nodal reentry in the dog. Amer. J. Cardiol. **35,** 370 (1975)
37. Paulay, K. L., Varghese, P. J., Damato, A. N.: Sinus node reentry. An in vivo demonstration in the dog. Circulat. Res. **32,** 455 (1973)
38. Puech, P.: Le traitement des arythmies cardiaques par le disopyramide. Journ. méd. Montpellier **4,** 132 (1969)
39. Reiffel, J. A., Bigger, Jr., J. T., Konstam, M. A.: The relationship between sinoatrial conduction time and sinus cycle length during spontaneous sinus arrhythmia in adults. Circulation **50,** 924 (1974)
40. Reiffel, J. A., Bigger, Jr., J. T., Reid, D. S.: The effect of atropine on sinus node function in adults with sinus bradycardia. Amer. J. Cardiol. **35,** 165 (1975), abstr.
41. Seipel, L., Breithardt, G.: Sinusknotenautomatie und sinu-atriale Leitung. Z. Kardiol. **64,** 1014 (1975)

42. Seipel, L., Breithardt, G., Both, A.: Elektrophysiologische Effekte der Antiarrhythmika Disopyramid und Propafenon auf das menschliche Reizleitungssystem. Z. Kardiol. **64,** 731 (1975)
43. Seipel, L., Both, A., Breithardt, G., Loogen, F.: Die Wirkung neuer Antiarrhythmika (Aprindin, Propafenon, CI 661) auf die intrakardiale Erregungsleitung und die Sinusknotenautomatie beim Menschen. In: Syposium His-Bündel-Elektrographie (Seipel, L, ed.), Stuttgart: Schattauer, 1975
44. Seipel, L., Breithardt, G., Both, A., Loogen, F.: Messung der „sinu-atrialen Leitungszeit" mittels vorzeitiger Vorhofstimulation beim Menschen. Dtsch. med. Wschr. **99,** 1895 (1974)
45. Seipel, L., Both, A., Breithardt, G., Gleichmann, U., Loogen, F.: Action of antiarrhythmic drugs on His bundle electrogram and sinus node function. Acta cardiol. (Brux.) Suppl. **18,** 251 (1974)
46. Seipel, L., Both, A., Gleichmann, U., Loogen, F., Sawowa, A.: Effects of antiarrhythmic drugs on sinus node and cardiac conduction in man. Presented at: VII World Congress of Cardiology, Buenos Aires, 1974
47. Strauss, H. C., Saroff, A. L., Bigger, Jr., J. T., Giardina, E. G. V.: Premature atrial stimulation as a key to the understanding of sinoatrial conduction in man. Presentation of data and critical review of the literature. Circulation **47,** 86 (1973)
48. Steinbeck, G., Lüderitz, B.: Comparative study of sinoatrial conduction time and sinus node recovery time. Brit. Heart J. **37,** 956 (1975)
49. Steinbeck, G., Körber, H.-J., Lüderitz, B.: Die Bestimmung der sinuatrialen Leitungszeit beim Menschen durch gekoppelte atriale Einzelstimulation. Klin. Wschr. **52,** 1151 (1974)
50. Spurrel, R. A., Thorburn, C. W., Camm, J., Sowton, E., Deuchar, D. C.: Effects of disopyramide on electrophysiological properties of specialized conduction system in man and on accessory atrioventricular pathways in Wolff-Parkinson-White syndrome. Brit. Heart J. **37,** 861 (1975)
51. Talbot, R. G., Nimmo, J., Julian, D. G., Clark, R. A., Neilson, J. M. M., Prescott, L. F.: Treatment of ventricular arrhythmias with mexiletine (Kö 1173). Lancet 339 (1973)
52. Wit, A. L., Cranefield, P. F.: Effect of verapamil on the sinoatrial and atrioventricular nodes of the rabbit and the mechanisms by which it arrests reentrant atrioventricular nodal tachycardia. Circulat. Res. **35,** 413 (1974)
53. Yek, B. K., Sung, P.-K., Scherlag, B. J.: Effects of disopyramide on electrophysiological and mechanical properties of the heart. J. Pharmac. Sciences **62,** 1924 (1973)

Evaluation of Suction Electrode Recording

J. CABASSON and P. PUECH

There is a gap between electrophysiologic events recorded by conventional or intracavitary electrocardiography, and the electrical activity of a single heart cell recorded *in vitro* by the microelectrode technique.

Suction electrode recording makes a link between these two kinds of tracings, permitting recording of the *in vivo* monophasic action potential (MAP) of the intact heart which is closely related to the transmembrane action potential of the isolated cell.

Suction electrode, recording introduced by Schütz in 1931 [17], enabled recording of good potentials from heart fibers for almost 20 years. It was supplanted in 1949 by the microelectrode technique [11], but gained new interest in 1964 with *in vivo* recording in animals and man [5, 7, 10, 12].

Since 1971 we have been working in Montpellier on suction electrode recording. We have developed a special catheter while the technical aspects have been developed elsewhere [3, 15].

MAP recording can be performed in human heart, and we have done it several times, but short suction periods must be observed in man to avoid myocardial damage. This limits the method and therefore we use mainly animals, e.g., the anesthetized dog. The figures illustrating this paper come from animal experiments.

Normal Monophasic Action Potentials of the Right Heart

Configuration. The usual type of potential that can be recorded in the right atrium is triangular, with preponderant phase 3, and is supposed to show the activity of the working myocardium.

Less frequently we record right atrial potential with a small plateau. The significance of such a potential, which looks somewhat like that of a Purkinje fiber, is controversal [9]. It testifies at the least to functional heterogeneity of the atrium.

At the upper part of the right atrium we can record a third type of potential, characterized by an early onset before the peripheral P wave, a slowly ascending phase 0, and a slightly ascending phase 4. This MAP is thought to translate the activity of the perisinusnodal region (Fig. 1) [3].

The usual right ventricular MAP shows a clear plateau and fairly rapid repolarization during phase 3, and exhibits the activity of the working myocardium.

Less frequently we record ventricular MAP with slightly ascending phase 4 (diastolic depolarization). This potential is supposed to show Purkinje cells activity.

Duration. Figure 2 illustrates how to measure total MAP duration. It is the A – B interval, point B being the crossing of the base line and the tangent of phase 3.

In the anesthetized dog (pentobarbital) right ventricular MAP duration is 180 ± 3 ms.

MAP duration is related to cycle length; both decrease at the same time, and there is a linear relation: $x = 0.17\,y + 102$ for the atrium and $x = 0.34\,y + 65$ for the ventricle in dog (x = MAP duration, y = cycle length) [3].

MAP duration varies also with the location of the electrode, the potential being slightly shorter at the base than at the apex [1].

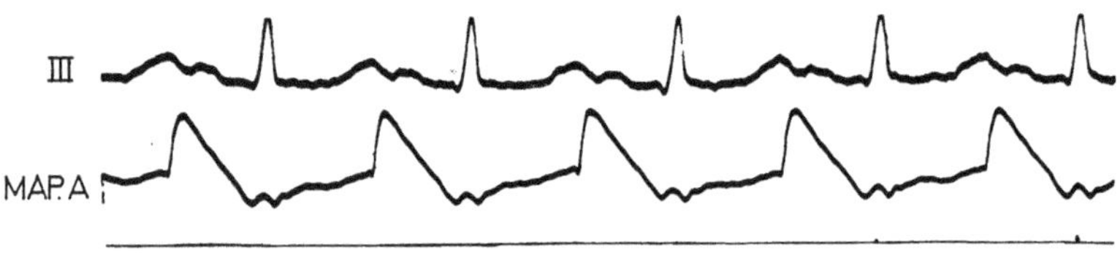

Fig. 1. Atrial MAP of perisinusnodal region. MAP is characterized by early onset before peripheral P wave, a slowly ascending phase 0, and a slightly ascending phase 4.

Amplitude. The amplitude of atrial MAP is between 3 and 18 mV, and the amplitude of ventricular MAP between 10 and 50 mV. This is much less than the amplitude of transmembrane action potential, and is mainly due to close bipolar electrode recording. MAP recorded with the unipolar catheter are higher, but not as much as the true cellular potential.

The difference between atrial and ventricular MAP magnitude may be explained by the different thicknesses of subendocardial layers [12].

Phase 0. Phase 0 of MAP lasts at least 3 – 4 ms and is not as rapid as in transmembrane action potential. This is due to the fact that suction electrode recording does not explore one cell, but a small group of cells, and MAP phase 0 is influenced not only by rapid depolarization but also by synchronization of these cells.

Phase 0 is best evaluated by its first derivative: the dv/dt (mV/s).

Potential Change. With long suction times (more than 20 min) we currently observe a plateau drop, but the MAP duration and the dv/dt remain unchanged.

MAP impairment by the peripheral electrocardiogram. With unipolar suction electrode catheter recording we encounter a notch on the descending limb of the atrial MAP. This is due to the QRS complex of the peripheral electrocardiogram and can be almost completely suppressed by close bipolar recording.

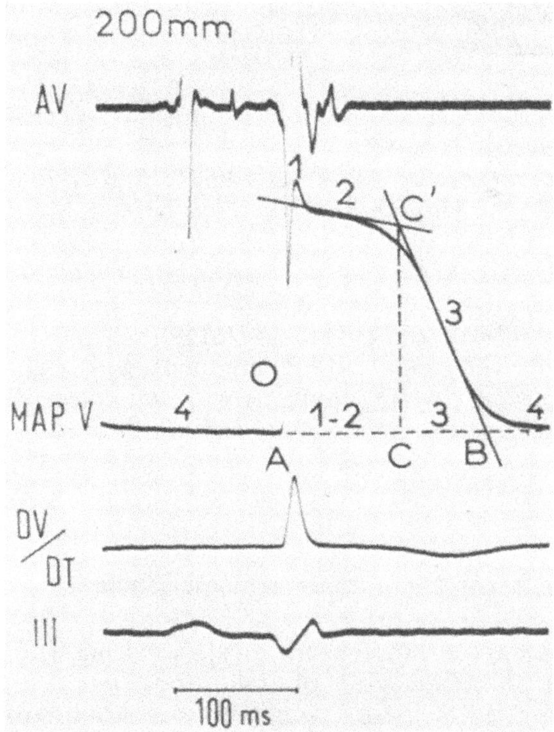

Fig. 2. Different phases of ventricular action potential (0 – 1 – 2 – 3 – 4) and their measurement. *AV* = His bundle potential, dv/dt of phase 0 and lead III.

Application of Suction Electrode Recording to the Study of Cardiac Arrhythmias

MAP recording allows a better understanding of local electrophysiologic events.

Early premature beats occurring during incomplete repolarization have a shorter duration and a slower dv/dt, while late premature beats have almost normal duration.

In recent atrial fibrillation the MAPs are well organized, due to patent good local depolarizations. Whereas in old atrial fibrillation the potentials are poorly organized, due to hypoxemia.

Similarly, recent ventricular fibrillation is accompanied by well-organized ventricular MAPs. In terminal tracing local MAPs persist after discernible electrical activity has disappeared on surface ECG.

During AV junctional tachycardia and ventricular tachycardia MAP durations are quite constant along the burst; only capture beats are of shorter duration.

Application of Suction Electrode Recording to the Study of Ventricular Repolarization Troubles

Metabolic and endocrine disorders which modify the QT interval, specifically distort the right atrial or ventricular MAP.

During hypocalcemia right ventricular MAP lengthens; this is due mainly to phase 2 prolongation [18]. Hypothyroïdism gives similar MAP lengthening [6].

On the other hand right ventricular MAP shortens during hypercalcemia and hyperthyroïdism.

Hyperkalemia gives short atrial MAP and reduced dv/dt [8].

During coronarography right ventricular MAP lengthens with right coronary injection, and left ventricular MAP lengthens with left coronary injection [18]. This might be due more to the effects of sodium in the contrast agent, than to hypoxemia.

Application of Suction Electrode Recording to Pharmacologic Studies

Antiarrhythmic drug study represents to our sense the most promising field. Few studies until now have been published [4, 13, 14, 16].

A special methodology is required including synchronous recordings of MAP, dv/dt, His potential and peripheral ECG. A basic pacing at atrial or ventricular level, and the extrastimulus method at various intensities allows determination of refractory periods and conduction times.

Evaluation of the MAP duration/effective refractory period ratio (MAP/ERP) is of special interest; it is recognized as one of the best criteria of antiarrhythmic effectiveness [2].

Electrophysiologic Properties of Amiodarone. This class III antiarrhythmic agent has been injected i.v. at 5 – 15 mg/kg in the anesthetized dog, and studied at four cardiac levels [4].

Atrial myocardium: MAP duration is increased by 9%; the dv/dt slightly decreases; the total refractory period is increased by 22%; the effective refractory period is increased by 26%; the functional refractory period is increased by 19%; facilitation of conduction disappears; the MAP/ERP ratio (1.20 at basic level) becomes inferior to 1.

Sinus node: cardiac frequency is decreased by 38%.

Atrioventricular junction: the AH interval is increased by 46%; the HV interval remains unchanged; the functional refractory period of the AV node is increased by 80%.

Ventricular myocardium (Fig. 3): MAP duration is increased by 21%; dv/dt is practically unchanged; the total refractory period is decreased by 9%; the effective refractory period is decreased by 13%.

Electrophysiologic Properties of Ajmaline. This class I antiarrhythmic drug has been injected i.v. at 1 – 3 mg/kg in the anesthetized dog.

Atrial MAP duration is unchanged; the dv/dt is strongly reduced; the total refractory period is increased by 16 – 25%; the effective refractory period is increased by 5 – 20%; the MAP/ERP ratio diminishes from 1.2 to 0.9.

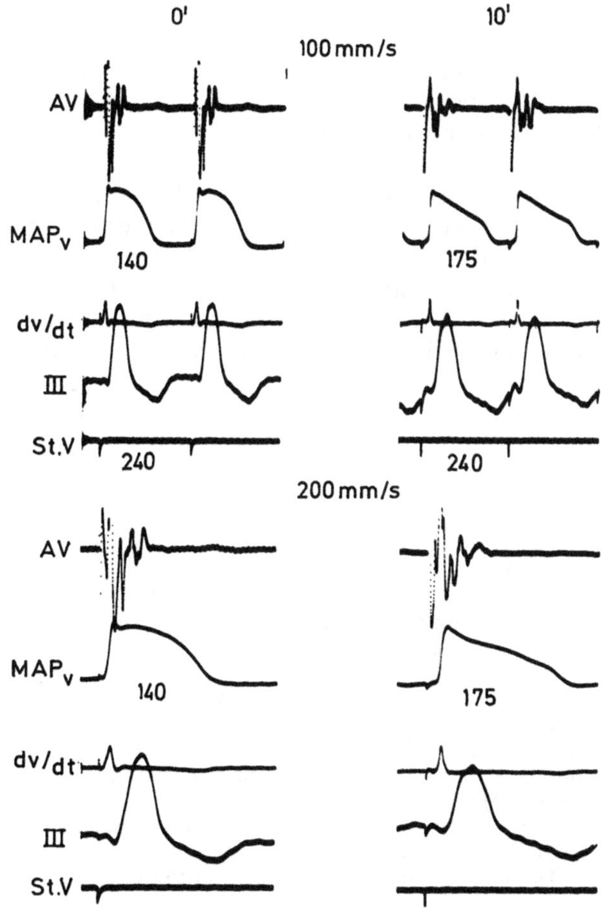

Fig. 3. Effects of i.v. amiodarone 10 mg/kg on right ventricular MAP. *Left:* before amiodarone; *right:* 10 min. after injection. MAP duration increases from 140 to 175 ms; dv/dt does not change.

Ventricular MAP duration slightly increases; the dv/dt is strongly reduced.

We can conclude that MAP recording permits the study of myocardial fibers in their physiologic medium, with all their neurohumoral connections, and allows accurate electrophysiologic assessment with antiarrhythmic drugs.

Summary

Suction electrode permits *in vivo* recording of the monophasic action potential (MAP) of the heart, which is closely related to the action potential recorded on isolated fiber by the microelectrode technique. We can record in atrial and ventricular chambers of the right heart various kinds of MAPs that suggest the electrical activity of the working myocardium and of the specialized myocardium.

Electrophysiologic events underlying cardiac arrhythmias are better understood by MAP recording. Metabolic and endocrine disorders which modify the QT interval specifically distort the right atrial or ventricular MAP.

Pharmacologic studies represent the most promising field of suction electrode recording. A special methodology is required including synchronous recording of MAP, dv/dt, His potential and ECG. A basic pacing at atrial or ventricular level and the extrastimulus method at various intensities, allow accurate evaluation of refractory periods and conduction times. The MAP/ERP (effective refractory period) is of special value for antiarrhythmic drug assessment.

References

1. Autenrieth, G., Surawicz, B., Kuo, C. S.: Sequence of repolarization on the ventricular surface in dog. Amer. Heart J., **89**, 463 (1975)
2. Bigger, J. T.: Arrhythmias and antiarrhythmic drugs. Advanc. intern. Med. **18**, 251 (1972)
3. Cabasson, J., Mellet, J. M., Guimond, C., Bachy, C., Sassine, A., Puech, P.: L'étude des potentiels d'action monophasiques du myocarde par voie endocavitaire et ses applications. Ann. Cardiol. Angéiol., **24**, n° 6 (1975)
4. Cabasson, J., Puech, P., Mellet, J. M., Guimond, C., Sassine, A.: Analyse des effets électrophysiologiques de l'amiodarone par l'enregistrement des potentiels d'action monophasiques et du faisceau de His. Soc. franç. Cardiol., 15 Novembre 1975
5. Churney, L., Ohshima, H.: An improved suction electrode for recording from the dog heart in situ. J. appl. Physiol. **19**, 793 (1964)
6. Cotoi, S., Constantinescu, L., Gavrilescu, S.: The effect of thyroid state on monophasic action potential in human heart. Experientia (Basel) **29**, 797 (1972)
7. Gavrilescu, S., Cotoi, S., Pop, T.: The monophasic action potential of the right atrium. Cardiology **57**, 200 (1972)
8. Gavrilescu, S., Streian, C., Comsulea, L., Luca, C.: Refractoriness of the right atrium and AV conduction system. Influence of practolol, chronic hypoxia and uremia. Rev. roum. Méd. interne **12**, 255 (1974)
9. Hoffman, B. F., Cranefield, P. F.: Electrophysiology of the Heart. New York: McGraw Hill Book Co., 1960
10. Korsgren, M., Leskinen, E., Sjostrand, U., Varnauskas, E.: Intracardiac recording of monophasic action potentials in the human heart. Scand. J. clin. Lab. Invest. **18**, 561 (1966)
11. Ling, G., Gerard, R. W.: The normal membrane potential of frog sartorius fibers. J. cell. comp. Physiol. **34**, 383 (1949)
12. Olsson, B.: Monophasic Action Potential of Right Heart. Göteborg: Elanders Bocktryckeri Aktienbolag 1971
13. Olsson, B., Brorson, L., Varnauskas, E.: Class 3 antiarrhythmic action in man. Observations from monophasic action potential recordings and amiodarone treatment. Brit. Heart J. **35**, 1255 (1973)

14. Olsson, B.: Atrial repolarization in man. Effects of betareceptor blockade. Brit. Heart J. **36,** 806 (1974)
15. Puech, P., Cabasson, J., Latour, H., Grolleau, R., Baissus, C., Mellet, J. M.: Étude des potentiels d'action monophasiques du myocarde par voie endocavitaire. Méthodologie. Arch. Mal. Coeur **67,** 1117 (1974)
16. Puech, P., Cabasson, J., Mellet, J. M., Guimond, C.: Effets de l'aprindine injectable chez le chien, avec mention spéciale à l'enregistrement des potentiels d'action monophasiques auriculaires et ventriculaires et de l'électrogramme hisien. Thérapie **29,** 731 (1974)
17. Schütz, E.: Monophasische Aktionsströme vom in situ durchbluteten Säugetierherzen. Klin. Wschr. **10,** 1454 (1931)
18. Shabetai, R., Surawicz, B., Hammil, W.: Monophasic action potential in man. Circulation **38,** 341 (1968)

The Recording of the Human Right Atrial Monophasic Action Potential

T. Pop, D. Fleischmann, and S. Effert

A great advance in electrophysiology was made in 1949 when Ling and Gerard [10] introduced the microelectrode technique for recording the transmembrane action potential. Unfortunately, the action potentials cannot be recorded from the intact human heart. This disadvantage can to a large extent be overcome by recording the monophasic action potentials (MAP) from the intact beating heart.

The suction electrode method for MAP recording was introduced in animal studies as early as 1931 by Schütz [16]. Only in 1966 did Korsgren et al. [9] develope a method to measure the MAP in the human heart. This technique was further developed and improved by Olsson et al. [11].

The MAP has a configuration similar to that of an action potential recorded in its immediate vicinity and their durations are identical [8]. The amplitude of the MAP is, however, lower than that of the action potential [8]. Because the MAP has the same configuration as the action potential, the same notations are used for the depolarization as well as the repolarization phases (Fig. 1), e.g., phase 0 indicates the time of excitation of the tissue under the exploring electrode [8].

Technique

The MAP is usually recorded by means of a bipolar suction electrode catheter [11]. This catheter is introduced percutaneously from an arm or a femoral vein, advanced to the right heart during fluoroscopy control, and manipulated into the desired position. After application of slight pressure an injury current is obtained. Suction is then applied and the recording of the MAP is made possible. With a satisfactory position no blood in withdrawn inside the catheter.

Olsson et al. [11] and Puech et al. [15] use a negative suction pressure of 350 mm Hg. Under this condition the MAP recording must be released within 2 min to avoid irreversible damage of the tissues [11, 15]. A reduction of this negative pressure to 100 mm Hg enables Gavrilescu et al. [1, 4, 5] and us to prolong the recording time up to 20 min.

The duration of the MAP is measured at 90% repolarization [11]. The normal values given by Olsson et al. [11, 16] are between 216 and 421 ms. The amplitude of the MAP recording during regular sinus rhythm ranges between 3 and 20 mV in our laboratory.

Right Atrial MAP During and After Conversion of Atrial Arrhythmias to Sinus Rhythm

1. During atrial fibrillation the MAP is irregular in frequency and duration [11]. Its amplitude is significantly lower than in sinus rhythm [3, 4, 11]. Re-

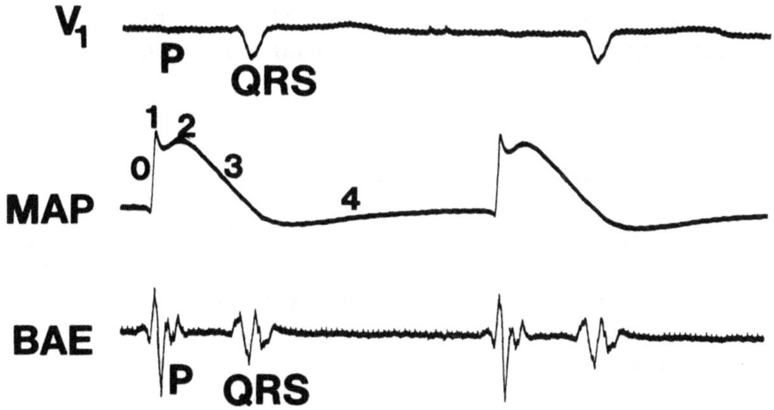

Fig. 1. Notation of depolarization and repolarization phases of MAP. *From top to bottom:* lead V_1, right atrial monophasic action potential (MAP), and a bipolar atrial electrogram (BAE).

cording of the MAP allows for amplification of electrical activity during atrial fibrillation [5]. The stability of the sinus rhythm after DC shock is correlated to the duration of the right atrial MAP recorded immediately after conversion [2, 12]. The relapse of atrial fibrillation occurs much earlier in the cases with short MAP duration than in patients with long MAP duration. This method thus gives prognostic information about the stability of the sinus rhythm [12].

2. During atrial flutter the phase 0 of the MAPs coincide in time with the flutter waves of the ECG [11]. The repolarization phase is terminated by the succeeding MAP and thus no phase 4 can be recorded [4, 11].

During the transitional phase from atrial flutter or fibrillation to sinus rhythm a progressive prolongation of the MAP duration is observed [7]. When a critical duration is reached sinus rhythm occurs spontaneously. These data are interpreted as an expression of the prolongation of the refractory period of the atrial muscle which may interrupt the reentry mechanism [7].

3. In contrast to atrial flutter, in paroxysmal supraventricular tachycardia the transition to sinus rhythm does not show any progressive prolongation of the MAP duration [5]. An explanation of this finding is the fact that the atrial tissue is not a part of the reentry pathway of the arrhythmia.

4. The recording of the MAP permits a differentiation between atrial flutter and atrial tachycardia with block in doubtful cases [6]. While in atrial flutter the duration of the MAP is allways shorter than 200 ms; in patients with atrial tachycardia with block a longer duration than 200 ms is constantly found.

5. Chaotic atrial rhythms. A significant difference of right atrial MAP duration could be observed by comparing the chaotic atrial mechanism with the chaotic atrial tachycardia [3]. In the first entity, a relatively long MAP duration was recorded which can explain the stability of this rhythm.

In the chaotic atrial tachycardia the duration of the MAP was rather short. This indicates a reduced refractoriness of the atrial tissue which favors reentry phenomena and development of atrial fibrillation and flutter.

Other Applications of the MAP Recording

1. Drug investigations. Olsson et al. [13] have measured the duration of the right atrial MAP before and 4 weeks after the beginning of an anti-arrhythmic treatment with amiodarone. This drug produces a delayed repolarization of the action potential. In all patients, a significant prolongation of the MAP duration was observed.

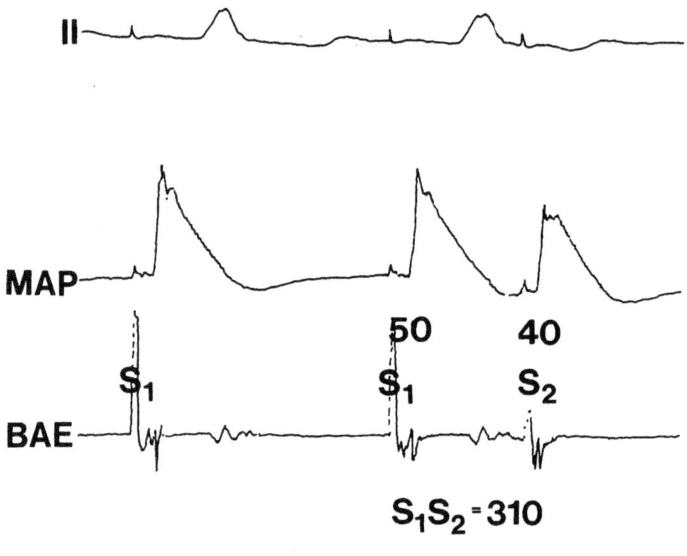

Fig. 2. Supernormal phase of intra-atrial conduction. *From top to bottom:* lead II, right atrial monophasic action potential (MAP), and a bipolar atrial electrogram (BAE). A premature atrial stimulus (S_2) is introduced 310 ms after the foregoing basic stimulus (S_1). S_1 is conducted within 50 ms to the low right atrium where the MAP was recorded. Paradoxically, S_2 needed only 40 ms to be conducted to the low right atrium. This phenomenon is compatible with a supernormal phase of intra-atrial conduction.

2. The MAP recording permits accurate measurement of the intra-atrial conduction time [14]. In this way, during programmed premature atrial stimulation we were able to demonstrate in 4 of 13 patients a supernormal phase of conduction (Fig. 2).

In conclusion, the MAP recording provides an interesting and useful method for analysis of the electrical events during sinus rhythm and atrial arrhythmias.

References

1. Cotoi, S., Pop, T., Gavrilescu, S.: Intracavitary ECG in the diagnosis and study of arrhythmias. Rev. roum. Méd. interne **8,** 219 (1971)
2. Cotoi, S., Gavrilescu, S., Pop, T., Vicas, E.: The prognostic value of right atrium monophasic action potential after conversion of atrial fibrillation. Europ. J. clin. Invest. **2,** 472 (1972)
3. Gavrilescu, S., Cotoi, S., Pop, T.: Chaotic atrial rhythms. Clinical and electrophysiological observations. G. Ital. Card. **1,** 388 (1971)
4. Gavrilescu, S., Cotoi, S., Pop, T.: L'enregistrement du potential monophasique d'action de l'oreillette et du ventricule droits chez l'homme. Rev. roum. Méd. interne. **9,** 23 (1972)
5. Gavrilescu, S., Cotoi, S., Pop, T.: The monophasic action potential of the right atrium. Cardiology **57,** 200 (1972)
6. Gavrilescu, S., Cotoi, S., Pop, T.: Explorarea electrocardiografica endocavitara in tahicardia atriala cu bloc. St. Cerc. Méd. interne. (Buc) **13,** 359 (1972)
7. Gavrilescu, S., Cotoi, S., Pop, T.: Monophasic action potential of the right atrium in paroxysmal atrial flutter and fibrillation. Brit. Heart J. **35,** 585 (1973)
8. Hoffman, B. F., Cranefield, P. F., Lepeschkin, E., Surawicz, B., Herrlich, H. C.: Comparison of cardiac monophasic potentials recorded by intracellular and suction electrodes. Amer. J. Physiol. **196,** 1297 (1959)
9. Korsgren, M., Leskinen, E., Sjöstrand, U., Varnauskas, E.: Intracardiac recording of monophasic action potentials in the human heart. Scand. J. clin. Lab. Invest. **18,** 561 (1966)
10. Ling, G., Gerard, R. W.: The normal membrane potential of frog sartorius fibers. J. cell. comp. Physiol. **34,** 383 (1949)
11. Olsson, B., Varnauskas, E., Korsgren, M.: Further improved method for measuring monophasic action potentials of the intact human heart. J. Electrocardiol. **4,** 19 (1971)
12. Olsson, B., Cotoi, S., Varnauskas, E.: Monophasic action potential and sinus rhythm stability after conversion for atrial fibrillation. Acta med. scand. **190,** 81 (1971)
13. Olsson, S. B., Brorson, L., Varnauskas, E.: Class 3 antiarrhythmic action in man. Observations from monophasic action potential recordings and amiodarone treatment. Brit. Heart J. **35,** 1255 (1973)
14. Pop, T., Fleischmann, D., de Bakker, J. M. T.: Demonstration of supernormal conduction in the human right atrium. Pflügers Arch. ges. Physiol. Suppl. **359,** – R 23 (1975)
15. Puech, P., Cabasson, J., Latour, H., Grolleau, R., Baissus, C., Mellet, J. M.: Étude des potentiels d'action monophasiques du myocarde par voie endocavitaire. Méthodologie. Arch. Mal. Coeur **67,** 1117 (1974)
16. Schütz, E.: Monophasische Aktionsströme vom in situ durchbluteten Säugetierherzen. Klin. Wschr. **10,** 1454 (1931)
17. Woie, L., Brorson, L., Olsson, S. B.: Syncope during sinus massage. Observations on conduction disturbances by atrial pacing, His-bundle and monophasic action potential (MAP) recordings. J. Electrocardiol. **6,** 263 (1973)

II. Atrioventricular Conduction

Contributions of Intracardiac Electrography to the Understanding of Normal and Disturbed AV Conduction

M. Schlepper

Tissues of different conduction properties are traversed by an impulse of nomotopic origin to activate the working myocardium. These tissues may differ in respect to refractoriness and conduction velocity and may be influenced to varying degrees by the autonomous nervous system. Although the process of excitation transmission is only poorly reflected by the surface ECG, a bulk of information has been collected during a 50-year period of clinical electrocardiography. Some of the more sophisticated explanations, as for instance the Mobitz "Interferenz Dissoziation," were not even based on proper animal experiments but still hold true, while many have been confirmed with newer techniques. The introduction of intracardiac electrography and especially recordings from specific conduction system components [6, 19] have contributed a great deal to the understanding of cardiac arrhythmias.

In the study of AV conduction and its abnormalities, it is generally sufficient to use two or three recording catheters, one being placed in the high atrium, one adjacent to the bundle of His at the right side of the ventricular septum, and one in the right ventricle. These catheters may also be used for programmed cardiac stimulation. This method seems to be well standardized with the exception of minor alterations based on the investigators' own experience. Usually the interelectrode distance is about 0.5 – 1 cm, with bipolar recordings being depicted. It is essential that a filter permitting recording in the frequency range of 40 – 200 Hz be employed with this system [20].

Provided a fast enough paper speed is chosen, the interpotential distances and the duration of the potentials can be measured with accuracy. The interval between the cranial atrial potential and that recorded in the vicinity of the AV node is usually 25 – 35 ms with a mean of 30, while AH duration is 50 – 100 ms, and the duration of the His potential 15 – 20 ms. About 15 ms later, a potential from the right bundle branch can be recorded with a duration of 10 ms, which further divides the HQ interval of normally 35 – 50 ms. A similar potential from the left bundle branch may be recorded just beneath the aortic valve in the left ventricle [8, 15]. The two branch potentials appear at almost the same time but may differ slightly. Damato et al. [3] have claimed the recording of potentials due to depolarization of the AV node proper, but this finding has not been subsequently confirmed.

The His spike reflects depolarization of the whole of the common bundle, as has been shown in animal experiments with simultaneous recordings from the surface of the bundle and by implanted microelectrodes [17, 23]. This exemplifies that the recording of the proper potential from the surface of a given cardiac structure not only depends on the magnitude of depolarization in the cells but also on the amount of tissue involved. Taking a normal length of the common bundle of about 2 cm, a 15 ms duration would represent a conduction velocity of about 1.5 m/s, whereas a widening and slurring of the His spike to 45-ms duration indicates a reduction of conduction velocity to one-third of normal.

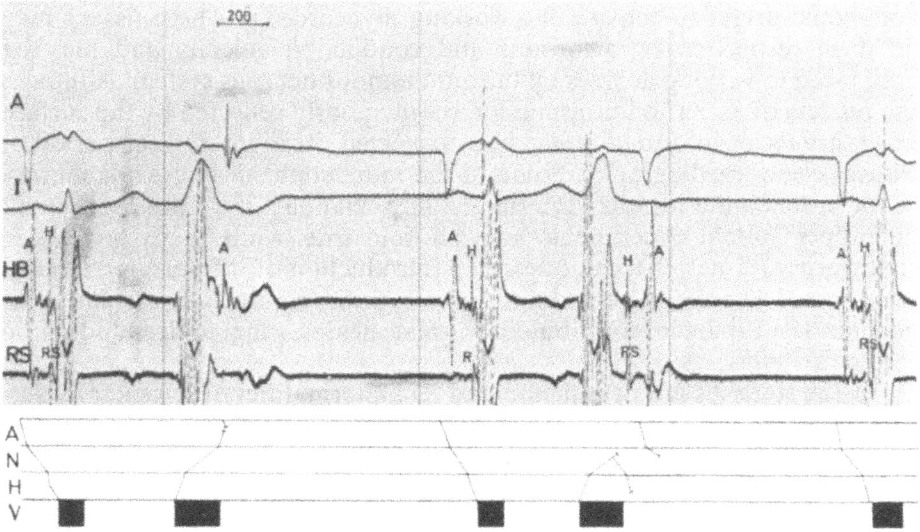

Fig. 1. Original record from 52-year-old patient. *Top to bottom: A* = cranial atrial electrogram. ECG I, His bundle electrogram, and right bundle branch electrogram. The first right ventricular ES with long coupling interval depolarizes atrium in retrograde fashion. Following second ES with shorter coupling interval retrograde conduction is delayed, so that H spike becomes visible. Right bundle is penetrated again (concealed reentry); atrium is normally depolarized. All time marks in ms. From Schlepper and Neuss [20].

The application of intracardiac electrography then allows a more detailed analysis of the impulse transmission from the atrium to the ventricles as shown in Figure 1, [20]. Since all structures involved are able to transmit in both orthograde and retrograde directions, the sequence of activation can give information as to the direction of impulse propagation. Monotopic extrasystoles with different coupling intervals lead to a retrograde activation of the atria when the coupling interval is long. The retrograde conduction velocity is fast so that a His spike is not visible. When the coupling interval of the right ventricular extrasystole is shorter, the retrograde conduction is delayed and the His and RS spikes become visible; however, the atrium is normally depolarized and there is physiologic interference at the level of the AV node.

Disturbances of AV impulse conduction can occur in any one of the structures involved. While the surface ECG only permits differentiation according to the P – R interval and as to the morphology of the QRS complex, intracardiac recordings allow a more exact localization of the site of block. Using the His potential as a point of reference, AV conduction disturbances may be localized above (suprahisian), in the bundle of His (intrahisian), or below (infrahisian) the recording site.

In a series of 383 patients with AV block studied by Puech [14], 37% showed isolated or combined suprahisian block while in 18% the conduction disturbances, either isolated or combined, were localized in the bundle of His. In the remaining 45% the lesion was below the recording site of the His spike.

Intra-atrial conduction disturbances may well be recognized in the surface ECG by widening of the P wave and only result in a prolongation in the P – R interval. Conduction defects confined to the AV node proper can lead to an increase in the AH interval while, in higher degrees, conduction is completely blocked so that no His spike occurs. In congenital complete AV block the block is always localized in the nodal structures. This was the case in 10 patients studied in our laboratory with the subsidiary pacemaker always being located in the bundle of His, i.e., with a foregoing His spike.

Block of type I, i.e., with Wenckebach periods, typically occurs in the AV node, although not strictly confined to that structure. This is especially true for those blocks which exhibit a rate dependency. In Figure 2, at a driving frequency of 70 (SS 850) there is 3 : 2 AV block with a Wenckebach period. The AH interval is prolonged 125 – 175 ms, with failure of conduction of the next atrial depolarization. By decreasing the SS interval to 800 ms (75/min) stable 2 : 1 block is achieved. The absence of the H spike following atrial depolarization indicates a suprahisian lesion.

Bradycardia-dependent AV block has been well documented and is thought to be due to an abnormal spontaneous diastolic depolarization

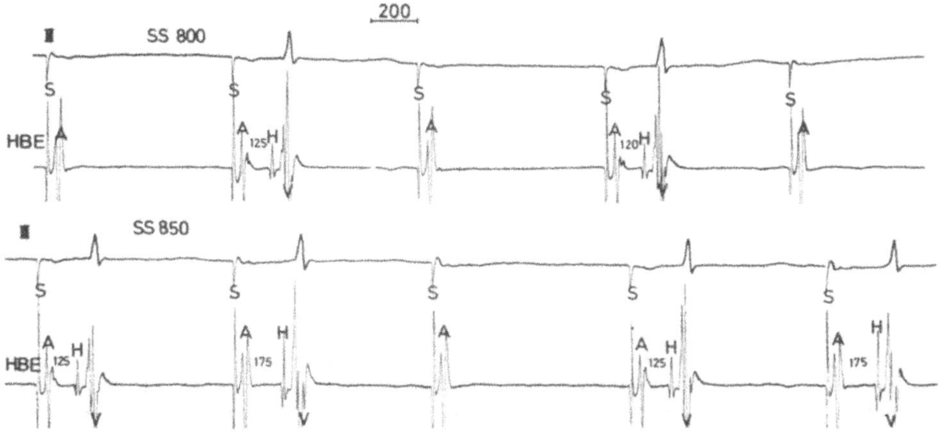

Fig. 2. Suprahisian AV block. Degree of blockage is rate-dependent. Original record from a 20-year-old patient with congenital high degree AV block.
All time marks in ms. From Neuss and Schlepper [10].

(phase 4 block) [16]. Subsequent spontaneous stimulation of cells with such a degree of abnormal diastolic depolarization results in an action potential characterized by a diminished upstroke velocity and decreased magnitude, both of which contribute to a failure of propagation. Conduction is restored by a spontaneous or induced escape beat leading to normal diastolic polarization. Cases reported in the literature were not studied during presence of this form of block, although conduction disturbances could be observed above the recording site of the His spike [2, 7]. This seems understandable in that it is more likely that enhanced automaticity occurs in a damaged His-Purkinje system.

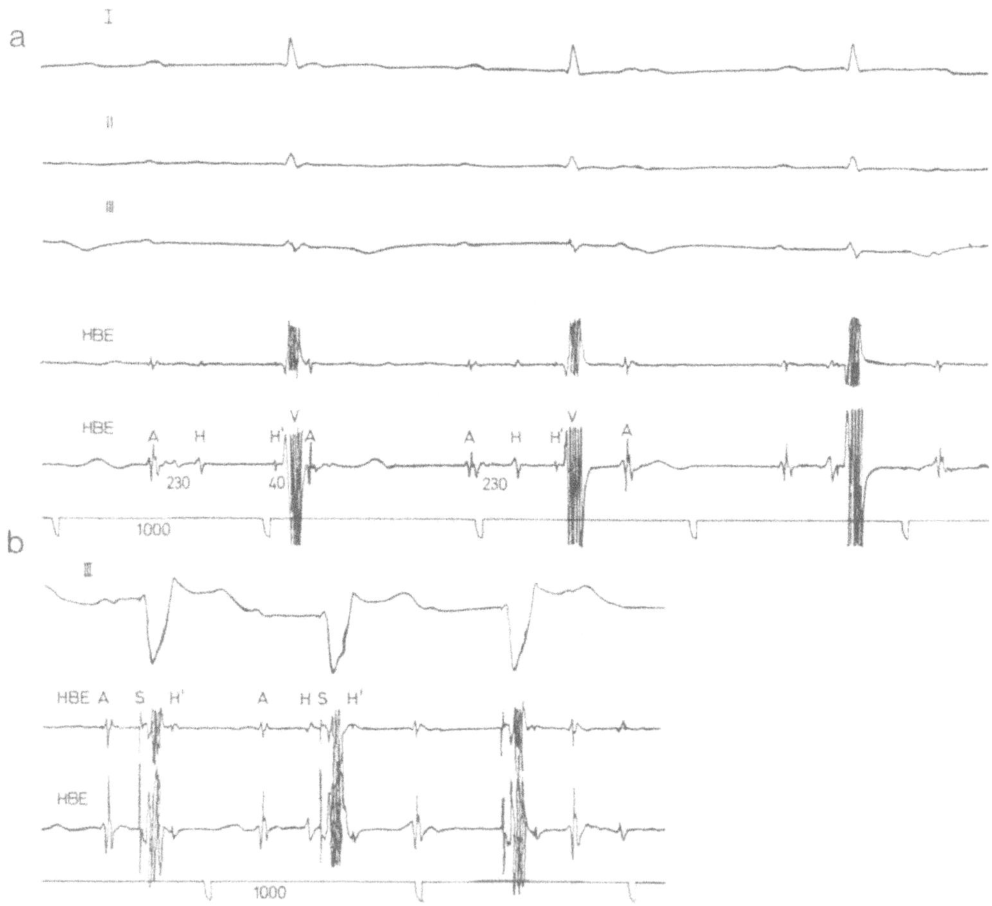

Fig. 3 a and b. Original record from 64-year-old patient with complete AV block. During spontaneous rhythm there is 2 : 1 suprahisian block with prolongation of AH interval to 230 ms during impulse conduction. His spike is widened and conduction is always blocked in bundle of His (*a*). During right ventricular pacing with rate of 65/min (*b*) the activation sequence above the bundle of His is maintained. Retrograde activation proceeds to the bundle of His as indicated by the occurrence of an H′ spike (see text).
All time marks in ms. From Neuss and Schlepper [10].

In patients with degenerative cardiac disease, multiple lesions in the specific conduction system may occur [9]. Figure 3 a and b represents a 3rd degree AV block with an escape rhythm of suprabifurcational origin. As judged by the surface ECG one would expect the lesion to be supra- or infrahisian. The HBE demonstrates a 2 : 1 suprahisian block with a conduction delay of 230 ms in the AV node when conduction is propagated. The His spike is slurred and widened to 45 ms, pointing to a conduction delay in the common bundle. However, there is also complete block in the same structure since the escape beats show a foregoing H′ potential with a constant HQ interval of 40 ms.

During right ventricular pacing the activation sequence of sinus node impulses are maintained (suprahisian 2 : 1 block with an AH interval of 230 ms). Each ventricular excitation is propagated with constant conduction velocity to the bundle of His, so that an H′ spike is always visible. Increase in atrial depolarization rate by atrial pacing prolonged the AH interval, but at a rate of 90/min complete suprahisian block occurred. The suprahisian block is substantiated by atrial pacing and the intrahisian block by ventricular pacing (Fig. 3 b).

The actual frequency of intrahisian conduction disturbances is probably higher than found in studies using His bundle electrography. Intracavitary recordings do not always allow the differentiation between high truncal blocks and intranodal blocks and between conduction disturbances in the vicinity of the branching portion and bilateral bundle branch block. The importance of proper recording technique for the verification of intrahisian block has recently been emphasized by Fishenfeld et al. [5].

A cardinal feature of the N zone of the AV node is decremental conduction. There is evidence that decremental conduction may be more pronounced during retrograde impulse transmission than during orthograde transmission [13]. In some cases there is complete orthograde AV block while under certain conditions retrograde conduction is simultaneously preserved. In Puech's [14] series, the incidence of such unidirectional blocks was higher with AV block below the bundle of His. A critical interval between the P wave of the sinus rhythm and the escape QRS has apparently to exist to permit VA conduction.

In Figure 4 a VA conduction with complete suprahisian AV block occurs at P – R interval of 400 ms, resulting in an R – P′ interval of 285 ms. The inverse relationship between the P – R and R – P′ interval as usually found suggests that refractoriness in a common pathway is responsible for this phenomenon. When ventricular pacing at a rate of 60/min is performed, the same relationship between orthograde atrial depolarizations, ventricular excitation, and the occurrence of VA conduction seems to exist (Fig. 4 b). The apparent existence of this critical relationship is, however, misleading. These time sequences are merely a reflection of two competitive excitation waves with physiologic interference at the level of a common pathway. When ventricular pacing is accelerated there is 1 : 1 VA conduction up to a rate of 125 and the normal sequence of atrial depolari-

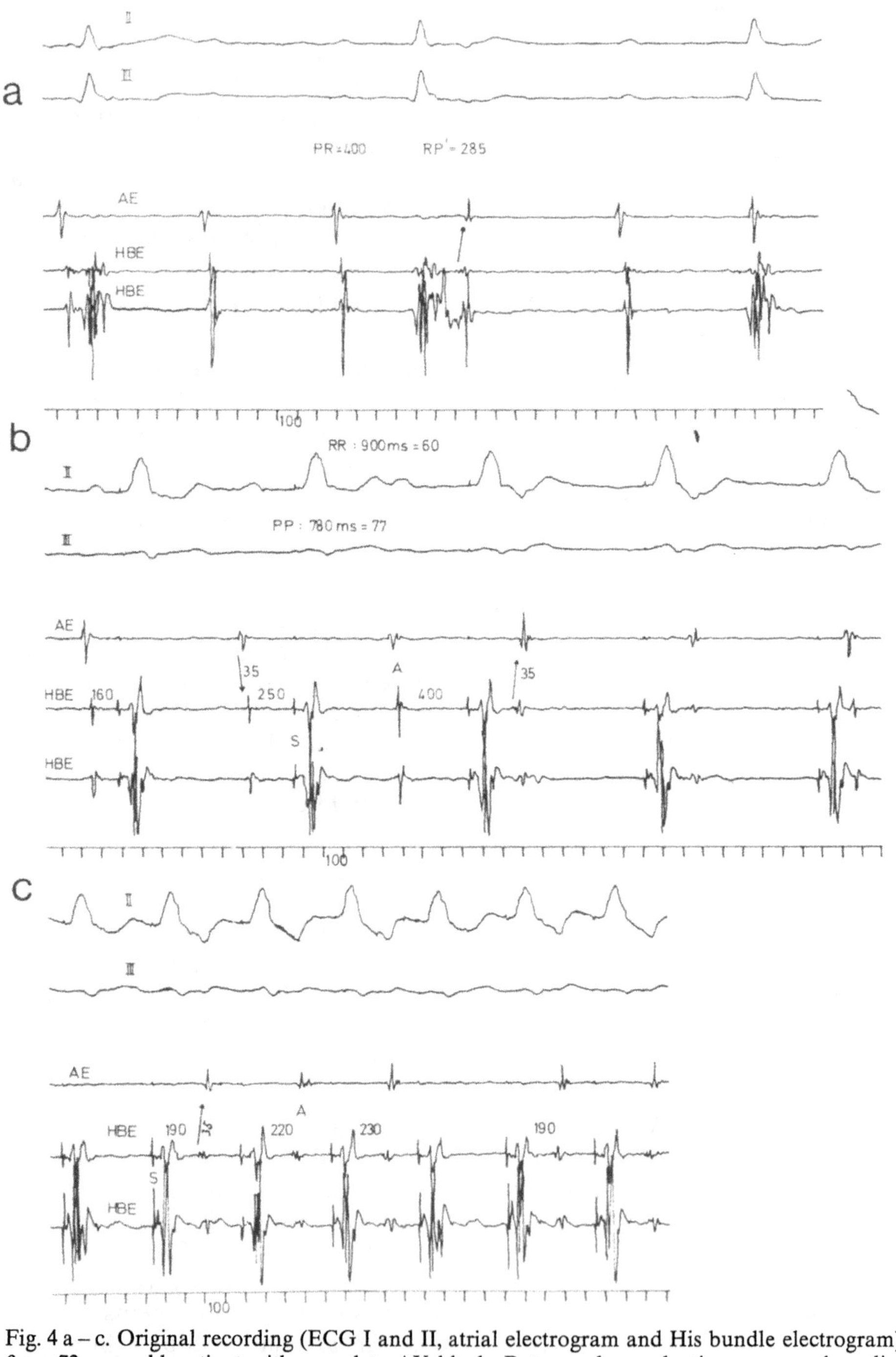

Fig. 4 a – c. Original recording (ECG I and II, atrial electrogram and His bundle electrogram) from 72-year-old patient with complete AV block. Retrograde conduction occurs when distance to proceeding P wave is between 280 and 530 ms (*a*). At ventricular pacing rate of 77/min (*b*) this relationship exists, orthograde and retrograde atrial activation time being 35 ms. At a ventricular pacing rate of 130/min (*c*) sinus rhythm is overridden. There is 4 : 3 retrograde AV block with Wenckebach period.
All time marks in ms.

zation is overriden. At a rate of 130 (Fig. 4 c), 4 : 3 VA block with Wenckebach period occurred. The occurrence of a Wenckebach period is a powerful argument against the theory of an accessory pathway being responsible for that type of unidirectional AV block [18]. Since only nodal structures seem to be involved, longitudinal dissociation with unidirectional block in one pathway is a more likely explanation. Since in this patient an H spike before the escape QRS is not present, there might be additional intrahisian lesions.

In infrahisian conduction disturbances the block is located below the recording site of the H spike. In 1st degree block there is an increase of

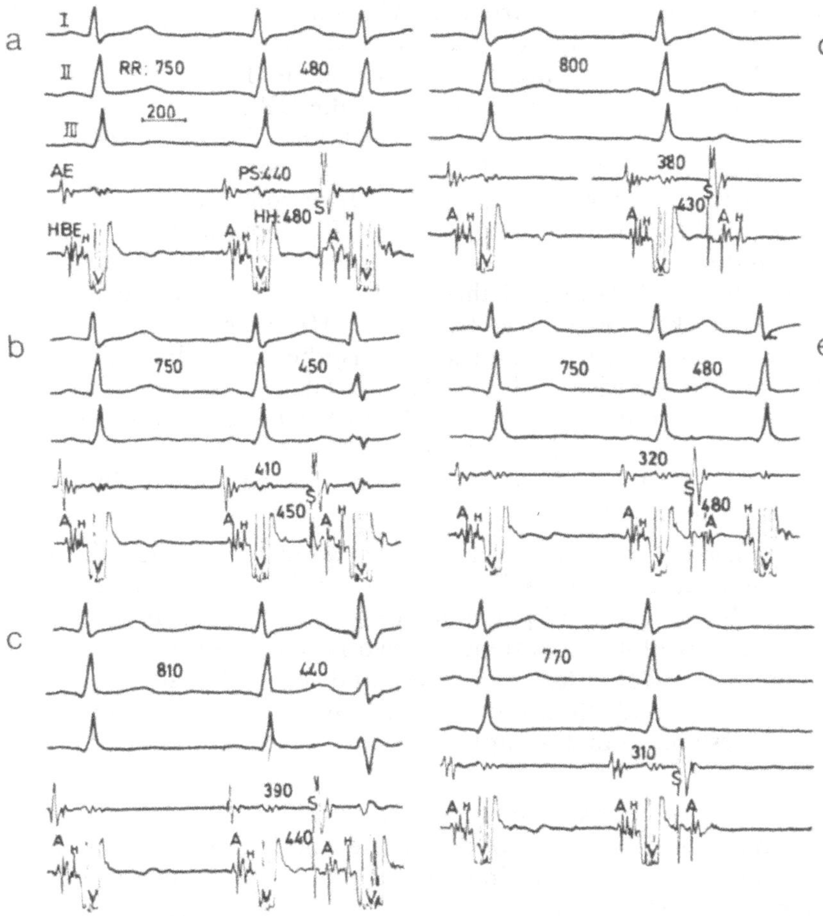

Fig. 5 a – f. Original recording (ECG I – III, atrial electrogram, His bundle electrogram), From 25-year-old patient are demonstrated in each panel the last two sinus impulses and premature atrial depolarization. Increasing prematurity leads at first to axis deviation, and RBBB. Impulses are then blocked below the bundle of His. Conduction is restored when at critical H_1H_2 interval structures below the bundle of His are out of their refractoriness.
All time marks in ms.

the HV interval to more than 55 ms. The QRS morphology is changed to either complete or incomplete right (RBBB) or left bundle branch block (LBBB) or, as indicated by additional axis deviation, to bifascicular forms of block. If an increase in HV interval is sufficient to lead to an augmentation of the P – R interval in the presence of normal QRS configuration, the lesion is most probably in the lower part of the trunk or else there must be an equal degree of delay in both branches. Type II block is much more common in infrahisian lesions. The intermittent interruption of conduction following the AH interval occurs in that branch not permanently blocked. In 3rd degree block complete dissociation of the AH groupings and a widened escape QRS is present, and the ventriculogram is not proceeded by an H potential.

In inapparent conduction disturbances with sinus rhythm, programmed cardiac stimulation may be necessary to provoke the block. In a 25-year-old patient a PAD with a coupling interval of 440 ms (Fig. 5 a) leads to an H_1H_2 interval of 480 ms. The HV interval and the QRS remain unaltered. By decreasing the coupling interval to 410 and 390 ms respectively (Figs. 5 b and 5 c), the H_1H_2 interval decreases by about the same amount (450 and 440 ms). Simultaneously, left axis deviation and RBBB occur, indicating that the functional refractory period (FRP) of the two fascicles is reached. When the coupling interval is further reduced by 10 ms, the effective refractory period (ERP) of all three fascicles is reached and impulse propagation is blocked below the bundle of His (Fig. 5 d). When the coupling interval is further shortened to 320 ms, there is nodal conduction delay with a sudden increase in the H_1H_2 interval from 430 to 480 ms. At this interval, the structures below the bundle of His are out of their refractory period and distal conduction is unimpaired (Fig. 5 e). At even shorter coupling intervals, the ERP of the AV node is reached and conduction is blocked above the level of the His spike (Fig. 5 f) [10].

The normalization of conduction at times when it is expected to be worse is is called supranormal AV conduction and is in such a case conventionally attributed to a gap I phenomenon [1]. In this case, however, the findings are indicative for the existence of two nodal pathways, one with a long refractory period and a fast conduction and one with a shorter refractory period and slow conduction velocity. This dual AV conduction is a prerequisite for the establishment of supraventricular tachycardias due to reentry mechanisms.

To evaluate the functional properties of the structures being traversed in AV conduction it is necessary to determine the refractory periods at varying heart rates with the extrastimulus method. In the atrium and in the His Purkinje system (HPS), refractory periods are decreased when heart rate is accelerated, while nodal refractoriness is prolonged with increasing rate [4]. Accessory pathways usually show a shortening of refractory periods with increasing heart rates, and in some cases this behavior has been observed with nodal structures. In these cases intranodal anomalous pathways have to be considered [11].

In a patient with dual AV conduction the α- and β-pathways may differentially alter their refractoriness with changing heart rates. This makes it understandable that an extrasystoly, able to initiate a tachycardia at a certain coupling interval, may not do so when heart rate has changed [11]. In Figure 6 the relationship between the coupling interval of a PAD (A_1A_2 or S_1S_2 respectively) and the resulting H_1H_2 and R_1R_2 interval is demon-

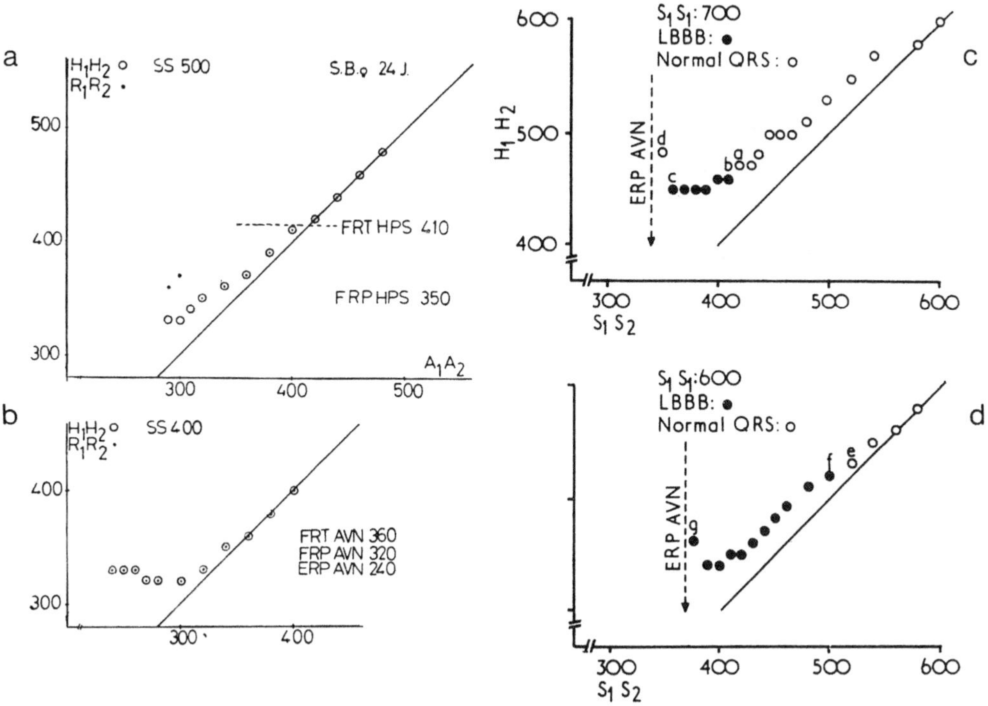

Fig. 6 a – d. Graph demonstrating relationship between coupling interval (A_1A_2 or S_1S_2) of premature atrial depolarization and resulting H_1H_2 interval. In a normal individual (*left*) increasing heart rate shortens effective refractory periods of atrium and of HPS while refractory periods of AV node are prolonged. In a patient with frequency-dependent LBBB refractory periods of left bundle branch as well as those of AV node are prolonged with increasing heart rates.
All time marks in ms.

strated. At a basic heart rate of 120/min the full recovery time of the HPS is 410 ms and the FRP 350 ms. Conduction is blocked at a coupling interval of 280 ms because of the effective refractoriness of the atrium. When heart rate was accelerated to 150/min (SS 400 ms, Fig. 6 b), conditions for conduction were determined by the refractoriness of the AV node, because refractory periods of the atrium and the HPS were shortened while they were prolonged in the AV node [21]. In contrast to this normal behavior, a different mode was found in a 67-year-old patient with coronary heart disease and a frequency-dependent LBBB. At a basic heart rate of 86/min

(SS 700 ms, Fig. 6 c), LBBB is present if H_1H_2 is below a critical value of 470 ms. Due to gap I phenomenon, intraventricular conduction is normalized, when at a shorter S_1S_2 interval the H_1H_2 interval exceeds this critical value again. When heart rate is accelerated to 100/min (S_1S_2 600 ms, Fig. 6 d), the critical H_1H_2 interval at which LBBB occurs is prolonged to 530 ms, with no gap phenomenon elicited. The ERP_{AVN} is again normally prolonged (330 – 380 ms).

When parts of the specific conduction system show a different behavior than that expected, its function can be considered impaired. In seven cases with rate dependent left bundle branch block, the expected shortening of refractory periods with increasing heart rates either did not occur or these parameters were prolonged [12].

In patients with dubious conduction disturbances the borderline between normal and abnormal can thus be established by evaluating the functional properties of the conduction system. This seems a more reliable approach than to attempt to define exact data for refractory periods. This applies particularly to the AV node, a structure greatly influenced by the autonomic nervous system. The diurnal changes in conduction properties of the AV node are exemplified in Figure 7. In two young male volunteers the conduction response to atrial pacing was studied over a 14-h period. Prior to

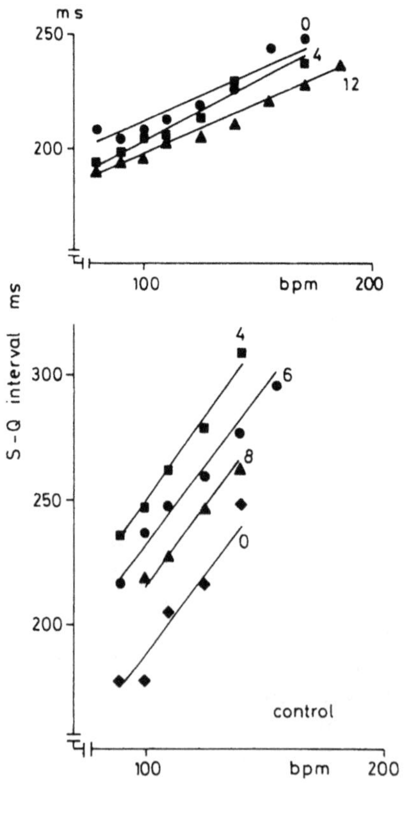

Fig. 7. Graph demonstrating relationship between increasing atrial pacing rate and resulting prolongation of SQ interval in two healthy volunteers. *Upper panel:* values for beginning, 4th and 12th hour; *lower panel:* beginning, 4th, 6th, and 8th hours, respectively. Regression lines and that paced rate at which 2nd degree AV block occurred (see text). *bpm* = beats per minute.

that study, the SQ prolongation seen with increasing atrial stimulation rate was proved to be confined to an AH prolongation. In one person the regression lines for pacing rate and SQ interval as well as the rate at which AV block occurred were essentially constant over the period of investigation. The other individual, highly disturbed by the procedure, was smoking and drinking coffee during the period of investigation, and showed extreme variations of these regression lines and of the critical heart rate at which AV-block became evident [22].

The simple method of atrial pacing useful in the detection of AV conduction disturbances in this example illustrates the influence of the mental state. These observations may be taken as an appropriate reminder of Durrer's characterization of the AV node as an "endorgan of the soul."

Summary

Intracardial electrography and especially recordings from the specific conduction system have contributed a great deal to the understanding of AV conduction and its disturbances. Although the method seems to be well standardized, some problems are yet unsolved. Using bipolar recordings the EG of the bundle of His reflects depolarization of the whole of the common bundle. Unipolar recordings have not revealed greater accuracy. In A – V block of all degrees His bundle electrograms allow the differentiation of the site of blockage into suprahisian, intrahisian and infrahisian structures. Since this knowlegde has widened the clinical electrocardiologic view of the problem, the diagnosis can in some cases now be assessed with greater accuracy by surface electrocardiography. In clinically inappearent disturbances of AV conduction intracardiac recordings together with programmed electrical stimulation may render further information as to the functional properties of the structures involved. Since the refractory parameters in different parts of the conduction system alter characteristically with changing heart rate their determination may provide additional diagnostic clues. However, the functional characteristics of the AV node proper are markedly influenced by changes in tone of the autonomic nervous system. Hence, it is almost impossible to give "normal" values for these specialized structures. The rate-dependent prolongation of the AH interval during atrial stimulation as well as the occurrence of 2nd degree block may or may not show diurnal alteration in healthy subjects.

References

1. Agha, A. S., Castellanos, A., Wells, D., Ross, M. D., Befeller, B., Myerburg, R. Y.: Type I, type II and type III gaps in bundle branch conduction. Circulation **47,** 325 (1973)
2. Barold, S. S., Ong, L. S., Young, J. A.: Electrocardiographic observations in bradycardia and tachycardia dependent atrioventricular block. Chest **67,** 450 (1975)
3. Damato, A. N., Lau, S. H., Berkowitz, W. D., Rosen, K. H., Lisi, K. R.: Recording of specialized conducting fibers (AV-nodal, His-bundle and right bundle branch) in man using an electrode catheter technic. Circulation **39,** 435 (1969)
4. Denes, P., Wu, D., Dhingra, R. C., Pietras, R. J., Rosen, K. M.: The effects of cycle length on cardiac refractory periods in man. Circulation **49,** 32 (1974)

5. Fishenfeld, J., Fleming, H., Desser, K. B., Benchimol, A.: False localization of atrioventricular block secondary to failure of "split His" recording. Chest **66,** 288 (1974)
6. Giraud, G., Puech, P., Latour, H., Hertault, J.: Variations de potentiel liées à l'activité du système de conduction auriculo-ventriculaire chez l'homme. Arch. Mal. Coeur **53,** 757 (1960)
7. Goodfriend, M. A., Barold, S. S.: Tachycardia dependent and bradycardia dependent Mobitz type II atrioventricular block within the bundle of His. Amer. J. Cardiol. **33,** 908 (1974)
8. Narula, O. S., Javier, R. P., Samet, P., Maramba, L. C.: Significance of His and left bundle recordings from the left heart in man. Circulation **42,** 385 (1970)
9. Narula, O. S., Scherlag, B. J., Samet, P., Javier, R. P.: Atrioventricular block. Localization and classification by His bundle recordings. Amer. J. Med. **50,** 146 (1971)
10. Neuss, H., Schlepper, M.: Befunde zur supranormalen ventrikulären Erregungsleitung. Z. Kardiol. **62,** 267 (1973)
11. Neuss, H., Schlepper, M., Spies, H. F.: Effects of heart rate and atropine on "dual AV conduction." Brit. Heart J. **37,** (1975)
12. Neuss, H., Thormann, J., Schlepper, M.: Electrophysiological findings in frequency-dependent left bundle branch block. Brit. Heart J. **36,** 888 (1974)
13. Paes de Carvallho, A.: Excitation of atrioventricular node during normal rhythm. In: Mechanism and Therapy of Cardiac Arrhythmias. Dreifus, L. S., Likoff, W. (eds.). New York – London: Grune and Stratton 1966
14. Puech, P.: Atrioventricular block: The value of intracardiac recordings. In: Cardiac Arrhythmias. Krikler, D., Goodwin, B. (eds.). London: Saunders, 1975
15. Rosen, K. M., Rahmtoola, S. H., Sinno, M. Z., Gunnar, R. M.: Bundle branch and ventricular activation in man. A study using catheter recordings of left and right bundle branch potentials. Circulation **43,** 193 (1971)
16. Rosenbaum, M. B., Elizari, M. V., Levi, R. J., Nau, G. L.: Paroxysmal atrioventricular block related to hypopolarization and spontaneous diastolic depolarization. Chest **63,** 678 (1973)
17. Sano, T., Nakai, M., Suzuki, F.: Nature of His potential in His electrogram. Jap. Heart J. **13,** 521 (1972)
18. Schamroth, L.: The Disorders of Cardiac Rhythms. Oxford – Edinburgh: Blackwell, 1971
19. Scherlag, B. J., Lau, S. H., Helfant, R. H., Berkowitz, W. D., Stein, E., Damato, A. N.: Catheter technique for recording His bundle activity in man. Circulation **39,** 13 (1969)
20. Schlepper, M., Neuss, H.: Die Elektrographie vom menschlichen Reizleitungssystem. Z. Kreisl.-Forsch. **61,** 865 (1972)
21. Schlepper, M., Neuss, H.: Changes of refractory period in the AV conduction system induced by antiarrhythmic drugs. A study using His bundle recordings. Acta cardiol. (Brux.) Suppl. **18,** 269 (1974)
22. Schlepper, M., Thormann, J., Schwarz, F.: The pharmacodynamics of orally taken verapamil and verapamil retard as judged by their negative dromotropic effects. Arzneimittel-Forsch. **25,** 1425 (1975)
23. Varghese, P. J., Elizari, M. V., Lau, S. N., Damato, A. N.: His bundle electrograms of dog: Correlation with intracellular recordings. Circulation **48,** 753 (1973)

Clinical Significance of AV Conduction Disturbances

K. Lang

Although experimental and clinical work has shown that the loss of coordinated atrial systole at rest leads to a reduction of cardiac output between 10 and 30% [4, 41, 45], the significant clinical symptoms of AV conduction disturbances are due to reduction of ventricular rate.

Since heart rate is one of the two determinants of cardiac output and since under normal conditions an increase in cardiac output, for example, with exercise, is achieved by increasing heart rate [41], bradycardia will have a deleterious effect in situations requiring an increase of output. Analysis of patients with congenital heart block has shown that the critical minimal heart rate is about 40/min [16]. This, of course, will depend much on the underlying disease, especially cardiac disease.

The fall of heart rate leads to two forms of clinical symptoms: a chronic form, consisting of congestive heart failure due to the bradycardia, and an acute form, Adams-Stokes attacks due to sudden drastic reduction of cardiac output. The treatment of both forms poses no real problem with the artificial pacemaker. There are still problems to be resolved in patients who still have a sufficiently high heart rate but in whom a sudden drop of rate might be expected, as it has been shown that some forms of low degree block and certain intraventricular conduction disturbances can lead to high degree or complete block in the distal portion of the conduction system with a ventricular pacemaker with slow onset and slow rate.

Before the introduction of the concept of fascicular block it has been demonstrated that certain forms of bundle branch block have a significant prognostic value, although, as Hiss and Lamb (1962) have pointed out, this depends very much on the underlying disease. A left anterior hemiblock (LAH), the most common form of monofascicular block (3 – 10%; [10, 30, 38]), has no unfavorable diagnosis according to the Tecumseh study [30] in contrast to the opinion of others [5].

The most common form of bifascicular block is right bundle branch block (RBBB) and LAH, seen in 0.8 – 1% of routine ECGs [10, 19, 23], with a risk of developing complete AV block being 10 – 30% [10, 19, 43]. This percentage depends on the time of observation and the presence of additional AV conduction disturbances.

In a retrospective study with an average observation time of 20 months we found a high degree or complete block in 23 out of 70 patients with RBBB and LAH [19] and in 24 out of 51 patients examined with the His-bundle electrogram (HBE).

Due to the anatomic structure and the blood supply to the posterior fascicle a left posterior hemiblock (LPH) is much less frequent [38]. Over half of the few patients with RBBB and LPH in our series developed a complete block. Rosenbaum et al. [39] found high degree or complete block in 63% of their 30 patients with Adams-Stokes attacks in all but one.

The significance of fascicular block for the development of high degree block is demonstrated in a review of 100 patients with artificial pacemakers, 62 of whom had fascicular block before onset of complete block, the largest group consisting of patients with RBBB and LAH (26 patients; Table 1).

Table 1. Fascicular block in 100 pacemaker patients

RBBB+LAH	26
RBBB+LPH	7
LBBB	13
RBBB	9
LAH	6
LPH	1
	62
No fasc. block	26
No record	12

The course of patients with fascicular block depends on the clinical setting which leads to the block. In 350 patients with acute myocardial infarct no patients with monofascicular block developed complete block (Table 2). This is in accordance with the observations of Lie et al. [24] in contrast to other authors [2, 32, 44]. Five out of 20 patients with bifascicular block and 3 out 4 with intermittent trifascicular block developed 3rd degree block. Complete block has been observed in 24 – 60% of patients with bifascicular block and acute myocardial infarction [2, 11, 19, 24, 29, 42, 43, 44]. The wide range may be due to the fact that in some series intraventricular conduction defects before onset of the infarct could not be excluded and that some patients had additional AV conduction disturbances. The prognosis also depends on the time of onset of block and on the persistence of block [4, 24]. On the other hand we could confirm the observation of other authors [11, 24, 29], that temporary pacing in those patients who developed complete block did not reduce mortality because these patients died from pump failure due to extensive myocardial damage.

It has been shown that a combination of AV conduction disturbance in combination with intraventricular block might have a significant impact on the clinical course. Analysis with the HBE has demonstrated that an abnormal slowing of conduction can be present even in patients with normal PQ interval [27, 31, 37, 47]. Of 37 patients with fascicular block and normal PQ interval, 10 had a conduction disturbance, and 7 of these had prolonged HV interval; 3 of whom proceeded to higher degree block (Table 3). Patients with left bundle branch block (LBBB) showed

Table 2. Fascicular block in 350 patients with infarct

	No. of Patients	Development of 3rd degree AV block	Deceased
LAH	11	0	0
LPH	4	0	0
RBBB	3	0	2
LBBB	12	0	6
RBBB + LAH	18	4	5
RBBB + LPH	2	1	1
RBBB + LAH – LBBB – RBBB + LPH	4	3	2

Table 3. Fascicular block with normal PQ interval

		Without conduction disturbance	Proximal conduction disturbance	Distal conduction disturbance	Development of higher degree AV block
RBBB + LAH	24	19	2	3[a]	1
RBBB + LPH	1	1	–	–	–
RBBB	2	2	–	–	–
LBBB	8	3	1	4[a]	2
LAH	2	2	–	–	–
Total	37	27	3	7	3

The one patient with RBBB + LAH and the two patients with LBBB who developed higher degree AV block came out of the groups of 3, and 4 patients (marked with [a]) respectively who had distal conduction disturbance

the highest percentage of distal conduction disturbance and development of high degree block. Of 57 patients with LBBB and varying PQ interval analyzed by Rosen et al. [34] 24% had a normal HV interval, 39% a definitively prolonged HV interval over 60 ms and 37% an "intermediate" HV interval of 50 – 60 ms. Although there was a wide overlap, some patients with normal PQ interval having prolonged HV time and some with prolonged PQ interval having normal HV interval, the AV conduction time recognizable on the surface ECG was significantly longer in patients with abnormal HV time (mean PQ interval for the group with normal HV time being 172 ± 13 ms, for the intermediate group, 185 ± 7 ms, for the group with prolonged HV time, 225 ± 14 ms). Two patients developed intermittent and one patient persistent complete block, each patient belonging to the group with abnormal HV interval. Puech and Grolleau [31] found an abnormal HV interval in 22 patients with normal PQ interval, most of them demonstrating bifascicular block. In accordance with these and other authors [28, 37] we found in most of our patients with 1st degree AV block a conduction disturbance proximal to the His bundle except for 10 of 26 patients who had fascicular block with distal block and, in some, additional AH prolongation. With the exception of one patient with RBBB and LPH with normal HV interval 9 of these patients developed high degree block (Table 4).

In patients with Mobitz type I block with and without fascicular block we found proximal conduction disturbance, whereas 29 of 35 patients with type II block had block distal to the His bundle (Table 5). This agrees well with the findings of Narula et al. [27], Rosen et al. [36] and Langendorf et al. [22]. In 13 a pacemaker had to be inserted due to development of high degree block. Langendorf and Pick [21] have pointed out that the differentiation of AV block into Mobitz type I and II has great prognostic significance. Our findings as well as others [22, 26, 36] demonstrate the close relation of type I block to functional disturbances in the AV node and of type II block to changes in the His-Purkinje system. On the other hand it has been shown in experimental and clinical work that type I can occur in the His-Purkinje system as well [1, 6, 8, 9, 40].

Mobitz in 1924 stated that his type II block "points to an organic disease of the conduction fibers and is the first step to Adams-Stokes attacks and total permanent dissociation." Since there has been some confusion about the definition of type I and II block in the recent past [3] it seems appropriate to review some of the fundamental differences. In type I a blocked atrial impulse is preceded by two or more impulses with changing PQ intervals. If there is a stepwise prolongation of AV conduction before the complete block, this constitutes a Wenckebach period, which in its classic form shows the longest PQ interval before the blocked beat, the shortest interval after the blocked beat, and the largest PQ increase after the first conducted beat. This in turn leads to a stepwise shortening of the R – R interval, the longest interval (due to the blocked beat) being shorter than the double of the shortest R – R interval. Of course this phenomenon will not be demonstrable in those cases where the blocked atrial impulse is situated before the last conducted QRS complex due to excessive PQ prolongation.

A schematic diagram modified after Barold and Friedberg [3] (Fig. 1) reveals that type I block can consist of atypical Wenckebach periods with fluctuation of the AV interval (A) or a constant AV interval for two or more beats (B) before the blocked beat, whereas a dropped beat without warning is typical of Mobitz type II block (C). If there is shortening of the AV conduction after the blocked beat with increase in the following beat it is a type I block, unless one assumes that it is simulated by an escape beat after the blocked beat, this then being a type II block (D). Langendorf et al. [22] believe that shortening of the PQ interval not exceeding 20 ms

Table 4. 1st degree AV block

	No. of patients	Block proximal to His bundle	Block distal to His bundle (with proximal conduction disturbance)	Development of higher degree block
Without intraventricular conduction disturbance	15	14	1	2
RBBB + LAH	15	11	4[a]	4
RBBB + LPH	5	4[a]	1[a]	2
LBBB	6	1	5[a]	3
Fascicular block (total)	26	16	10	9

All 4 patients with RBBB + LAH and the 3 patients with LBBB, who developed higher degree block came out of the groups of 4 and 5 patients respectively with distal conduction disturbance (marked with [a]), whereas 1 of the 2 patients with RBBB + LPH who developed higher degree block had proximal block (group of 4 marked with [a]) and 1 had distal block (marked with [a]).

Table 5. 2nd degree AV block

	No.	Proximal block	Distal block	Development of high degree block
Mobitz type I				
RBBB + LAH	2	2	–	–
without intraventricular conduction disturbance	5	5	–	–
Mobitz type II				
without intraventricular conduction disturbance	13	3[a]	10[a]	2
RBBB + LAH	10	–	10[a]	7
RBBB + LPH	1	1[a]	–	1
LBBB	8	–	8[a]	4
RBBB	1	–	1[a]	1
	20	1	19	13

One of the 2 patients without intraventricular conduction disturbance who developed high degree block came out of the group of 3 with proximal block (marked with [a]), all having had 2 : 1 block (see text), and 1 came out of the group of 10 with distal block (marked with [a]). All 7 patients with RBBB + LAH and all 4 patients with LBBB who developed high-degree block came out of the groups of 10, and 8 respectively with distal block (marked with [a]), whereas the 1 patient with RBBB and LPH with high-degree block had proximal block (marked with [a]).

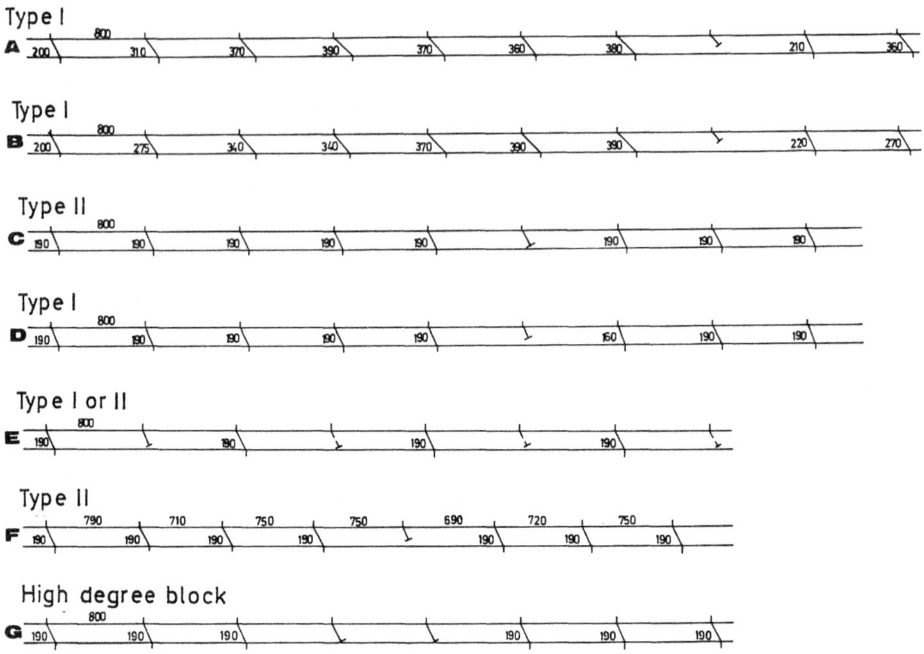

Fig. 1. (A) Atypical Wenckebach period with decrease and increase of PQ interval before blocked beat. (B) Type I block with increasing AV conduction time and constant PQ interval for 2 (or more) beats before blocked impulse. (C) Type II block with constant PR interval before and after sudden block. (D) Type I block with shortening of first conducted beat about 30 ms after blocked beat with increase of conduction time of second conducted beat. Type II block cannot be ruled out if escape beat is assumed. (E) Constant 2 : 1 block does not allow classification into type I or II block. (F) Type II block with constant PQ interval of conducted beats with sinus arrhythmia which could simulate type I block. (G) High degree block with complete block of 2 (or more) atrial impulses with constant PQ interval of conducted beats (modified after Barold and Friedberg [3]).

after the blocked beat can occur in type II block, a concept then has been challenged recently by Narula [26] with the following argument: If one assumes that the conduction time through the abnormal region is independent of the number of impulses transmitted and therefore constant, as is typical for type II block, there seems no logical reason for the PQ interval to shorten even slightly in the first conducted beat after the intermittance, whereas type I block shows time-rate dependence of conduction time, a phenomenon that is easily demonstrated by increasing the atrial rate by artificial pacing.

Since type I block can only be diagnosed or ruled out by presence or absence of progressing lengthening of the PQ interval in consecutive beats, a 2 : 1 block can not be classified as either type I or II, regardless of the presence or absence of fascicular block and regardless of the site of the block [3]. Three of our patients with normal QRS complex had 2 : 1 conduction with block proximal to the His bundle (marked with [a] in Table 5), whereas 11 out of 12 patients with intraventricular conduction defects and

2 : 1 conduction had distal block. Narula [26] found block in the AV node in 35%, in the His bundle in 12%, and below the His bundle in 53% of 17 patients with 2 : 1 block. A definitive statement of the type of block in those patients should only be made when review of long strips demonstrate conduction of two or more conducted beats. It is evident that change of sinus rate will not affect the constant PQ interval in true type II block (F). Sudden block of two or more beats with constant AV conduction time before and after the blocked beats can occur in the more advanced form of type II block [21], a type which is referred to as "high degree block" [3] (G).

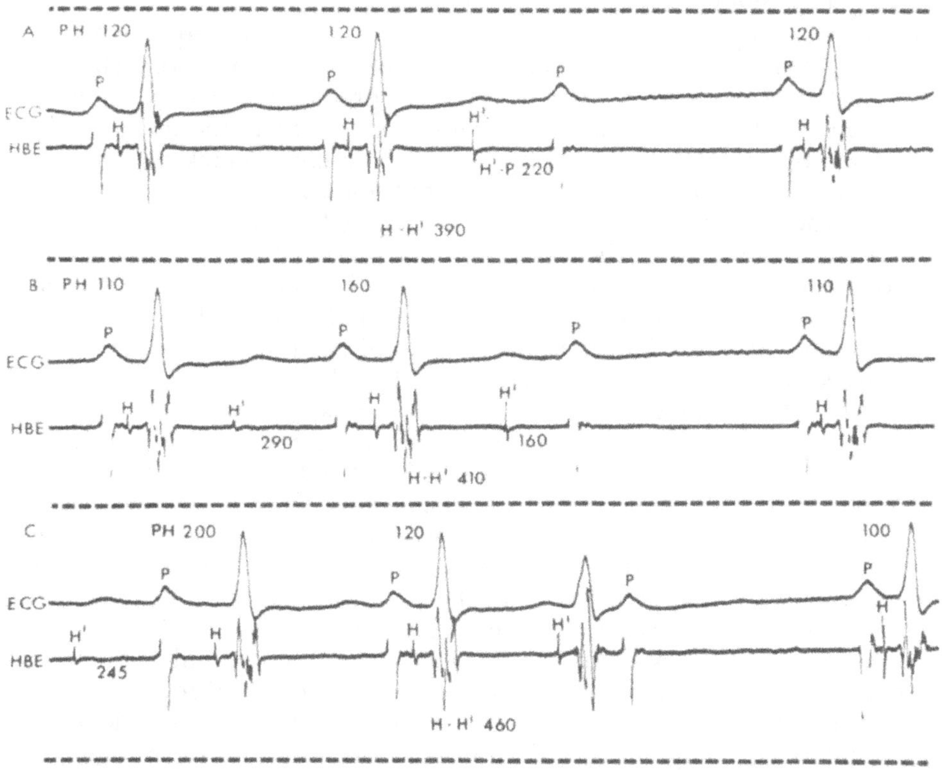

Fig. 2. Lead II ECG and HBE of patient with multiple premature His bundle depolarizations. P-H intervals are listed at top, H′-P intervals are noted under the HBE and H-H′ intervals on the bottom of each strip. In strip A there is a blocked P wave due to a premature His bundle depolarization (H′) occurring 220 ms before the atrial impulse with ante- and retrograde block. The consecutive conducted beats have a constant P-H (and P-Q) interval, the ECG resembling Mobitz type II block. In strip B the prolonged P-H interval (160 ms) of the second beat and the following blocked P wave are due to H′ occurring 290 ms and 160 ms before the atrial impulse, the ECG resembling a Wenckebach period. In strip C the first P-H interval is prolonged to 200 ms due to an H′-P interval of 245 ms. The second H′ is propagated to ventricles with aberrant conduction because of sufficient long distance to preceding His bundle depolarization (H-H′ interval) of 460 ms. From: Rosen et al.: Pseudo a-v block secondary to premature nonpropagated His bundle depolarizations. Documentation by His bundle electrocardiography. Circulation **42,** 367 – 373 (1970). By permission of The American Heart Association, Inc.

Kaufman et al. [15] described ECGs of two patients with 3 : 2, 4 : 3, and 5 : 4 block with constant PQ interval of the conducted beats with Adams-Stokes attacks. They mentioned the frequent association of this type of block with intraventricular conduction defects. Indeed, one of their patients had RBBB and LAH and the other RBBB and LPH. Spang in 1957 reported a similar case.

Type I as well as type II block can be simulated by concealed conduction as was demonstrated as early as 1947 by Mehlman and Langendorf. Nonpropagated premature beats can be visualized with the HBE, as has been shown by Rosen et al. [33]. They demonstrated in a patient that premature His bundle depolarizations generally undetectable on the ECG because of antegrade and retrograde block can effect subsequent AV conduction by virtue of concealed conduction into the AV junction. The effect was related to the time of occurrence of the premature beats in relation to the subsequent atrial impulses producing more or less pronounced PQ prolongation or complete block of the P wave, thereby mimicking type I and II block (Fig. 2). Prognosis was considered good in this type of "pseudoblock," whereas Grolleau et al. [12] who observed six cases and Narula [26] who described 10 cases believe that concealed premature His bundle extrasystoles are a manifestation of disease in the His bundle, especially since Narula observed a prolonged HV interval in the conducted beats in his patients and distal block even in the absence of extra beats.

The significance of distal conduction disturbances is demonstrated in patients with complete AV block, as in almost all of those with acquired complete block this block is located distal to the His bundle [18, 28, 35]. Of our 74 patients with complete block, 58 showed distal block, associated with additional proximal conduction disturbance in 25%, whereas patients with congenital block had proximal block. Although this type of block in general is associated with a much better prognosis, we could confirm the observation of Rosen et al. [35] that there are exceptions to the rule: after 2 years observation one of our patients with congenital block which changed to Mobitz type I block with exercise had to be treated with an artificial pacemaker due to Adams-Stokes attacks. Rosen et al. [35] found syncopal attacks in 29% of their patients with complete or high degree block with proximal block, compared with 25% of those with intra-His block and 71% of those with distal block.

We tried to test AV conduction in patients with (bi)fascicular block by atrial stimulation, increasing the rate until block occurs. All but 2 of the 28 patients showed proximal block. Block occurred at a wide range of atrial stimulation rates (Table 6) which did not correlate with the occurrence of syncope on clinical observation of the patients.

Our results demonstrate that especially in patients with fascicular block a distal AV conduction disturbance leads to high degree block with clinical symptoms requiring the insertion of a pacemaker in a high percentage (27 out of 46 patients). This percentage depends on the kind of fascicular block, the accompanying AV conduction defects, and the clinical setting in which the block occurred. On the other hand it has been shown that a

Table 6. Atrial stimulation of patients with (bi)fascicular block

		HV prolongation	
RBBB+LAH	21	1	
RBBB+LPH	5	–	
LBBB	2	1	
	28	2	
onset of block		Patients	Patients with syncope
at rate:	80 – 100	3	2
	100 – 120	1	–
	120 – 140	9	6
	140 – 160	12	3
	160 – 200	3	2
		28	13

normal distal AV conduction time with or without proximal conduction disturbance does not exclude the possibility of development of high degree block, just as a conduction disturbance distal to the His bundle will not necessarily lead to complete block, at least in our series with a limited observation time up to 3 years.

Denes et al. [7] analyzed 119 patients with bifascicular block manifested by RBBB with LAH with an average observation time of 1½ years. Progression of conduction disease occurred in a rather small percentage in those with normal (4%) as well as in those with prolonged HV interval (14%). But distal conduction disturbance was associated more frequently with serious myocardial dysfunction, i.e., congestive heart failure cardiomegaly, and higher mortality. This seems logical if one assumes that distal conduction disturbance is a manifestation of organic disease in the His-Purkinje system which generally does not seem to be limited to the conduction fibers [17]. It seems doubtful that the mortality in this group can be reduced by pacemaker treatment. A definitive answer will only be possible after observation of a greater number of patients over a longer period of time.

Summary

Clinical symptoms of AV block mainly are due to reduction of ventricular rate. Certain forms of intraventricular conduction disturbance with or without low-degree block seem to bear the risk of sudden onset of complete block, which also depends on the clinical situation in which the conduction disturbance occurs.

None of our patients with acute infarct and monofascicular block but most of the ones with intermittend trifascicular and bifascicular block developed 3rd degree block. Of 88 patients with fascicular block 74% of those with conduction disturbance distal to the His bundle in the His bundle electrogram progressed to high-degree block, the percentage differing with the kind of intraventricular conduction disturbance and the degree of AV block. The differentiation between atypical Mobitz type I and II as well as the recognition of concealed conduction leading to pseudo-AV block is stressed. With atrial stimulation in patients with bifascicular block nonconduction of the artificial impulse occurred at a wide range of stimulation rate which did not correlate with occurrence of syncope due to high-degree block. Development of significant clinical symptoms due to progressing AV block seems difficult to predict.

References

1. Anderson, G. J., Greenspan, K., Fisch, C.: Electrophysiological studies of Wenckebach structures below the AV junction. Amer. J. Cardiol. **30,** 232 – 236 (1972)
2. Atkins, J. M., Leshin, S. J., Blomquist, G., Mullins, C. B.: Ventricular conduction blocks and sudden death in acute myocardial infarction. New Engl. J. Med, **288,** 281 – 284 (1973)
3. Barold, S. S., Friedberg, H. D.: Second degree atrioventricular block. A matter of definition. Amer. J. Cardiol. **33,** 311 – 315 (1974)
4. Benchimol, A., Ellis, J. G., Dimond, E. G.: Hemodynamic consequences of atrial and ventricular pacing in patients with normal and abnormal hearts. Amer. J. Med. **39,** 911 – 922 (1965)
5. Borden, H. H., Ibrahim, M. A.: The epidemiology of the QRS axis measurements. Amer. J. publ. Hlth. **60,** 722 – 730 (1970)
6. Cerqueira-Gomes, M., Vasconelos Texeira, A.: Wenckebach phenomenon in the posterior division of the left bundle branch. Amer. Heart J. **82,** 377 – 381 (1971)
7. Denes, P., Dhingra, R. C., Wu., D., Chuquimia, R., Amat-y-Leon, F., Windham, C., Rosen, K. M.: H-V interval in patients with bifascicular block (right bundle branch block and left anterior hemiblock). Clinical, electrocardiographic and electrophysiologic correlations. Amer. J. Cardiol. **35,** 23 – 29 (1975)
8. El-Sherif, N., Scherlag, B. J., Samet, P.: Analysis of second degree a-v block following acute myocardial ischemia of the canine His-Purkinje system (abstr.) Clin. Res. **21,** 417 (1973)
9. Friedberg, H. D., Schamroth, L.: The Wenckebach phenomenon in the left bundle branch block. Amer. J. Cardiol. **24,** 591 – 593 (1969)
10. Gleichmann, U., Seipel, L., Grabensee, B., Loogen, F.: Häufigkeit und klinische Bedeutung uni-, bi- und trifaszikulärer Blockbilder. Dtsch. med. Wschr. **97,** 539 – 544 (1972)
11. Godman, M. J., Lassers, B. W., Julian, D. G.: Complete bundle branch block complicating acute myocardial infarction. New Engl. J. Med. **282,** 237 – 240 (1970)
12. Grolleau, R., Puech, P., Latour, H.: Les dépolarisations Hissiennes ectopiques non propagées. Arch. Mal. Coeur **65,** 1069 – 1080 (1972)
13. Hiss, R. G., Lamb, L. E.: Electrocardiographic findings in 122, 043 individuals. Circulation **25,** 947 – 961 (1962)
14. Hunt, D., Sloman, G.: Bundle-branch block in acute myocardial infarction. Brit. med. J. **1,** 85 – 88 (1969)
15. Kaufman, J. G., Wachtel, F. W., Rothfield, E., Bernstein, A.: The association of complete heart block and Adams-Stokes syndrome in two cases of Mobitz type of block. Circulation **23,** 253 – 256 (1961)

16. Kelly, D. T., Brodsky, S. J., Mirowski, M., Krovetz, L. J., Rowe, R. D.: Bundle of His recordings in congenital complete block. Circulation **45**, 277 – 281 (1972)
17. Knieriem, H.-J., Effert, S.: Morphologische Befunde beim kompletten Herzblock. Klin. Wschr. **44**, 349 – 360 (1966)
18. Lang, K. F., Just, H. G.: Das Konzept des fasciculären Blocks. Klassifizierung, Genese und Differenzierung mit Hilfe des Hisbündel-EKG's. Klin. Wschr. **51**, 791 – 800 (1973)
19. Lang, K. F., Rosellen, E., Limbourg, P., Recke, S., Just, H.: Prognostische Bedeutung ventrikulärer Erregungsausbreitungsstörungen vom Typ des fasciculären oder Hemiblocks. Verh. Dtsch. Ges. Inn. Med. **78**, 1107 – 1109 (1972)
20. Langendorf, R., Mehlman, J. S.: Blocked (nonconducted) a-v nodal premature systoles imitating first and second degree a-v block. Amer. Heart J. **34**, 500 – 506 (1947)
21. Langendorf, R., Pick, A.: Atrioventricular block, type II (Mobitz): its nature and clinical significance. Circulation **38**, 819 – 821 (1968)
22. Langendorf, R., Cohen, H., Gozo, E. G.: Observations on second degree atrioventricular block, including new criteria for the differential diagnosis between type I and type II block. Amer. J. Cardiol. **29**, 111 – 119 (1972)
23. Lasser, R. P., Haft, J. I., Friedberg, C. K.: Relationship of right-bundle-branch block and marked left axis deviation (with left parietal or peri-infarction block) to complete block and syncope. Circulation **37**, 429 – 437 (1968)
24. Lie, K. I., Wellens, H. J. J., Schuilenburg, R. M., Becker A. E., Durrer, D.: Factors influencing prognosis of bundle branch block complicating acute antero-septal infaction. The value of His bundle recordings. Circulation **50**, 935 – 941 (1974)
25. Mobitz, W.: Über die unvollständige Störung der Erregungsüberleitung zwischen Vorhof und Kammer des menschlichen Herzens. Zschr. ges. exp. Med. **41**, 180 – 237 (1924)
26. Narula, O. S.: Wenckebach type I and type II atrioventricular block (revisited). In: Complex Electrocardiography 2. Cardiovascular Clinics. Brest, A. N. (ed.) Philadelphia: F. A. Davies, 1974, Vol. VI, pp. 138 – 167
27. Narula O. S., Samet, P.: Right bundle branch block with normal left or right axis deviation. Amer. J. Med. **51**, 432 – 455 (1971)
28. Narula, O. S., Scherlag, B. J., Samet, P., Javier, R. P.: Atrioventricular block: localization and classification by His bundle recordings. Amer. J. Med. **50**, 146 – 165 (1971)
29. Norris, R. M., Croxson, M. S.: Bundle branch block in acute myocardial infarction. Amer. Heart J. **79**, 728 – 733 (1970)
30. Ostrander, L. D.: Left axis devation: prevalence, associated conditions and prognosis. An epidemiologic study. Ann. intern. Med. **75**, 23 – 28 (1971)
31. Puech, P., Grolleau, R.: L'activité du faisceau de His normale et pathologique. Paris: Editions Sandoz, 1972
32. Rizzon, R., Rossi, L., Beissus, C., Demoulin, J. C.: Die Biase, M.: Left posterior hemiblock in acute myocardial infarction. Brit. Heart J. **37**, 711 – 720 (1975)
33. Rosen, K. M., Rahimtoola, S. H., Gunnar, R. M.: Pseudo a-v-block secondary to premature nonpropagated His bundle depolarizations. Documentation by His bundle electrocardiography. Circulation **42**, 367 – 373 (1970)
34. Rosen, K. M., Ehsanie, A., Rahimtoola, S. H.: H-V intervals in left bundel-branch block. Circulation **46**, 717 – 723 (1972)
35. Rosen, K. M., Dhingra, R. C., Loeb, H. S., Rahimtoola, S. H.: Chronic heart block in adults. Arch. intern. Med. **131**, 663 – 672 (1973)
36. Rosen, K. M., Loeb, H. S., Gunnar, R. M., Rahimtoola, S. H.: Mobitz type II block without bundle-branch block. Circulation **44**, 1111 – 1119 (1971)
37. Rosen, K. M., Rahimtoola, S. H., Chuquimia, R., Loeb, H. S., Gunnar, R. M.: Electrophysiological significance of first degree atrioventricular block with intraventricular conduction disturbance. Circulation **43**, 491 – 502 (1971)
38. Rosenbaum, M. B., Elizari, M. V., Lazzari, J. O.: The Hemiblocks. Oldsmar, Fla.: Tampa Tracings, 1970
39. Rosenbaum, M. B., Elizari, M. V., Lazzari, T. O., Halpern, M. S., Rypa, D.: QRS patterns heralding the development of complete heart block with particular emphasis on right bundle branch block with left posterior hemiblock. In: Symposium on Cardiac Arrhyth-

mias. Sandøe, E., Flenstedt-Jensen, E., Olesen, K. H. (eds.): Södertälje Astra, 1970, pp. 249 – 269

40. Rosenbaum, M. B., Nau, G. J., Levi, R. J., Halpern, M. S., Elizari, M. V., Lazzari, J. O.: Wenckebach periods in the bundle branches. Circulation **40,** 79 – 88 (1969)
41. Rushmer, R. F.: Cardiovascular Dynamics, 2nd ed. Philadelphia: Saunders, W. B., 1961
42. Scanlon, P. J., Pryor, R., Blount, S. G.: Right bundle branch block associated with left superior of inferior intraventricular block. Clinical setting, prognosis and relation to complete block. Circulation **42,** 1123 – 1133 (1970)
43. Scanlon, P. J., Pryor, R., Blunt, S. G.: Right bundle branch block with left superior of inferior intraventricular block associated with acute myocardial infarction. Circulation **42,** 1135 – 1142 (1970)
44. Scheinman, M., Brenman, B.: Clinical and anatomical implications of intraventricular conduction blocks in acute myocardial infarction. Circulation **46,** 753 – 760 (1972)
45. Sowton, G. E.: Haemodynamic studies in patients with artificial pacemakers. Brit. Heart J. **26,** 737 – 746 (1964)
46. Spang, K.: Rhythmusstörungen des Herzens. Systematik, Ursache und klinische Bedeutung. Therapie. Stuttgart: Thieme, 1957, pp. 241 – 245
47. Touboul P., Ibrahim, M.: Atrioventricular conduction defects in patients presenting with syncope and normal PR interval. Heart J. **34,** 1005 – 1011 (1972)

Fascicular Block Patterns – Observations on Differential Diagnosis

M. GERTSCH and D. BERNOULLI

Fascicular block patterns merit clinical interest because they are the most frequent precursors of acquired complete atrioventricular block [6, 16, 22, 24, 26, 28]. In the present paper we lay stress on differential diagnostic aspects. The behavior of the intrinsicoid deflection and the presence of mirror image effects may be helpful for diagnosis whereas interferences between fascicular blocks and infarction patterns may render a correct diagnosis more difficult. The anatomical variations of the intraventricular conduction system, as well as the age, the physical constitution, and the clinical diagnosis of a patient are always to be considered. The difficulties in recognition of the left anterior fascicular block are shown on the basis of 100 consecutive ECGs with left axis deviation.

I. Typical Pattern of Fascicular Blocks

Typical *left anterior fascicular block* (LAFB) shows the following principal signs (Fig. 1 a and b): (1) delay of intrinsicoid deflection in the bipolar leads aVL and/or I (step or slurring in the descending foot of the R wave) of 15 ms or more in relation to the unipolar lead V6; (2) left axis deviation with qR in aVL/I and rS in lead III/aVF/II ($\hat{A}QRS_F$ situated between $-30°$ and $-70°$); (3) RS or qRs in lead V6; (4) relatively high R waves in lead V2/V3 (not compulsory); (5) positive asymmetric T waves in lead III/aVF/II (not compulsory).

Isolated *left posterior fascicular block* (LPFB) is very rare and can be diagnosed based on the following alterations (Fig. 1 c): (1) delay of intrinsicoid deflection (step or slurring in the descending foot of the R wave) in lead III/aVF/II and often in lead V6 (18) of 15 – 20 ms or more, compared to lead aVL/I; (2) right axis deviation ($\hat{A}QRS_F$ between $+70°$ and $+100°$) with rS in lead aVL and qR in lead III/aVF/II; (3) qR or qRs in lead V6; (4) relatively deep S waves in lead V2/V3 (not compulsory); (5) negative asymmetric T waves in lead III/aVF/II.

In *bilateral bifascicular block* the characteristics of left fascicular block are joined to those of right bundle branch block (RBBB). In general each block pattern can be recognized separately, since the signs of left fascicular block are projected mainly on the frontal plane, whereas the marks of

---

The authors wish to express their appreciation and gratitude to Miss Th. Minder for her technical assistance.

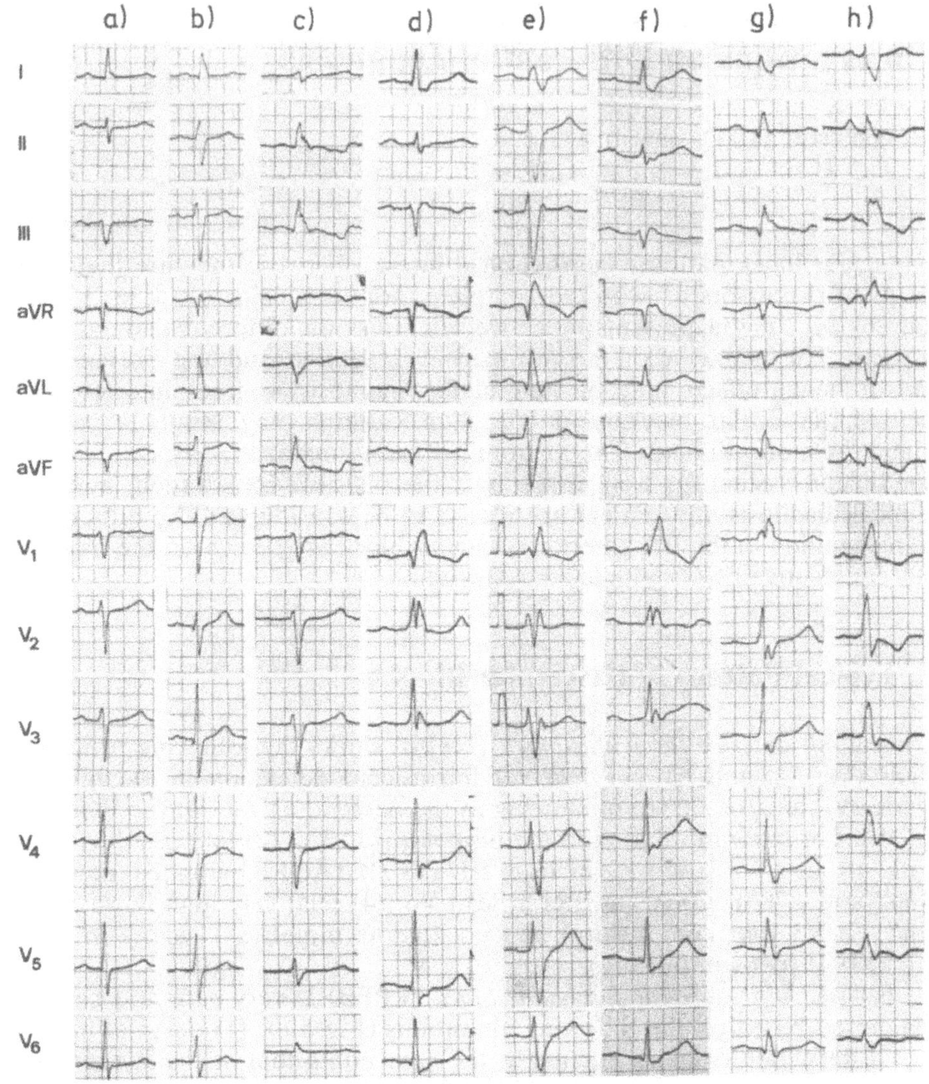

Fig. 1. (a) Left anterior fascicular block (LAFB). (b) LAFB with q wave in anteroseptal leads. (c) Left posterior fascicular block (LPFB), atrial fibrillation, artifacts by muscular tremor and alternating current. (d) Isolated right bundle branch block (RBBB), slight left ventricular hypertrophy. Possible right ventricular hypertrophy. (e) RBBB + LAFB, left ventricular hypertrophy. (f) RBBB + LAFB. The delayed intrinsicoid deflection caused by LAFB is scarcely visible in lead aVL. (g) RBBB = LPFB, infarction of posterior and inferior wall. (h) RBBB, excessive right ventricular hypertrophy. For detailed explanation, see text. Paper speed 50 mm/s

RBBB are directly visible in lead VI (sometimes we find an enlarged slurred R wave in lead V1 instead of an rsR′ configuration).

The more frequent pair *RBBB + LAFB* are shown in Fig. 1 e, the pattern of isolated RBBB in Fig. 1 d.

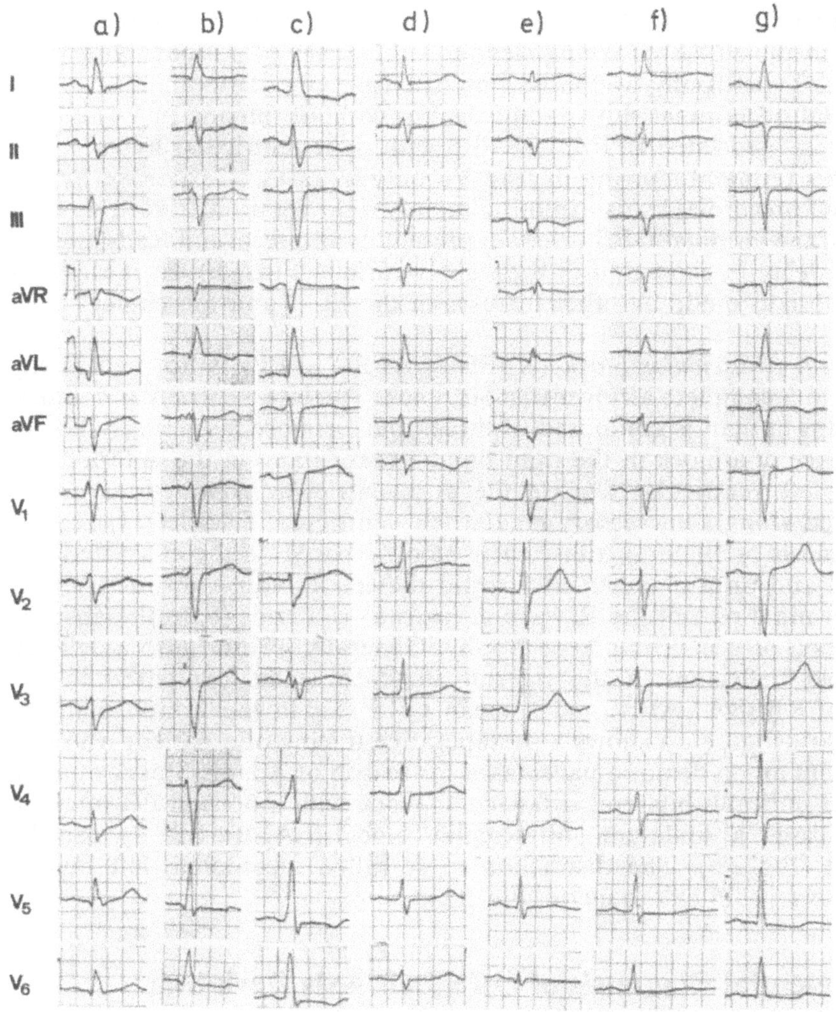

Fig. 2. (a) RBBB (morphologically incomplete) + LAFB + LPFB without atrioventricular block. (b) LAFB + LPFB. (c) Incomplete left bundle branch block. (d) LAFB with mirror-image effect of delayed intrinsicoid deflection in lead III. (e) Pseudo-LAFB produced by infarction of posterior and lateral wall. (f) LAFB without left axis deviation (associated to incomplete LPFB?). (g) Left axis deviation without LAFB, left ventricular hypertrophy. (Detailed explanations see text). Paper speed 50 mm/s

The difference between bilateral bifascicular block of type RBBB + LAFB and isolated RBBB may be minimal in the ECG. Occasionally the only manifestation of an associated LAFB is a slight step at the end of the R wave (Fig. 1 f) or at the beginning of the s wave in lead aVL, or there is simply a delayed slope of the R wave in aVL with a consecutive small s wave, compared to V6. This type probably corresponds to an anatomical small left anterior fascicle.

The pair *RBBB + LPFB* (Fig. 1 g) are rather rare. This pattern may be imitated in the ECGs of young slender individuals, of patients with right ventricular hypertrophy, and those with extensive anterolateral infarction. A preterminal or terminal slurring in lead V6 (without slurring in V4) is suggestive of an associated LPFB. In RBBB with right ventricular hypertrophy we see this terminal slurring in lead V6 only in cases of excessive hypertrophy, the precordial leads exploring mainly right ventricular vectors; here a delay of the terminal QRS forces in present in all precordial leads and indicates a delay in excitation of the right ventricle (Fig. 1 h). In most cases the diagnosis is made by other features of the ECG and the clinical findings.

Bilateral trifascicular block (RBBB + LAFB + LPFB) is not necessarily identical to a complete atrioventricular block. The intraventricular conduction system in man is composed of three, four or more fascicles [7, 19]. In the presence of a block in the right bundle branch and in the anterior and posterior left ventricular fascicle the atrioventricular conduction can be maintained along a successory medial left ventricular fascicle [11, 12, 19]. The diagnosis of bilateral trifascicular block is based on the characteristics of RBBB and on a delayed intrinsicoid deflection with a distinct step in the preterminal part of the R wave in leads aVL/I and V6, in the absence of infarction or ventricular hypertrophy. Generally we find also a delayed intrinsicoid deflection in the inferior standard leads (compared to the pattern of RBBB + LAFB) and a mean QRS axis in the frontal plane at about $-30°$. Figure 2 a shows a postoperative tracing of a patient who was treated with an on demand pacemaker for reason of Adams-Stokes attacks. The ECG indicates bilateral trifascicular block with a normal PR interval. In rare cases a unilateral bifascicular block (LAFB + LPFB) can be identified (Fig. 2 b). The distinction to so-called incomplete left bundle branch block is difficult to made (Fig. 2 c).

II. Differential Diagnosis of QRS Left Axis Deviation

Cardiologists, internists as well as general practicioners will meet frequently an ECG with left axis deviation. Many authors [e.g., 3, 14, 23, 27] equate a left axis deviation ($\hat{A}QRS_F$ beyond $-30°$) to a left anterior fascicular block (or "left anterior hemiblock"). In agreement with others [2, 10, 20, 21] we do not share this opinion. In our experience a left axis deviation with an rS in the inferior bipolar leads is possible without LAFB [12, 13]. However, the differentiation between LAFB and "simple" left axis deviation may be difficult or even impossible in an individual case. Mirror-image patterns and the imitation or covering up of an infarction by an LAFB (and vice versa) must be considered in the interpretation.

Mirror-Image Effect of Delayed Intrinsicoid Deflection in LAFB

Sometimes a delayed intrinsicoid deflection is projected on a lead line in the frontal plane between $-60°$ and $-90°$ and therefore is not captured directly by means of a conventional lead. In these cases the delayed excitation of high lateral portions of the left ventricle produces a mirror-image effect in the inferior lead III and/or aVF, where we can detect a step in the ascending foot of the S wave (Fig. 2 d).

Mirror-Image Effect of "Peri-Infarction Block" in Inferior Infarction

We use the term "peri-infarction block" for the intraventricular conduction disturbance caused by necrotic myocardial tissue, regardless of QRS duration and in absence of a left fascicular block. The distinction between peri-infarction-block and left fascicular block should be made. The combination of both block patterns is not rare.

An inferior infarction may imitate the pattern of LAFB in lead aVL by mirror-image effect, especially if an initial small r wave is preserved in lead III. The correct diagnosis is sometimes made only by alterations of repolarization or by ECG series. A posteroinferior infarction (Fig. 2 e, where also the lateral wall is compromised) may imitate LAFB as well.

Imitation of an Anteroseptal Infarction in LAFB

In about 30% of cases LAFB leads to a qrS or a qRS configuration in leads V2 and V3, thus imitating an anteroseptal infarction (Fig. 1 b). McHenry et al. [15] indicate that the disappearence of the q waves in leads placed one intercostal space lower excludes infarction. In rare cases the LAFB conceals the Qr or QS configuration of a lateral infarction in lead V5 and V6 by a rS complex [12]. On the other hand the covering up of an anteroseptal infarction by LAFB is more common [1].

Concealing of Inferior Infarction in LAFB

In the combination of an old or subacute inferior infarction with LAFB we miss the typical Q waves of the infarction in lead III and aVF as well as the signs of subepicardial ischemia; the pattern of LAFB predominates with an rS configuration and a positive asymmetric T wave in leads III and aVF [1]. Occasionally there is a small q wave in lead II. However, the other clinical data are of more important diagnostic value.

In combination with an inferior infarction the LPFB (without or with RBBB) tends to narrow the q waves due to infarction (Fig. 1 g) [17].

QRS Left Axis Deviation Without LAFB

A QRS left axis deviation with rS in leads III, aVF, and II (and in absence of an RBBB or left bundle branch block) *without* direct or indirect signs of delayed excitation of the high lateral left ventricular portions include the following possibilities: (1) Incomplete LAFB; (2) block within a small left anterior fascicle; (3) association of LAFB to incomplete LPFB; (4) posterior infarction with extension to the inferior wall; (5) *isolated left axis deviation* (without LAFB).

The presence of QRS left axis deviation without LAFB has been reported in ostium primum atrial septal defect, as a familiar variation of the intraventricular conduction system in healthy individuals as well as in abnormal position of the heart, in combination with left ventricular hypertrophy, and in association with obesity [2, 4, 5, 8, 9, 12, 13]. The ECG in Figure 2 g is an example of left axis deviation without LAFB. The intrinsicoid deflection in lead aVL/I shows a delay of only 5 ms compared to that in lead V6. Moreover the QS in lead V2 associated to a qR in lead V6 and the negative T wave in lead III/aVF make LAFB improbable. The differentiation between LAFB and left ventricular hypertrophy on the one hand, and between LAFB and LAFB + left ventricular hypertrophy on the other is sometimes difficult or impossible.

LAFB Without QRS Left Axis Deviation

On rare occasions LAFB is accompanied by a mean QRS vector in the frontal plane between +30° and −30° (Fig. 2 f). The alteration may be caused by pulmonary emphysema (which in other instances may itself cause LAFB) or by an associated incomplete LPFB.

III. Electrocardiographic and Clinical Diagnosis in 100 Cases of QRS Left Axis Deviation

According to the above-mentioned criteria for LAFB we have analyzed 100 consecutive ECGs with QRS left axis deviation and made the correlation to the clinical diagnosis [1]. The ECGs come from the department of internal medicine (in about two-thirds of the cases) and from our department (in about one-third of the cases).

In a first group of 59 ECGs (59%) we made the diagnosis of LAFB. The left anterior fascicular block was predominantly associated to coronary heart disease with or without myocardial infarction and to "idiopathic fibrosis of the ventricular conduction system" (Lenègre's disease [16, 25]). In a second group of 26 ECGs (26%) we were able to exclude an LAFB. The clinical diagnoses were myocardial infarction, left ventricular hypertrophy, RBBB, obesity, other diseases, and a normal heart. Inferior infarction was the most frequent diagnosis. In 15 ECGs (15%) we could neither exclude nor diagnose LAFB with certainty. Especially the differentiation

[1] Detailed data will be communicated in another publication [13].

between LAFB and a peri-infarction-block caused problems. In other cases we could only assume the association of LAFB to incomplete LPFB.

Our results allow the following conclusions. LAFB seems to be the most frequent reason for left axis deviation in patients of an internalmedical/cardiological center. Left axis deviation may be present without LAFB. The electrocardiographic interpretation of left axis deviation is not without problems. The difficulties in diagnosis may be best illustrated by the words of Breall [5]: "When is a cat not a cat?"

Summary

The principal electrocardiographic criteria for the diagnosis of left fascicular block are the behavior of the intrinsicoïd deflection in the high lateral and inferior leads and the shift of the mean QRS axis in the frontal plane. Mirror-image effects in the standard leads may be helpful for the diagnosis of left anterior fascicular block; preterminal slurring in V_6 (in the absence of high degree right ventricular hypertrophy or inferolateral infarction) may indicate left posterior fascicular block. The patient's age, habitus, and clinical findings as well as earlier ECGs are important for interpretation. Myocardial infarction may obscure or imitate left fascicular block. Anatomical variations of the left ventricular conduction system occasionally allow the identification of bilateral trifascicular block without complete atrioventricular block; on the other hand they may render the diagnosis of left fascicular block difficult if not impossible.

The difficulties in the recognition of left anterior fascicular block are discussed based on 100 consecutive ECGs with left axis deviation.

References

1. Altieri, P., Schaal, S.: Inferior and anteroseptal myocardial infarction concealed by transient left anterior heimiblock. J. Electrocardiol. **6,** 257 (1973)
2. Arriaga, J. J., Scampardonis, G., Watanabe, Y.: Comparison of the 12-lead and orthogonal electrocardiograms, with special reference to the frontal QRS-axis. J. Electrocardiol. **5,** 47 (1972)
3. Beck, O. A., Hochrein, H.: Häufigkeit und Prognose des linksanterioren Hemiblocks als Komplikation des akuten Myokardinfarktes. Dtsch. med. Wschr. **99,** 77 (1974)
4. Borkon, A. M., Pieroni, D. R., Varghese, P. J., Ho, Ch. S., Rowe, R. D.: The superior QRS axis in ostium primum ASD: A proposed mechanism. Amer. Heart J. **90,** 215 (1975)
5. Breall, W. S.: Fascicular block vs. left ventricular hypertrophy. Amer. Heart J. **84,** 575 (1972)
6. Castellanos, A. Jr., Maytin, O., Arcebal, A. G., Lemberg, L.: Significance of complete right bundle branch block with right axis deviation in absence of right ventricular hypertrophy. Brit. Heart. J. **32,** 85 (1970)
7. Demoulin, J. C., Kulbertus, H. E.: Histopathological examination of concept of left hemiblock. Brit. Heart J. **34,** 708 (1972)
8. Dougherty, J. D.: The relation of the frontal QRS axis to the anatomic position of the heart. J. Electrocardiol. **3,** 267 (1970)
9. Durrer, D., Roos, J. P., van Dam, R. Th.: The genesis of the electrocardiogram of patients with ostium primum defects. Amer. Heart J. **71,** 642 (1966)

10. Durrer, D.: Personal communication
11. Gertsch, M., Medrano, G. A., de Micheli, A.: Schenkelblock, bilateraler bifaszikulärer und bilateraler trifaszikulärer Schenkelblock. Schweiz. med. Wschr. **104**, 1623 (1974)
12. Gertsch, M.: Die linksfaszikulären Blockierungen („Hemiblocks"). Bull. schweiz. Akad. med. Wiss. **31**, 59 (1975)
13. Gertsch, M., Bernoulli, D.: 100 konsekutive EKGs mit überdrehter QRS-Linkslage, In preparation.
14. Grayzel, J., Neyshaboori, M.: Left-axis deviation: etiologic factors in one-hundred patients. Amer. Heart J. **89**, 419 (1975)
15. McHenry, P. L., Phillips, J. F., Fisch, Ch., Corya Betty R.: Right precordial QRS pattern due to left anterior hemiblock. Amer. Heart J. **81**, 498 (1971)
16. Lenègre, J.: Etiology and pathology of bilateral bundle branch block in relation to complete heart block. Progr. Cardiovasc. Dis. **6**, 409 (1964)
17. Medrano, G. A., de Micheli, A., Brenes, C., Alatriste, V. M., Sodi-Pallares, D.: Necrosis posterior complicada con bloquéos bifascicular y trifascicular. Arch. Inst. Cardiol. Méx. **40**, 375 (1972)
18. Medrano, G. A., Brenes, P. C., de Micheli, A., Sodi-Pallares D.: Block of the posterior subdivision of the left bundle branch of His. J. Electrocardiol. **3**, 309 (1970)
19. Medrano, G. A., Brenes, C., de Micheli, A., Sodi-Pallares, D.: El bloquéo simultaneo de las subdivisiones anterior y posterior de la rama izquierda del Haz de His (bloquéo bifascicular) y su asociación con bloquéo de la rama derecha (bloquéo trifascicular). Arch. Inst. Cardiol. Méx. **40**, 752 (1970)
20. Medrano, G. A., Brenes, C., de Micheli, A., Sodi-Pallares, D.: Clinical electrocardiographic and vectorcardiographic diagnosis of the left anterior subdivision block, isolated or associated with RBBB. Amer. Heart J. **83**, 447 (1972)
21. Ostrander, L. D.: Left axis deviation: Prevalence, associated conditions and prognosis. Ann. intern. Med. **75**, 23 (1971)
22. Rosenbaum, B. M., Elizari, M. V., Lázzari, J. O: Los Hemibloquéos. Buenos Aires: Ed. Paidos, 1967
23. Rosenbaum, M. B., Elizari, M. V., Lazzari, J. O., Nau, G. J., Levi, R. J., Halpern, M. Susana: Intraventricular trifascicular blocks. Review of the literature and classification. Amer. Heart J. **78**, 450 (1969)
24. Rosenbaum, M. B., Elizari, M. V., Lázzari, J. O.: The Hemiblocks: New Concepts of Intraventricular Conduction Based on Human Anatomical, Physiological and Clinical Studies. Oldsmar, Fla.: Tampa Tracings, 1970.
25. Rosenbaum, M. B., Elizari, M. V., Kretz, A., Taratuto, A. L.: Anatomical basis of A-V conduction disturbances. In: Symposium on Cardiac Arrhythmias, Elsinore, Denmark. Sandøe E., Flensted-Jensen, E., Olesen K. H. (eds.), Södertälje, Sweden, Astra, 1970
26. Scanlon, P. J., Prior, R., Blount, S. G. Jr.: Right-bundle-branch block associated with left superior or inferior intraventricular block. Clinical setting, prognosis and relation to complete heart block. Circulation **42**, 1123 (1970)
27. Talbot, S.: Electrical axis and voltage criteria of left ventricular hypertrophy. Amer. Heart J. **90**, 420 (1975)
28. Trevino, A. J. and Beller, B. M.: Conduction disturbances of the left bundle branch system and their relationship to complete heart block. II. A review of differential diagnosis, pathology and clinical significance. Amer. J. Med. **51**, 374 (1971)

AV Nodal Tachycardias

Ph. Coumel

Writing an article about nodal tachycardias was certainly much easier some years ago, before the great progress of clinical electrophysiology. As a matter of fact, Moe and Mendez [11] had shown that a reentry mechanism was present every time a tachycardia could be initiated and terminated by programmed stimulation. Experimental work in animals had suggested the presence of at least two functionally separate pathways within the AV node [10, 11] which therefore appeared anatomically and electrophysiologically predisposed to be the site of a closed circuit of conduction. It was admitted that such theory could be extended to human cases of paroxysmal junctional tachycardia every time a pre-excitation pattern was not present during sinus rhythm. In fact, things have progressively become more complicated, as more exceptions were found to the rules initially formulated. If it remains true that the nonparoxysmal type of junctional tachycardia is probably due to an increase in AV junctional automaticity both clinical pattern and exact location of junctional circus movements should be reviewed.

I. Theoretical Considerations

It is widely admitted that three conditions are required to establish reentry: closed circuit of conduction, unidirectional block and slowed conduction. These three conditions are indeed present every time a circus movement is operating. But it does not mean that in every case the presence of both conditions is overt.

Closed Circuit of Conduction

One should appreciate the limitations of experimental techniques with respect to the concept of dual pathways in the AV node, because activation of the entire isolated AV node in three dimensions during junctional tachycardia has not yet been mapped. Reflection phenomena, responsible for isolated echo beats, are mainly observed in animals, and do not suppose the existence of a *closed* circuit of reentry. Two cases only of sustained reciprocating tachycardia have been studied by microelectrode techniques, and these very few observations are to be opposed to the relative frequency of the disease in humans. Hence, it is probably abusive to extend readily to humans, in whom extranodal pathways are known to be frequent, what is observed rarely, and not absolutely proved, in animals. As electrophysiologic evaluation of the reentry circuit is becoming more and more precise, latent accessory pathways instead of true intranodal longitudinal dissociation are found to be the very anatomic basis for reentry [4, 12, 13, 18, 19].

Unidirectional Block

A unidirectional block is necessarily present in a point of the circuit for establishing reentry. It does allow an impulse to engage a conducting pathway anterogradely without entering the alternate one, so that the latter can be conductive in the retrograde direction, setting the stage for reentry. The occurrence of the unidirectional block is easily recognized when it happens in an overtly present pathway: thus the disappearance of a delta wave at the beginning of an attack of junctional tachycardia obviously means that the bundle of Kent has been blocked anterogradely and will permit retrograde conduction of the impulse having reached the ventricle. But this condition is obvious only if the accessory pathway is permeable entirely, from the atrium to the ventricle. Conceivably, a concealed conduction may well be present in this pathway, preventing it from being entered retrogradely but without a pre-excitation pattern during sinus rhythm. Then this concealed anterograde conduction may well disappear at the onset of the tachycardia without being responsible for any modification of the QRS pattern. Hence, conversely, the absence of any changing pattern of R when the tachycardia starts, does not allow in any way the conclusion that no pre-exciting pathway is present. Misknowledge of such possibility has frequently led to erroneous conclusions concerning the supposed intranodal location of the reentry circuit.

Slowed Conduction

After the impulse has engaged the anterograde pathway and returned via the retrograde one, it must encounter a responsive anterograde pathway to perpetuate the reentry process. Therefore, the time needed for the impulse to traverse the whole circuit must exceed the duration of the refractory period in both pathways. Though such a condition is obviously mandatory, it does not need necessarily to be always apparent. Prolongation of the conduction time can concern P′ – R intervals as well as R – P′ during the tachycardia, knowing that in fact these intervals reflect only indirectly anterograde and retrograde conduction times since an initial and a final common pathway are supposed to be present. If the requisite prolongation [9] of the conduction time does concern the anterograde pathway, it is apparent as soon as the tachycardia starts, and the prolongation of the first P – R interval is indeed an overt necessary condition for reentry to appear. However, if this prolonged P – R is not present at the onset of the tachycardia, it does not mean at all that it is not due to a reentrant mechanism.

It means only that the retrograde instead of the anterograde conduction time is prolonged. This situation is very rare in paroxysmal forms of reciprocating tachycardia, but it is always present in the permanent (or chronic relapsing) form of the tachycardia [1, 2].

To summarize, our experience of junctional reciprocating tachycardia involving about 200 cases studied by programmed stimulation, leads us to consider that the vast majority of the reentry circuits, in human patients, is related to the presence of an accessory pathway. Its existence may be overt during sinus rhythm, with a delta wave in case of Kent bundle or a short P – R interval in case of atrio-His bypass. Unidirectional block of the accessory pathway [6] is indeed a frequent phenomenon, so that the direct proof of the pre-excitation may well be missing. Then the precise study of the localization of the reentry circuit relies upon indirect arguments: endocavitary or epicardial mapping of the atrium [16], study of the capture phenomena during the tachycardia, study of the bundle branch block – dependent rate of the tachycardia, etc. Most of these tachycardias are paroxysmal, with or without Wolff-Parkinson-White (WPW) syndrome, and a few are permanent.

II. Clinical Pattern of Intranodal Reciprocating Tachycardias

The question arises, as to whether true intranodal reciprocating tachycardias do exist, once the different forms of overt or latent, partial or complete pre-excitation syndromes are eliminated. The problem is precisely, before exploring the possibility of an intranodal reentry, to rule out the possibility of a concealed WPW syndrome. Indeed, this is not easy as the techniques become more and more sophisticated, and in any case the diagnosis of intranodal reentry cannot rely only on negative arguments. We shall see, with the following examples, which positive arguments can be gathered in favor of this diagnosis.

Two clinical patterns of nodal tachycardias should be distinguished in as much as the tachycardia is paroxysmal or permanent.

Paroxysmal Tachycardias

These tachycardias are always initiated by an atrial premature beat, and the extra-stimulus technique (Fig. 1) shows that a prolongation of P – R is always present at the beginning of the tachycardia. Denes et al. [7] have studied this mode of initiation extensively, and they have shown how a sudden increase of the A – H interval with only a slight increase in the prematurity of atrial stimulation is often present in this kind of tachycardia. This observation, however, does not constitute definite proof that the reentry pathway of tachycardia is confined only to the AV node, but Wellens [18] made a further observation of great interest about the relation between this phenomenon and the pattern of the tachycardia.

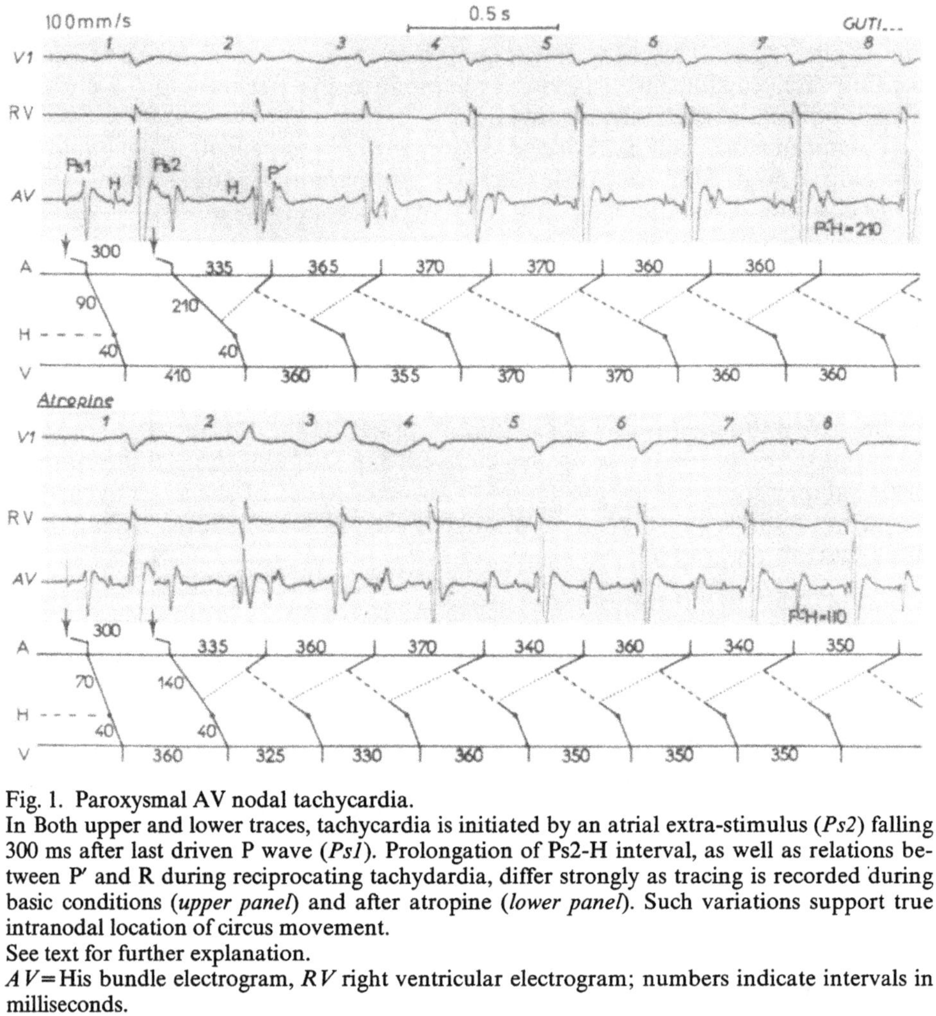

Fig. 1. Paroxysmal AV nodal tachycardia.
In Both upper and lower traces, tachycardia is initiated by an atrial extra-stimulus (*Ps2*) falling 300 ms after last driven P wave (*Ps1*). Prolongation of Ps2-H interval, as well as relations between P′ and R during reciprocating tachydardia, differ strongly as tracing is recorded during basic conditions (*upper panel*) and after atropine (*lower panel*). Such variations support true intranodal location of circus movement.
See text for further explanation.
AV=His bundle electrogram, *RV* right ventricular electrogram; numbers indicate intervals in milliseconds.

In 21 out of 49 Wellens' patients (group I) the beginning of atrial activation at the onset and in subsequent beats of the tachycardia *preceded* or was simultaneous with the beginning of ventricular activation. In addition, 19 of these 21 patients showed during application of atrial test stimuli, a *sudden* increase in A – H interval conduction time (50 ms or more) at the time of initiation of tachycardia. Obviously in group I a P or A wave superimposed with the onset of the QRS or actually preceding it, clearly excludes the WPW syndrome, but not an atrio-His bypass with anterograde block [3]. In contrast, the other 28 patients without WPW syndrome (group 2) demonstrated atrial activation following ventricular activation in the first and subsequent beats of the tachycardia. None of these 28 patients in group 2 exhibited sudden increase of A – H time (50 ms or more as seen in group I) at the onset of tachycardia. The striking difference in behavior of these two groups (both classified as AV nodal reentry) with regard to the A – H interval at the onset of the tachycardia appears more than coincidental and surely points to a different mechanism in group 2 which remains to be more clearly defined. Indeed, some patients in group 2 might well represent concealed WPW syndrome with anterograde block in the accessory pathway.

On the other hand, the existence of an R – P′ interval shorter than the P′ – R interval can only be considered as suggestive, but not indicative of a WPW syndrome; Figure 1 shows how positive arguments in favor of an intranodal reentry can be drawn from P′ and R relationships. The upper panel shows the initiation of the tachycardia during basic conditions: Psl is the last of the regularly driven beats at a rate of 80/min, with a Ps-H of 90 ms, and Ps2 is the atrial extrastimulus (Ps1 – Ps2 = 300 ms). Ps2 – H is prolonged to 210 ms, and the first P′ of the tachycardia follows immediately beat R2. Then the tachycardia is established, with a cycle length of 360 ms and a constant P′ – H interval of 210 ms. From these data, no conclusion is possible concerning the localization of the circus movement, which can be either extra- or intranodal. The lower panel of Figure 1, however, proves that the circuit is indeed intranodal, according to the modifications induced by atropine on the P′ and R relationships. The similarly given atrial extrastimulus starts the tachycardia in the same manner, but with an anterograde conduction time much shorter than in the upper panel : 140 ms. The shortening of anterograde conduction is confirmed by an R2 – R3 cycle shorter in the lower panel than in the upper one (325 ms instead of 360). The important fact is that, once the tachycardia is established, with a cycle length almost unchanged (350 ms instead of 360), the P′ and R relationships have been strikingly modified : P′ – H interval has been shortened by 100 ms while H – P′ has been proportionally lengthened. Such modifications of the intervals with a constant cycle length of the tachycardia imply that neither P′ nor H are part of the circuit, and that both of them are only linked to it by a common upper and lower avenue.

Even though the phenomena are not always as obvious as in Figure 1, it is very important to examine carefully the AV relationships during the first beats of the induced tachycardia. Slight changes in the P′H intervals are frequent indeed and confirm that the AV nodal-His conducting system does constitute the anterograde pathway. But the important point to consider is the H – P′ or R – P′ interval the variability of which supports an intranodal retrograde pathway while His fixity (much more frequent) strongly suggests the presence of an accessory pathway [14].

In the same way, retrograde VA conduction at various pacing rates should always be studied (and compared to the AV conduction time at the same cycle length) when the patient is in sinus rhythm to detect concealed retrograde pre-excitation [5, 8, 12, 18, 19]. VA conduction times during ventricular pacing (at cycle lengths compared to the SVT) should be comparable to the R – P′ interval during the tachycardia if an accessory pathway is used. Overall, the constancy of the retrograde conduction time [17] is a strong argument in favor of an accessory conducting pathway. On the other

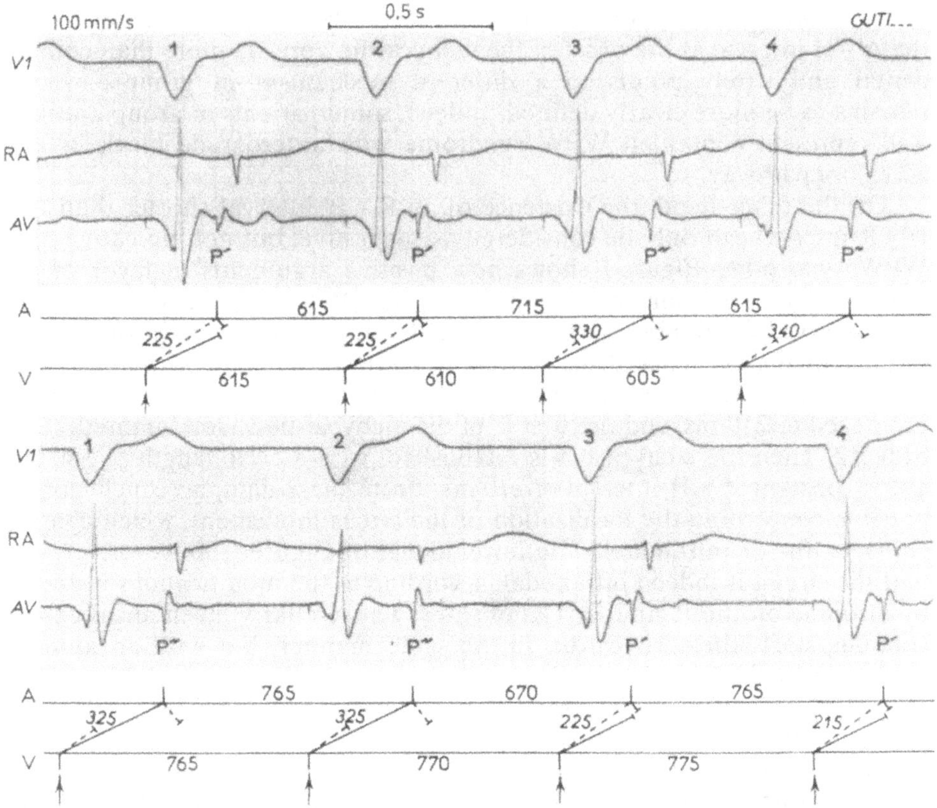

Fig. 2. Retrograde VA conduction (same patient as Fig. 1).
Studying the retrograde VA conduction provides further argument in favor of a functional longitudinal dissociation of AV node. Upper panel shows sudden increase in VA conduction time (225 – 330 ms) between beats 2 and 3 as the cardiac cycle length has been slightly reduced by 5 ms. Reverse phenomenon is observed in the lower panel, as a much longer cycle length is slightly increased.
See text for discussion.
RA = right atrial electrogram.

hand, the findings shown in Figure 2 (same patient as in Fig. 1) are rare indeed and confirm the coexistence of two functional nodal pathways. In the upper panel, the cycle length of the ventricular driving is shortened by 5 ms from beat to beat, and a sudden increase of the R – P′ interval occurs at beat 3, without any modification in the P′ pattern and the low to high right atrial spread of activation. This suggests that the nodal pathway with the shorter (though rather long) conduction time has also the longer refractory period. Conversely, the lower panel shows that the reverse phenomenon is observed only when the pacing cycle length is brought back to 770 ms. The difference between R2 – R3 intervals in both panels (160 ms) indicates the existence of a concealed conduction from the conductive pathway to the alternate one, analogous to what is observed in case of self-sustained functional bundle branch block.

Recording an even transient AV block in the course of a reciprocating tachycardia is certainly the best way to rule out the existence of bundle of Kent as part of the circuit. But it is rare indeed, in Wellens' experience [18] as in ours [3]. In addition, most often the block is distal to the His bundle, so that the possibility of a retrograde atrio-His bypass is not excluded but, on the contrary, in our opinion, suggested. In only two of our cases (case of Fig. 1 being one of them) and in three of Wellens' cases was the AV block proximal to the His bundle, proving undoubtedly the true intranodal location of the circuit.

Permanent Tachycardia

This form of tachycardia is rare, as we observed only 16 cases, half of them in children [1, 2]. It is characterized by a constant clinical pattern: an almost permanent supraventricular tachycardia, ending from time to time, particularly at rest, and starting again after the interposition of a few sinus beats [1 – 3]. The analysis of both pattern and timing of the P waves is very valuable in the diagnosis because of their constant characteristics: (1) P waves display the "classical" pattern of retrograde activation with negativity in leads II, III, and aVF. (2) They occur closer to the succeeding QRS than to the preceding one, but the apparent P – R interval is not necessarily short, as its absolute value depends on the cardiac rate (never less than 120 and up to 250/min). A rather characteristic feature is the abortive onset of tachycardia by an isolated atrial echo beat.

The triggering mechanism of this form of tachycardia is its most important characteristic, and the reason why it recurs so frequently, ending in a permanent tachycardia. Prolongation of the P – R interval is not required to initiate the tachycardia, suggesting that the speed of conduction is already slow enough to allow reentry in a potential pathway. Unidirectional block in the retrograde pathway is the only required condition, and this depends only on the cardiac rate, as shown in Figure 3. In the upper panel, the atrial pacing is progressively accelerated, with a cycle length gently reduced from 640 to 600 ms. A – H interval remains constant at 80 ms, particularly after the sixth stimulus after which occurs the first P′ wave of the tachycardia. The pattern of this first P′, and its time relationship with the following QRS is exactly the same as during the tachycardia, making it very difficult to interpret as an atrial premature beat because the phenomenon can be reproduced at will.

The critical value of the cycle length for the initiation of the tachycardia means that the unidirectional (anterograde) block of the retrograde pathway is present after every sinus beat and lasts just a few milliseconds more than 640 ms in this case. This rather long duration indicates that the unidirectional block is not related to the refractory period of this pathway for retrograde conduction, which is indeed normal permitting the reentry to occur.

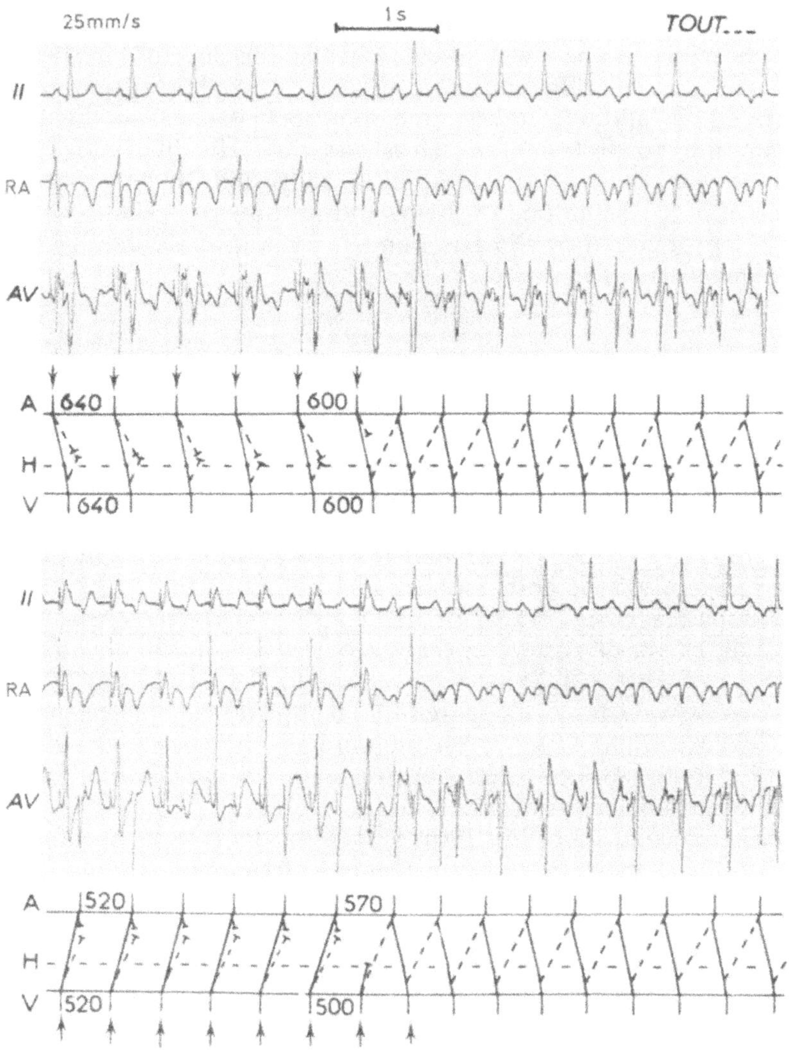

Fig. 3. Permanent AV nodal tachycardia.
Upper panel: Progressively accelerated atrial driving starts tachycardia as cycle reaches 600 ms, without prolongation of P-H or P-R, proving that triggering mechanism of tachycardia is occurrence of unidirectional block in retrograde pathway of circuit.
Lower panel: Tachycardia can be started also by progressive accleration of ventricular pacing. This time, the triggering mechanism is prolongation of retrograde VA conduction time (by 50 ms between first and the last driven beats).
See text for further explanation.

Studying the retrograde conduction (Fig. 3, lower panel) in this patient shows that a sudden increase in the retrograde conduction time triggers the tachycardia, in a way not so different from what happens in the paroxysmal forms mentioned above. The cycle length of the ventricular

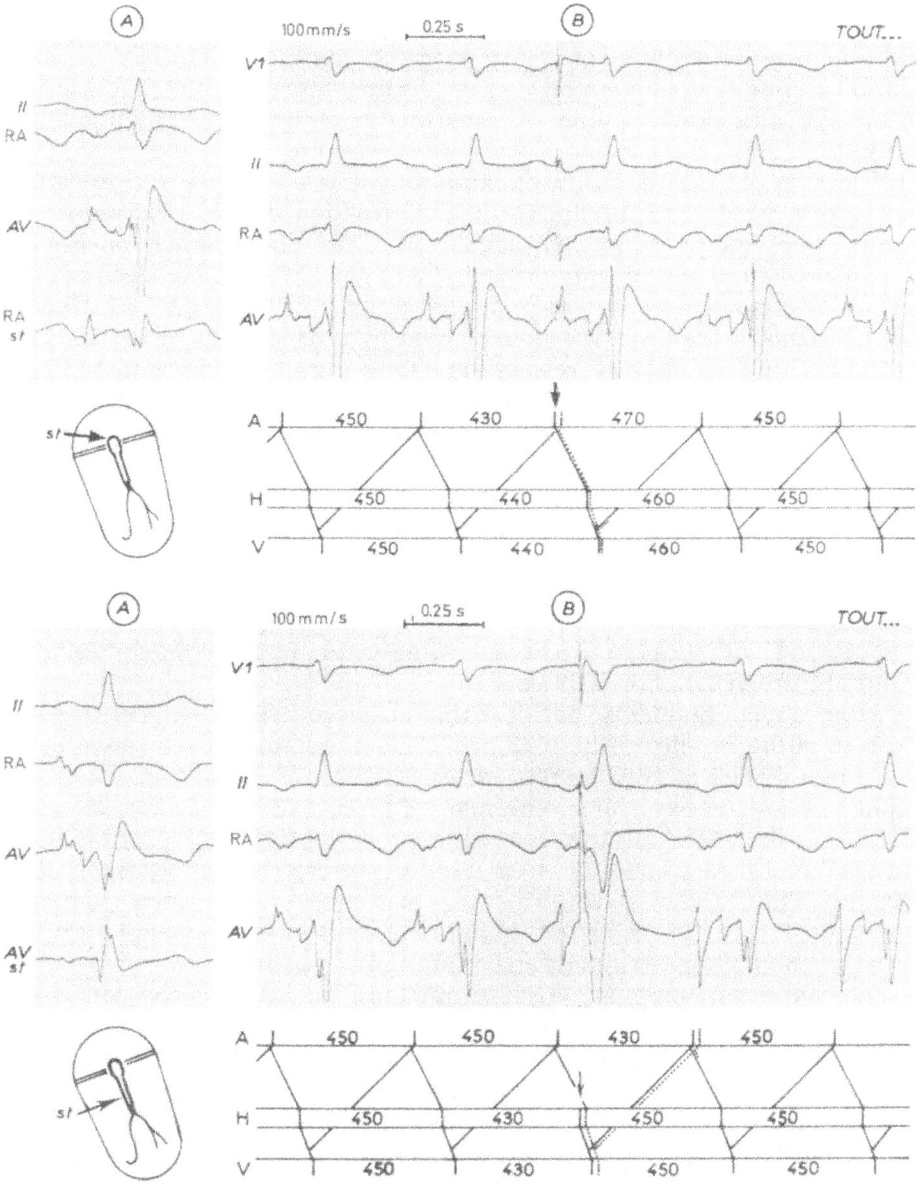

Fig. 4. Location of the upper and lower junctions of reentry circuit.
Above: In panel (A) electrogram (*RAst*) is recorded from pacing electrode, showing that first intrinsic deflexion of retrograde P′ wave of tachycardia occurs at AV junction. Stimulation given there (panel B) with a prematurity of 20 ms does produce a P wave identical to that of the tachycardia, but captures the His bundle and the ventricle by 10 ms (instead of 20). This difference favors an initial common pathway between the AV node and the atrium, as it proves that stimulation has been given outside the circuit.
Below: In panel (A) the electrogram (*AV st*) of His bundle pacing electrode is recorded. In (B) His bundle stimulation, premature by 20 ms captures both ventricle *and atrium* with the *same* prematurity, thus proving that stimulation has been given *within* the circuit and hence that lower junction is *distal* to His bundle.

pacing is gently reduced from 520 to 500 ms, and the retrograde conduction time increases after the 7th beat: then the third condition for reentry (slowed conduction) is met and it is not surprising to start the tachycardia, as the last atrial cycle length (570 ms) makes present the unidirectional block.

The very particular mode of initiation of this form of reciprocating tachycardia yields a means for further information on the location of the circuit. The first cycle of the tachycardia (in both panels of Fig. 3) is *shorter* than the following ones by 20 – 40 ms. The shortness of the first atrial cycle if present (which is often more difficult to decide than for the ventricular one) is obviously explained by a conduction speed in both pathways, anterograde and retrograde, faster during the first atrial cycle than during the following ones, according to the rate. But such an explanation cannot be applied to the first ventricular cycle, as the conduction velocity in the anterograde pathway between the first P′ and the following R has been necessarily slowed according to the prematurity of the first reentrant impulse. Therefore, the first R – R interval of the tachycardia should be longer than the first atrial one, and its paradoxically short duration cannot be explained other than by the the existence of an upper junction of the circuit situated *below* the atrium: thus the first ventricular cycle is shortened with respect to the following ones by the conduction time within the initial common pathway [2].

More direct arguments (but probably no more reliable) concerning the location of the circuit can be obtained from stimulation of various precise areas in the heart. The interest in these methods is that they can be applied in both paroxysmal and permanent forms of reciprocating tachycardia. Their limitation, as always, is due to the fact that only positive findings (exact or paradoxically premature captures) should be taken into account. Thus, Figure 4 confirms the existence of an initial common pathway in the case presented in Figure 3, and gives some light on the lower junction of the circuit and the final common pathway.

In Figure 4 (*above*), an atrial stimulation is given in the low right atrium thanks to the catheter located at the AV junction. The stimulation is thus delivered in the area where atrial depolarization is first recorded during the tachycardia. In addition, the stimulation is given very late in the cardiac cycle to avoid as much as possible any prolongation of the conduction time according to the prematurity. In spite of these conditions, Figure 4 (*above*) shows that it is not possible to obtain a His bundle and a ventricular capture having the same prematurity (20 ms) than the stimulation: the timing of H and R waves following the stimulation is 10 ms longer. This fact leads to the conclusion that the stimulation has not been given within the circuit, but *outside,* and that it is separated from the atrium by the final common pathway.

On the other hand, Figure 4 *(below)* shows that stimulating the His bundle can obtain an "exact" ventricular and atrial capture, i.e., a capture having the same prematurity as the His bundle stimulus (20 ms). This means that the stimulation has been given *inside* the circuit, i.e., *above* or at least at the level of the lower junction. This fact implies that this lower junction cannot be considered as strictly intranodal, and that the longitudinal dissociation might well concern also the His bundle itself.

Another way to prove that the lower junction of the reentry circuit is situated below the AV node, i.e., within the His bundle or even in the ventricle is to stimulate they very upper part of the interventricular septum [3]. If it appears possible to capture the atrium by a ventricular stimulation given late in the cardiac cycle, when the His bundle is refractory, then the takeoff of the retrograde pathway can be considered as certainly extra nodal.

III. Conclusion

The diagnosis of intranodal reciprocating tachycardia should be made step by step, because it relies upon negative and positive arguments. Negative arguments are only suggestive of an intranodal reentry circuit, while positive ones can confirm the diagnosis.

Negative arguments are mainly intended to eliminate as carefully as possible the possibility of an extranodal accessory pathway. The problem is that a negative argument can be due either to the absence of an important sign or to an incomplete or even incorrect exploration:

1. The absence of a pre-excitation pattern is obviously the weakest argument in favor of the intranodal location of a circus movement. Even its presence does not prove for some authors [17, 19] that the circus movement involves indeed the accessory pathway, though in our experience we have no proof of such a possibility, and some published cases can be challenged.
2. The absence of the following signs is obviously necessary to the diagnosis of intranodal reciprocation; their presence can be considered as pathognomonic of a WPW syndrome:

2.1. A short and all-or-none retrograde conduction.

2.2. The existence of paradoxically premature atrial captures by ventricular stimulation [1 – 3].

2.3. Influence of functional bundle branch block on the rate of the tachycardia: The absence of this sign does eliminate the possibility of a Kent bundle located laterally on the same side as the bundle branch block, but it does not rule out a controlateral or a septal accessory pathway [4, 8, 15].

2.4. A first retrograde atrial depolarization during reciprocating tachycardia recorded elsewhere than in the His bundle recording electrode: of course neither does this sign eliminate the possibility of a septal preexcitation.

Some positive signs allow us to rule out accurately the possibility of a Kent bundle as a part of the circuit:

1. An even transient AV block, provided its proximal location be proved by the His bundle electrogram.
2. The variability of the relationships between P' and R during the tachycardia, whatever its cause, overall if it does not influence the rate of the tachycardia.
3. A retrograde VA conduction having the characters of the conduction through the AV node, particularly the type I 2nd degree AV block.

If one takes into account both negative and positive signs in favor of true intranodal reentry, this diagnosis becomes much less frequent than commonly admitted. On the other hand, the permanent form of the tachycardia becomes not so rare with respect to the paroxysmal one.

Summary

Stimulation techniques have demonstrated a reciprocating mechanism in all junctional tachycardias, a term which should be preferred to AV nodal tachycardias. Three conditions are required for the creation of a circus movement: a potential circuit pathway, unidirectional block in this circuit, and slowed conduction. While all three conditions are readily apparent in reciprocating tachycardias of the WPW syndrome, two or even all of these factors may be concealed in the other forms.

Paroxysmal reciprocating tachycardias are characterized by prolongation of the P – R interval in the beat immediately preceding the tachycardia, and are generally accepted as being related to longitudinal dissociation of the AV node, though the possibility of unidirectional (anterograde) block of an extranodal accessory pathway should be appreciated. Precise technique for localizing the lower junction of the reentry circuit shows that in most cases where the retrograde P′ waves occur after QRS a unidirectionally-blocked AV accessory pathway is present. Even in cases where P′ and R waves are superimposed, the circuit cannot be considered in many cases as strictly intranodal: either a dissociation of the His bundle itself, or the presence of an atrio-His accessory pathway should be suspected.

The same situation is met in the permanent form of reciprocating tachycardia. Though rare in adults, chronic reciprocating tachycardia is in children the underlying mechanism of about one-third of idiopathic chronic supraventricular tachycardias. The 16 cases studied have in common [1] a tachycardia usually permanent (130 – 250/min) or rapidly recurring after a few sinus beats, [2] a 1/1 AV ratio with P′ – R intervals always shorter than R – P′, and typical retrograde P′ waves, [3] an initiation of the tachycardia without prolongation of P – R but provoked by the shortening of the atrial period, [4] termination always possible by stimulating the atrium and/or the ventricle, and prevention always possible by driving both of them simultaneously.

References

1. Coumel, Ph.: Junctional reciprocating tachycardias. The permanent and paroxysmal forms of A-V nodal reciprocating tachycardias. J. Electrocardiol. **8,** 79 – 90 (1975)
2. Coumel, Ph.: Supraventricular tachycardias. In: Cardiac Arrhythmias. The Modern Electrophysiological Approach. Krikler, D. M., Goodwin, J. F. (eds.), London: W. B. Saunders, 1975, pp. 116 – 143
3. Coumel, Ph.: Les tachycardies jonctionelles paroxystiques. Evaluation du point de jonction inférieur du circuit de réentrée. Démembrement des soi-disant rythmes réciproques intra-nodaux. Arch. Coeur **68,** 1255 – 1268 (1975)
4. Coumel, Ph., Attuel, P.: Reciprocating tachycardia in overt and latent pre-excitation. Influence of functional bundle branch block on the rate of the tachycardia. Europ. J. Cardio. **1,** 423 – 436 (1974)
5. Coumel, Ph., Barold, S. S.: Mechanisms of supraventricular tachycardia. In: His Bundle Electrocardiography and Clinical Electrophysiology. Narula O. S. (ed.), Philadelphia: F. A. Davis, 1975, pp. 203 – 241
6. De la Fuente, D., Sasyniuk, B., Moe, G. K.: Conduction through a narrow isthmus in isolated canine atrial tissue. A model of the W. P. W. Circulation **46,** 803 – 809 (1971)
7. Denes, P., Wu, D., Dhingra, R., Chuquimia, R., Rosen, K. M.: Demonstration of dual A-V nodal pathways with paroxysmal supraventricular tachycardias. Circulation **48,** 549 –555 (1973)
8. Gallagher, J. J., Gilbert, M., Svenson, R. H., Sealy, W. C., Kasell, J., Wallace, A. G.: Wolff-Parkinson-White syndrome. The problem, evaluation and surgical correction. Circulation **51,** 767 – (1975)
9. Goldreyer, B. N., Damato, A. N.: The essential role of A-V conduction delay in the initiation of paroxysmal supraventricular tachycardia in man. Circulation **43,** 679 – 687 (1971)
10. Janse, M. J., Van Capelle, M. J. L., Freud, G. E., Durrer, D.: Circus movement within the A-V node as a basis for supraventricular tachydardia as shown by multiple microelectrode recording in the isolated rabbit heart. Circulat. Res. **28,** 403 – 414 (1971)
11. Moe, G. K., Mendez, C.: Physiological basis of reciprocal rhythm. Progr. Cardiovasc. Dis. **8,** 461 – 481 (1966)
12. Narula, O. S.: Retrograde “pre-excitation”: comparison of antegrade and retrograde conduction intervals in man. Circulation **50,** 1129 – 1143 (1974)
13. Neuss, H., Schlepper, M., Thormann, J.: Analysis of reentry mechanism in three patients with concealed Wolff-Parkinson-White syndrome. Circulation **51,** 75 – 81 (1975)
14. Spurrell, R. A. J., Krikler, D. M., Sowton, E.: Effects of verapamil on electrophysiological properties of anomalous atrio-ventricular connection in Wolff-Parkinson-White syndrome. Brit. Heart, J. **36,** 256 – 262 (1974).
15. Spurrell, R. A. J., Krikler, D. M., Sowton, E.: Retrograde invasion of the bundle branches producing aberration of the QRS complexes during supraventricular tachycardia studied by programmed electrical stimulation. Circulation **50,** 487 – 495 (1974)
16. Svenson, R. H., Miller, H. C., Gallagher, J. J., Wallace, A. G.: Electrophysiological evaluation of the Wolff-Parkinson-White syndrome. Problems in assessing antegrade and retrograde conduction over the accessory pathway. Circulation **52,** 552 – 562 (1975)
17. Wellens, H. J. J., Durrer, D.: Patterns of ventriculo-atrial conduction in the Wolff-Parkinson-White syndrome. Circulation **49,** 22 – 31 (1974)
18. Wellens, H. J. J., Durrer, D.: The role of an accessory atrio-ventricular pathway in reciprocal tachycardia. Observations in patients with and without the Wolff-Parkinson-White syndrome. Circulation **52,** 58 – 72 (1975)
19. Zipes, D. P., De Joseph, R. L., Rothbaum, D. A.: Unusual properties of accessory pathways. Circulation **49,** 1200 – 1211 (1974)

Drug Effects on AV Conduction

H. NEUSS, H.-J. SCHAUMANN, and B. STEGARU

I. Drug Effects on the Normal AV Conduction System

On Methods

In recent years His bundle electrography has proved to be a valuable method for analysis of conduction disorders. In addition, drug effects on AV conduction and the preferential site of drug action can be evaluated with this method. Its accuracy, however, is limited. Pharmacologically induced changes of the conduction intervals must exceed at least 5 or 10 ms for reliable measurement at a recording paper speed of 100 mm/s (0.5 – 1 mm). Therefore, 10 or even 20% changes of the P – A and H – R intervals (normal values about 30 and 40 ms, respectively) may excape recognition.

In contrast to this, evaluation of drug effects on AV nodal conduction — as represented by the A – H interval — seems to be an easier task. Atrial pacing can reveal a negative dromotropic effect on AV nodal conduction that is not evident at sinus rhythm. A more pronounced increase in the A – H interval and the earlier occurrence of 2nd degree AV block at frequency stress are the definite parameters.

The determination of refractory periods of the AV conduction system (AVCS) according to Wit et al. [46] is a complementary procedure for the evaluation of drug effects. By applying the extrastimulus method it is possible to elicit conduction disorders due to incomplete recovery at different levels of the AVCS. As the refractory periods of the AVCS are a function of the heart rate, pharmacologically induced changes can only be identified if refractory periods are determined at identical heart rates.

In a recent paper [26] we have pointed out a methodical problem: A marked prolongation of the functional refractory period of the AV node (FRP AVN) by a drug may prevent determination of refractory periods of the His-Purkinje system (HPS). This is demonstrated in Figure 1: In a 56-year-old female patient with a history of paroxysmal tachycardias refractory periods of the AVCS were determined at a basic heart rate of 120/min ($S_1S_1 = 500$ ms). From left to right the coupling intervals of premature atrial depolarizations (PAD) were shortened successively. In the control period (upper panel) FRP AVN (shortest possible H_1H_2 interval) measured 370 ms, and the effective refractory period of the AV node (ERP AVN) was reached at an A_1A_2 interval of 250 ms. No conduction disturbances within the HPS were noticed.

Atropine (0.5 mg i.v.) shortened the FRP AVN to 300 ms (middle panel). At an H_1H_2 interval of 310 ms full recovery time of the right bundle

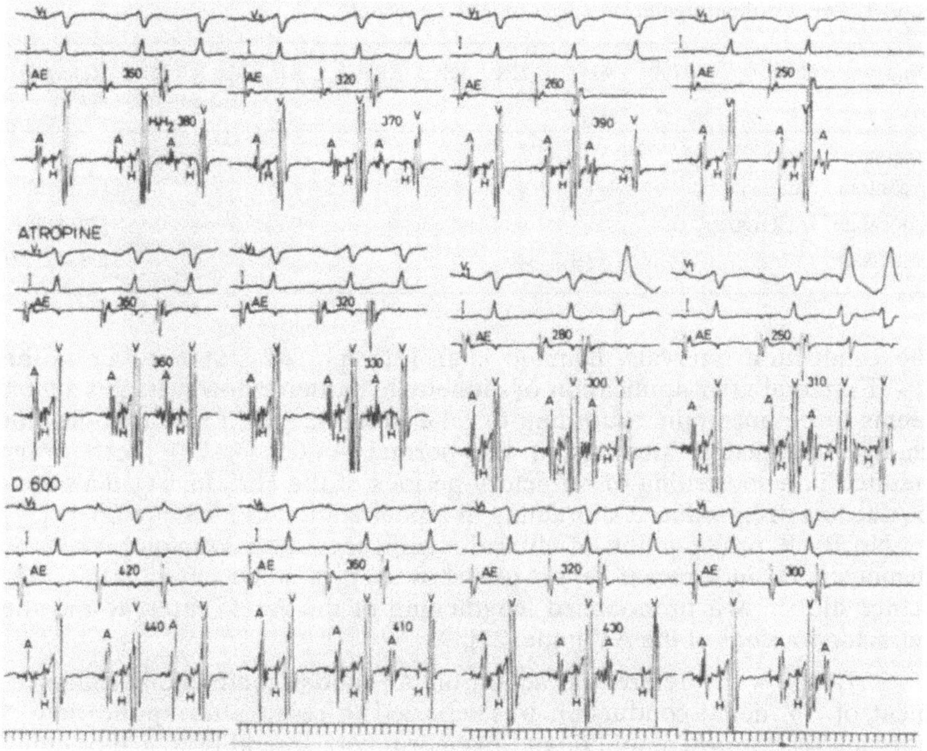

Fig. 1. ECG (lead I, V_1), atrial electrogram (*AE*), and His bundle electrogram in 56-year-old patient. Basic heart rate: 120/min (S_1S_2 : 500 ms). Paper speed: 100 mm/s. *A*: atrial potentials; *H*: His bundle potentials; *V*: ventricular potentials. *Left to right:* decreasing coupling intervals of test stimuli (S_2). Coupling intervals (S_1S_2) are given in ms above the AE, and the resulting H_1H_2 intervals are listed above the His bundle electrogram. *Upper panel:* control; *middle panel:* after administration of 0,5 mg atropine; *lower panel:* after administration of 2 mg D 600.

branch was reached, and right bundle branch block patterns became apparent.

Application of 2 mg D 600 (lower panel) prolonged the FRP AVN to 410 ms and ERP AVN to 310 ms. At the shortest possible H_1H_2 interval of 410 ms conduction in the HPS was undisturbed. Due to enhancement of AV nodal conduction, atropine unmasked conduction disturbances in the HPS, while D 600 had the opposite effect.

Results

The results of His bundle studies dealing with the effects of antiarrhythmic drugs on AV conduction allow a classification in three different groups.

1. Drugs without marked effects on AV conduction: The potent antiarrhythmic drugs — as listed in Table 1 — produce no significant effects on

Table 1. Drugs without significant effects on AV conduction

Drug	Dose	PA	AH	HR	QRS	ERP A	RP AVN	RP HPS	References
Diphenyl-hydantoin	5 mg/kg	Φ	– (?)	Φ	Φ	?	Φ	–	[7, 10, 6]
Lidocaine	1 – 2 mg/kg	?	Φ	Φ	Φ	Φ	Φ	–	[29, 4, 16]
Practolol	15 mg	Φ	Φ (+)	Φ	Φ	?	(+)	?	[38, 42, 27]

the conduction intervals. Damato et al. [7] reported a shortening of the P – H interval after application of diphenylhydantoin; however, this action seems to be uncertain, according to other authors [10]. Lidocaine did not change conduction intervals in the normal AVCS [4, 29]. Both drugs resulted in a shortening of refractory periods of the HPS [6, 14]. This may be due to a drug-induced shortening of repolarization in Purkinje fibers [37].

No P – R prolongation of clinical significance after Practolol could be demonstrated in a recent report [42]; however, in some patients this substance did show a pronounced lengthening of the A – H interval and the refractory periods of the AV node [27].

2. Drugs with preferential action on AV nodal conduction: Enhancement of AV nodal conduction was reported to result after application of atropine [1], isoproterenol [9], and oxyfedrin [24]. In addition, a shortening of the H – R interval was observed after administration of isoproterenol [9]. Atropine and isoproterenol led to a shortening of AV nodal refractory periods [1, 9]. While the enhancement of AV nodal conduction is easily explained by the anticholinergic action of the first and the adrenergic stimulation of the second and the third drugs, it is debatable whether the negative dromotropic effects of the three agents — listed in Table 2 — on

Table 2. Drugs with preferential action on AV nodal conduction

Drug	Dose	PA	AH	HR	QRS	ERP A	RP AVN	RP HPS	References
Atropine	0,5 mg	Φ	–	Φ	Φ	Φ	–	Φ	[1]
Isopro-terenol	0,2 mg in 200 ml	Φ	–	Φ	Φ	Φ	– Φ	Φ	[9]
Oxyfedrin	8 mg	Φ	–	Φ	Φ	?	?	?	[24]
Propra-nolol	0.1 mg/kg	?	+	Φ	Φ	?	?	?	[5]
Pindolol	0.5 mg	Φ	+	Φ	Φ	?	?	?	[21]
Ox-prenolol	4 mg	Φ	+	Φ	Φ	Φ	+	Φ	[27]
Verapamil	10 mg	Φ	+	Φ	Φ	?	?	?	[19, 10, 13]
D 600	2 mg	Φ	+	Φ	Φ	Φ	+	Φ	[34]
Digoxin	0.75 mg	?	+	Φ	Φ	?	+	Φ	[28]

AV nodal conduction are only due to their specific antiadrenergic action. These drugs resulted in a marked increase of A – H intervals. Second degree AV block occurred at a significantly lower basic cycle length and — as demonstrated in a yet unpublished study on the effects of oxprenolol [27] — the refractory periods of the AV node were distinctly prolonged. This is demonstrated in Figures 2 and 3. At a basic cycle length of 400 ms (heart rate = 150/min) FRP AVN was found to be 320 ms. ERP AVN could not be measured because it was shorter than the shortest possible A_1A_2 interval (FRP A) (Fig. 2). After i.v. application of 4 mg oxprenolol FRP AVN is prolonged to 350 ms and ERP AVN to 260 ms (Fig. 3).

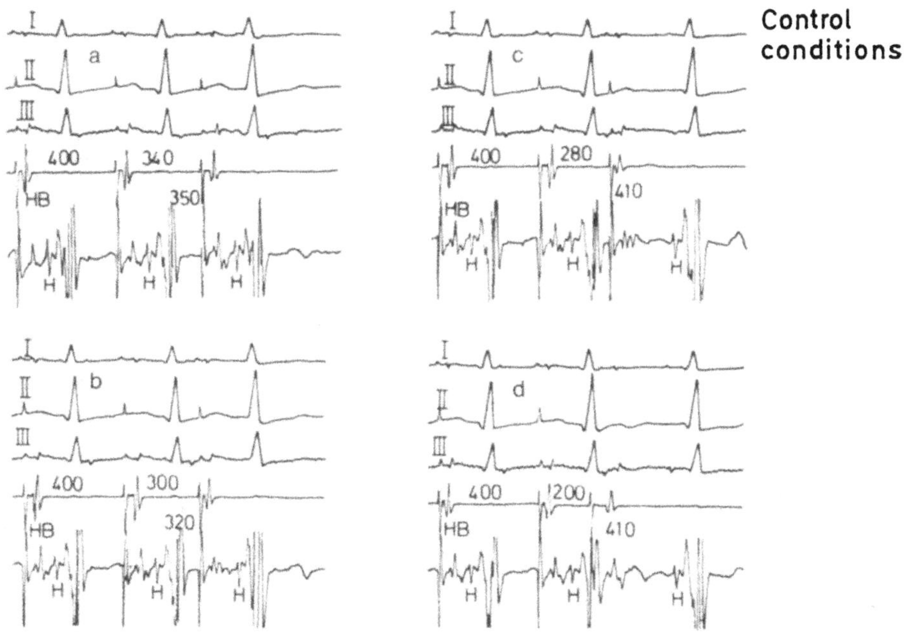

Fig. 2. ECG (lead I, II, III), atrial electrogram, and His bundle electrogram (*HB*) in a 34-year-old patient. Control conditions. Basic heart rate 150/min (S_1S_1 = 400 ms). A_1H_1 about 65 ms. FRP AVN is given at H_1H_2 interval of 320 ms (panel b). ERP of AV conduction is determined by the ERP A (panel d).

The negative dromotropic effect of verapamil on AV conduction is the established therapeutic principle in reducing ventricular rate during episodes of atrial tachycardias such as atrial flutter and fibrillation. The preferential site of action of verapamil was found to be the AV node [10, 13, 19]. Another compound with calcium antagonistic properties had a selectively depressant effect on AV nodal conduction [34]. The question that remains to be resolved is whether the inhibition of the inward calcium current in the heart by verapamil and D 600 is relevant to the antiarrhythmic action of these drugs.

Table 3. Drugs with preferential action on His-Purkinje system

Drug	Dose	PA	AH	HR	QRS	ERP A	RP AVN	RP HPS	References
Ajmaline	100 mg	+	+	+	+	Φ	+	–	[20, 10]
Aprindine	2 mg/kg	+	+	+	+	Φ	+	Φ	[34, 17, 35]
Quinidine	600 – 800 mg i.m.	?	–	+	+	+	–	+	[15]
Disopyramide	2 mg/kg	Φ	+	+	+	+	+	Φ	[3, 36]
Procainamide	500 mg	?	(+)	+	Φ	+	–	+	[16]
Propafenone	2 mg/kg	+	+	+	+	+	+	?	[2, 36, 27]

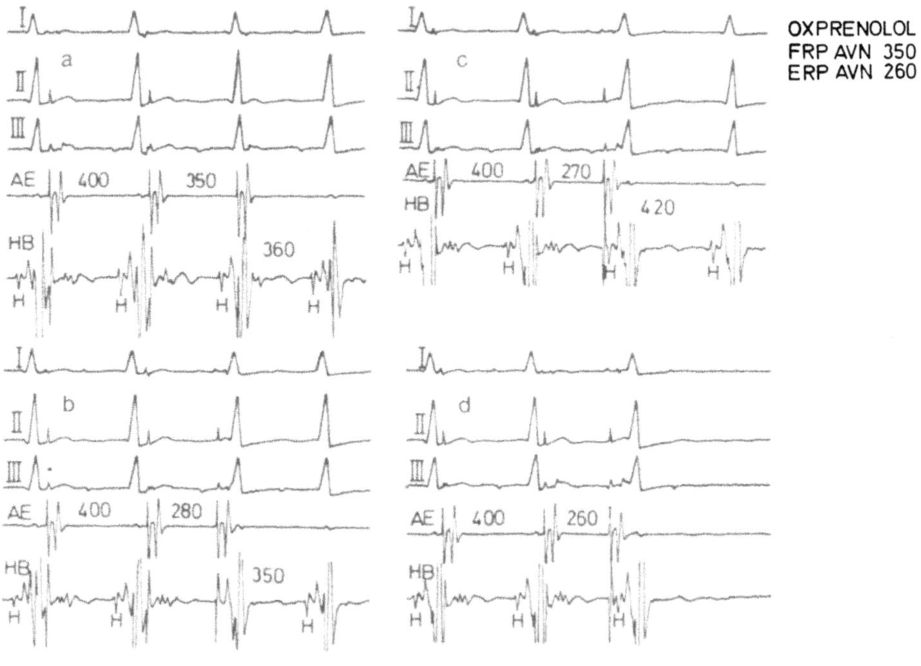

Fig. 3. ECG (lead I, II, III), atrial electrogram (*AE*), and His bundle electrogram (*HB*). Same patient as in Fig. 2. After administration of 4 mg oxyprenolol i.v. A_1H_1 is prolonged to 275 ms. FRP AVN is given at an H_1H_2 interval of 350 ms (panel b). ERP of AV conduction is determined by ERP AVN = 260 ms (panel d).

3. Drugs with preferential action on the HPS: The drugs listed in Table 3 hold in common a distinct prolongation of the H – R interval. With the exception of procainamide [16, 33] these drugs resulted in a broadening

of QRS. In comparison to group 2 the effects on AV nodal conduction are less pronounced. In contrast to its depressant effects on intraventricular conduction, quinidine exhibits an enhancement of AV nodal conduction [15]. The latter is thought to be due to its anticholinergic action. Ajmaline [10, 20], aprindine [17, 34, 35], and propafenone [2, 22, 36] depressed intra-atrial conduction (as represented by the P – A interval) and prolonged ERP A. A prolongation of AV nodal refractory periods was established for ajmaline [20], aprindine [34], disopyramide [36] and propafenone [22, 36]. Refractory periods of the HPS were significantly prolonged by quinidine [15] and procainamide [16].

Since the methods applied are restricted to phenomena of AV conduction the results will not provide us with a differentiated insight into the mode of antiarrhythmic drug action. It would be presumptuous to derive therapeutic recommendations from these data. This is at best possible for drugs whose negative dromotropic effects on AV nodal conduction may be used for termination of reentry tachycardias confined to the AV junction or for reduction of ventricular rate in atrial tachycardias.

II. Drug Effects on Conductivity in the Diseased AVCS

Data on drug effects on the diseased AVCS are of considerable practical importance. These findings are of value for the diagnosis of latent conduction disorders and their use in prognosis. As reported by Guérot et al. [11] a paroxysmal bundle branch block can be provoked by the application of ajmaline. Drug studies in patients with rate dependent left bundle branch block [23] emphasize these findings. The provocation of a latent conduction disorder in the right bundle branch by ajmaline is demonstrated in Figure 4. In a 17-year-old patient with a small ventricular septal defect ajmaline changed incomplete right bundle branch block patterns to complete right bundle branch block. The rate-dependency of this pattern is inconsistent with the normal behavior of conduction in the HPS, and this most likely unmasks a pathologic substrate. Analogous to this, latent conduction defects in the HPS may be uncovered, and already apparent conduction defects may be aggravated by lidocaine [12] and amiodarone [32]. The diagnostic value of these drug effects in the evaluation of patients with the risk of heart block in the HPS remains to be established. However, these findings provide us with important data for contraindications to antiarrhythmic therapy.

As recently proposed by Rosenbaum [31] analysis of drug effects on the diseased AVCS provides us with an important clinical model for the study of antiarrhythmic compounds. It is likely that drug effects on depressed AV conduction differ considerably from effects on the normal AVCS. These effects may represent a most important therapeutic principle, as a number of ventricular arrhythmias are possibly due to depressed conduction in the HPS [47].

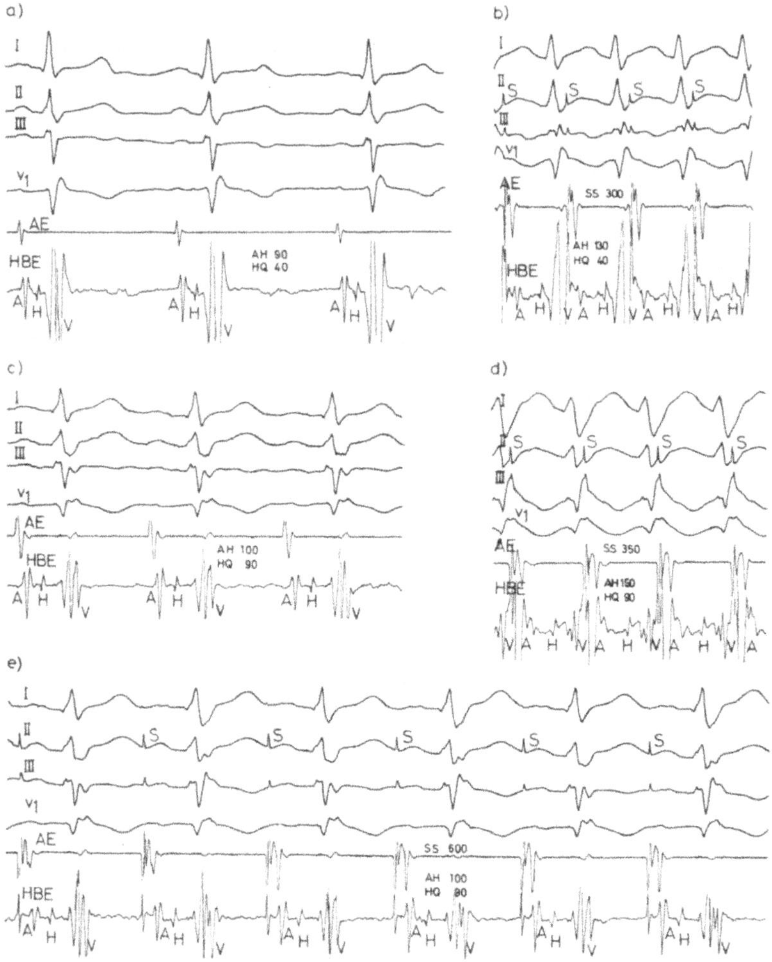

Fig. 4. ECG (lead I, II, III, V_1), atrial electrogram (*AE*), and His bundle electrogram (*HBE*) in a 17-year-old female patient (panel a, b). Control period, normal conduction intervals, and patterns of incomplete right bundle branch block. At atrial pacing there was 1 : 1 AV conduction up to a rate of 200/min without significant changes in QRS configuration. After application of 50 mg ajmaline there is prolongation of H – Q (90 ms) and increase in right bundle branch block patterns (panel c). At pacing stress there was a rate-dependent further increase of conduction delay in right ventricle (panel d, and e).

III. Drug Effects in the Evaluation of Supraventricular Reentry Tachycardias

Different drug action on the normal AVCS and on accessory AV connections has to be considered in patients with paroxysmal supraventricular tachycardias. Selective blockade of the accessory pathway could be achieved by ajmaline, quinidine, procainamide [44, 45], amiodarone [32], and aprindine [21, 25] in patients with the patterns of Kent bundle conduction. Supraventricular reentry tachycardias were terminated by block of accessory VA conduction. Contrary to this, verapamil [41] and digoxin [43] were efficacious through their depressant action on AV nodal conduction.

Recently Spurrell et al. [41] suggested that accessory paranodal bypass fibers may be identified by pharmacologic intervention. In some of their patients verapamil did not result in a prolongation of the H – A′ interval during supraventricular tachycardia and retrograde conduction time during ventricular pacing. This seems to be an argument for VA conduction via a paranodal bypass. In a study on the effects of propafenone in patients with AV junctional tachycardias [22] we found that this drug reliably terminated the paroxysms by blockade of VA conduction. Since VA conduction time did show a negligible increase at pacing stress and VA block was of Mobitz type II, we feel reasonably safe in dealing with accessory VA conduction via a paranodal bypass that could be selectively blocked by propafenone.

Summary

His bundle electrography combined with programmed atrial and ventricular pacing has proved to be a valuable procedure in the clinical evaluation of drug effects on AV conduction. The following points are stressed:

1. Conduction velocity can be affected by different drugs at different levels of the AV conduction system in normal subjects. The findings provide evidence regarding the preferential site of action of antiarrhythmic drugs. Additional information may be gained by determination of refractory periods of the AV conduction system.

2. Drug effects on AV conduction may differ in respect to quantity or quality under pathologic conditions. Evaluation of these often unwanted side-effects in patients with latent defects of AV conduction may provide us with a better understanding of indications and contraindications of antiarrhythmic therapy.

3. Drug effects in arrhythmias due to conduction disorders are analyzed. The results provide us with a better insight into the involved pathophysiologic conditions and an approach to a more rational therapy.

References

1. Akhtar, M., Damato, A. N., Caracta, A. R., Batsford, W. P., Josephson, M. E., Lau, S. H.: Electrophysiologic effects of atropine on atrioventricular conduction studied by His bundle electrogram. Amer. J. Cardiol. **33**, 333 – 343 (1974)
2. Beck, O. A., Witt, E., Hochrein, H.: Der Einfluß des Antiarrhythmikums Propafenon auf die intrakardiale Erregungsleitung. Klinische Untersuchungen mit Hilfe der His-Bündel-Elektrographie. Z. Kardiol. **64**, 179 – 187 (1975)
3. Befeler, B., Castellanos jr., A., Wells, D. E., Celeste Vagueiro, M., Yeh, B. K.: Electrophysiologic effects of the antiarrhythmic agent disopyramide phosphate. Amer. J. Cardiol. **35**, 282 – 287 (1975)

4. Bekheit, S., Murtagh, J. G., Morton, P., Fletcher, E.: Effect of lignocaine on conducting system of human heart.Brit. Heart J. **35**, 305 – 311 (1973)
5. Berkowitz, W. D., Wit, A. L., Lau, S. H., Steiner, Ch., Damato, A. N.: The effects of propranolol on cardiac conduction. Circulation **40**, 855 – 862 (1969)
6. Bisset, J. K., De Soyza, N. D. B., Kane, J. J., Murphy, M. L.: Improved intraventricular conduction of premature beats after diphenylhydantoin. Amer. J. Cardiol. **33**, 493 – 497 (1974)
7. Damato, A. N., Berkowitz, W. D., Patton, R. D., Lau, S. H.: The effect of diphenylhydantoin on atrioventricular and intraventricular conduction in man. Amer. Heart J. **79**, 51 – 56 (1970)
8. Denes, P., Wu, D., Dhingra, R., Pietras, R. J., Rosen, K. M.: The effects of cycle length on cardiac refractory periods in man. Circulation **49**, 32 – 41 (1974)
9. Dhingra, R. C., Winslow, E., Pouget, J. M., Rahimtoola, S. H., Rosen, K. M.: The effect of isoproterenol on atrioventricular and intraventricular conduction. Amer. J. Cardiol. **32**, 629 – 636 (1973)
10. Gleichmann, U., Seipel, J., Loogen, F.: Der Einfluß von Antiarrhythmika auf die intrakardiale Erregungsleitung (His-Bündel-Elektrographie) und Sinusknotenautomatie beim Menschen. Dtsch. med. Wschr. **98**, 1487 – 1994 (1973)
11. Guérot, C., Coste, A., Valère, P. E., Tricot, R.: L'épreuve à l'Ajmaline dans le diagnostic du bloc auriculo-ventriculaire paroxystique. Arch. Mal. Coeur **66**, 1241 – 1253 (1973)
12. Gupta, P. K., Lichstein, E., Chadda, K. D: Lidocaine-Induced heart block in patients with bundle branch block. Amer. J. Cardiol. **33**, 487 – 492 (1974)
13. Husaini, M. H., Kvasnicka, J., Rydén, L., Holmberg, S.: Action of verapamil on sinus node, atrioventricular, and intraventricular conduction. Brit. Heart J. **35**, 734 – 737 (1973)
14. Josephson, M. E., Caracta, A. R., Lau, S. H., Gallagher, J. J., Damato, A. N.: Effects of lidocaine on refractory periods in man. Amer. Heart J. **84**, 778 – 786 (1972)
15. Josephson, M. E., Seides, S. F., Batsford, W. P., Weisfogel, G. M., Akhtar, M., Caracta, A. R., Lau, S. H., Damato, A. N.: The electrophysiological effects of intramuscular quinidine on the atrioventricular conducting system in man. Amer. Heart J. **87**, 55 – 64 (1974)
16. Josephson, M. E., Caracta, A. R., Ricciutti, M. A., Lau, S. H., Damato, A. N.: Electrophysiologic properties of procainamide in man. Amer. J. Cardiol. **33**, 596 – 603 (1974)
17. Kulbertus, H., Collignon, P.: Action des antiarythmiques sur la conduction intracardiaque. Acta cardiol. (Brux.) Suppl. **18**, 241 – 250 (1974)
18. Lichstein, E., Chadda, K. D., Gupta, P. K.: Atrioventricular Block with Lidocaine therapy. Amer. J. Cardiol. **31**, 277 – 281 (1973)
19. Neuss, H., Schlepper, M.: Der Einfluß von Verapamil auf die atrio-ventrikuläre Überleitung. Lokalisation des Wirkungsortes mit His-Bündel-Elektrogrammen. Verh. dtsch. Ges. Kreisl.-Forsch. **37**, 433 – 438 (1971)
20. Neuss, H., Schlepper, M.: Die Aussagefähigkeit verschiedener Stimulationsverfahren bei Untersuchungen über die AV-Überleitung – dargestellt an der Einwirkung von Ajmalin. Verh. dtsch. Ges. Kreisl.-Forsch. **39**, 222 – 227 (1973)
21. Neuss, H., Schlepper, M.: Influence of various antiarrhythmic drugs (aprindine, ajmaline, verapamil, oxprenolol, orciprenaline) on functional properties of accessory A – V pathways. Acta cardiol. (Brux.) Suppl. **18**, 279 – 288 (1974)
22. Neuss, H., Schlepper, M.: Propafenone in patients with paroxysmal supraventricular tachycardias. In preparation
23. Neuss, H., Schlepper, M., Thormann, J.: Klinisch-experimentelle Befunde bei frequenzabhängigem Linksschenkelblock. Verh. dtsch. Ges. Kreisl.-Forsch. **40**, 402 – 405 (1974)
24. Neuss, H., Nowak, F. G., Schlepper, M., Wüsten, B.: The effects of anti-anginal drugs on AV-conduction in normal subjects. Arzneimittel-Forsch. (Drug Res.) **24**, 213 – 216 (1974)
25. Neuss, H., Schulze, V., Schlepper, M.: Beeinflussung der Leitungseigenschaften akzessorischer AV-Verbindungen durch Aprindin. Herz/Kreisl. **6**, 476 – 484 (1974)
26. Neuss, H., Spies, H. F., Schlepper, M.: Beeinflussung der Refraktärzeiten in den einzelnen Abschnitten des Reizleitungssystems durch Antiarrhythmika. In: Symposion über His-Bündel-Elektrographie. Stuttgart: Schattauer Verlag, 1975, p. 207
27. Neuss, H., Thormann, J.: Unpublished data

28. Przybyla, A. C., Paulay, K. L., Stein, E., Damato, A. N.: Effects of Digoxin on Atrioventricular conduction patterns in man. Amer. J. Cardiol. **33**, 344 – 350 (1974)
29. Rosen, K. M., Lau, S. H., Weiss, M. B., Damato, A. N.: The effect of lidocaine on atrioventricular and intraventricular conduction in man. Amer. J. Cardiol. **25**, 1 – 5 (1970)
30. Rosen, K. M., Barwolf, Ch., Ehsani, A., Rahimtoola, S. H.: Effects of lidocaine and propranolol on the normal and abnomalous pathways in patients with preexcitation. Amer. J. Cardiol. **30**, 801 – 809 (1972)
31. Rosenbaum, M. B.: A new clinical and experimental model for studying the effects of antiarrhythmic drugs upon automaticity and conduction. Acta cardiol. (Brux.) Suppl. **18**, 289 – 296 (1974)
32. Rosenbaum, M. B., Chiale, P. A., Ryba, D., Elizari, M. V.: Control of tachyarrhythmias associated with Wolff-Parkinson-White syndrome by amiodarone hydrochloride. Amer. J. Cardiol. **34**, 215 – 223 (1974)
33. Scheinman, M. M., Weiss, A. N., Shafton, E., Benowitz, N., Rowland, M.: Electrophysiologic effects of procaine amide in patients with intraventricular conduction delay. Circulation **49**, 522 – 529 (1974)
34. Schlepper, M., Neuss, H.: Changes of refractory periods in the A – V conduction system induced by antiarrhythmic drugs. A study using His bundle recordings. Acta cardiol. (Brux.) Suppl. **18**, 269 – 277 (1974)
35. Seipel, L., Gleichmann, U.: Die Wirkung des Antiarrhythmikums Aprindin (AC 1802) auf Erregungsleitung und Spontanautomatie des menschlichen Herzens. Z. Kardiol. **63**, 426 – 434 (1974)
36. Seipel, L., Breithardt, G., Both, A.: Elektrophysiologische Effekte der Antiarrhythmika Disopyramid und Propafenon auf das menschliche Reizleitungssystem. Z. Kardiol **64**, 731 – 740 (1975)
37. Singh, B. N., Hauswirth, O.: Comparative mechanisms of action of antiarrhythmic drugs. Amer. Heart J. **87**, 367 – 382 (1974)
38. Smithen, Ch. S., Balcon, R., Sowton, E.: Use of bundle of His potentials to assess changes in atrioventricular conduction produced by a series of beta-adrenergic blocking agents. Brit. Heart J. **33**, 955 – 961 (1971)
39. Spies, H. F., Neuss, H.: Funktionsdiagnostik der AV-Überleitung bei Schenkelblock. Herz/Kreisl. **7**, 34 – 41 (1975)
40. Spurrell, R. A. J., Krikler, D. M., Sowton, E.: Concealed Bypasses of the atrioventricular node in patients with paroxysmal supraventricular tachycardia revealed by intracardiac electrical stimulation and verapamil. Amer. J. Cardiol. **33**, 590 – 595 (1974)
41. Spurrell, R. A. J., Krikler, D. M., Sowton, E.: Effects of verapamil on electrophysiological properties of anomalous atrioventricular connexion in Wolff-Parkinson-White syndrome. Brit. Heart J. **36**, 256 – 264 (1974)
42. Thormann, J., Schwarz, F., Zimmermann, H.: Effects of practolol on A – V conduction during atrial stimulation in 50 patients with and without coronary heart disease. Basic Res. Cardiol. **70**, 299 – 306 (1975)
43. Wellens, H. J., Durrer, D.: Effect of digitalis on atrioventricular conduction and circus-movement tachycardias in patients with Wolff-Parkinson-White syndrome. Circulation **47**, 1229 – 1233 (1973)
44. Wellens, H. J., Durrer, D.: Effect of procaine amide, quinidine, and ajmaline in the Wolff-Parkinson-White syndrome. Circulation **50**, 114 – 120 (1974)
45. Wellens, H. J.: Effect of drugs in the Wolff-Parkinson-White syndrome. In: Recent Advances in Ventricular Conduction, Cerqueira-Gomes, M. (ed.) Basel: Karger, 1975, Vol. XIV, pp. 230 – 240
46. Wit, A. L., Weiss, M. B., Berkowitz, W. D., Rosen, K. M., Steiner, Ch., Damato, A. N.: Patterns of atrioventricular conduction in the human heart. Circulat. Res. **27**, 345 – 352 (1970)
47. Wit, A. L., Hoffman, B. F., Cranefield, P. F.: Slow Conduction and reentry in the ventricular conducting system. Circulat. Res. **30**, 1 – 10 (1972)

Split His

M. Runge and O. S. Narula

His bundle electrocardiography has considerably enlarged our knowledge of the functions of the normal and the diseased conduction system of the human heart. Based on the methodology of Narula and Scherlag, the technique has been standardized to a large extent. However, interpretation of the findings sometimes is lacking in the necessary caution and critical reserve. The limitation of this technique and its difficulties of interpretation become particularly clear where the His bundle potential itself is concerned. Before discussing the clinical implications we will first have to consider a few general questions.

Although bipolar recording catheters are widely used it is unclear whether the His bundle electrogram really represents a bipolar recording in every case. According to the animal studies of Alanis [1] who carried out direct unipolar and bipolar recordings along the entire His bundle, the H deflection has a duration of 20 ms and independent of the kind of recording and the recording site the His potential always had the same morphology. In this respect the results of Sano [30] are partly identical. Scherlag and his coworkers [11, 31] examined this question further with dog experiments. They first carried out a bipolar recording of the His bundle potential and then transformed this into a unipolar one by grounding one pole. Thus the recording was carried out either from the proximal or distal pole with the catheter in an unchanged position. From these experiments the authors conclude that the His bundle electrogram is basically a unipolar recording and represents a real bipolar recording only in isolated cases.

The second problem of importance for our subject is the question of how accurately the technique of extracellular potential recordings from the conducting system translates the electrical activity of these structures [19, 38, 40]. For the His bundle potential itself this means whether the electrical activity of the whole bundle is registered or just individual parts of the structure. And what is even more important is whether this question is to be answered differently for healthy and diseased His bundles. According to results in dogs the extracellular recordings (unipolar and bipolar) translate the electrical activity of the structures in relation to the temporal and directional course of the impulses correctly when a healthy conduction system is stimulated not faster than with frequencies of 250/min [19, 38]. These are frequencies rarely used in humans so that we may generally trust the information received by the extracellular recordings. However, consideration should be given to sources of error in the intrepretation of data obtained by extracellular recordings, even in the range of low frequencies. When a bipolar recording is carried out with electrodes arranged parallel to the direction of impulse propagation we receive electrograms whose morphologies may be monophasic or multiphasic. When the electrodes are revolved by 90° the amplitude is considerably reduced and it is possible that multiwave potentials appear which persist over a large distance and thus give the impression of a prolongation of the potential duration.

The amplitude of the extracellular recordings depends decisively on the distance of the electrodes from the structure from which recording is to take place. The fact that the amplitude of the extracellular recording decreases exponentially with the distance of the electrodes from the tissue applies equally to regular beats and extrasystoles. At an electrode distance of more than 0.5 mm from the recording site the electrogram is hardly identifiable and no longer measurable in a reliable way [19]. Moreover, extracellular recordings only reflect the electrical activity of the superficial layers of tissue and not of those deeper than $200-250\,\mu$ [19]. Since the human His bundle is a structure with a diameter of several millimeters this means that despite lesions in deeper layers the recordings of the His potential may still be normal. For extrabeats it is important to know that when they are introduced with great prematurity their deflections may show a decrease in amplitude, broadening, or even fragmentation which must not be attributed to a change in catheter position. In addition, in very premature beats the polarity and morphology of their extracellular electrogram may change without any change in the direction of impulse propagation or of the poles. Meyerburg observed this behavior in 15% of his dog experiments [19]. There is no explanation for this, but it is important to know that the possibility exists, for otherwise one might misinterpret it as a recording from different structures.

The question raised in the beginning — whether the His bundle deflection represents the activity of the whole His bundle or just of a part of it — can not be answered for the healthy structure, nor is it relevant from the clinical point of view. Alanis [1], who carried out simultaneous recordings from various sites along the His bundle, obtained potentials of identical morphology and amplitude from all sites over the total length of the structure with the corresponding delays. Thus, on the basis of morphology alone he could not decide whether the recording had taken place from the proximal or the distal His bundle. If we take these results into consideration and apply them to clinical conditions with the necessary caution, we must assume that the recording is carried through from any site of the His bundle. With a healthy structure this deflection is representative for the whole His bundle. Sano [30], however, presumes that the H potential can not be considered as the local activity of that part of the His bundle which happens to be particularly near the catheter, but that the H potential comprises the electrical field of the whole bundle. But at least with a diseased human His bundle the activity of the entire structure is not always registered; otherwise one could not explain why one or the other component in cases of "split His" is often missed. Technical reasons, e.g., the kind of filter frequency chosen, can not be held solely responsible for it, and an electrode distance of 1 cm from the recording catheter should be sufficient to cover the whole structure, since the penetrating and the branching portions of the human His bundle together are not longer than 0.5 cm.

The biggest problem with extracellular potential recording is to identify the structure from which the recording is carried out and above all to prove that the recorded potential really represents this special structure [24, 34]. This holds true especially for the validation of the two potentials in split His. In this special case the possibility must be excluded that the proximal His deflection is an atrial repolarization wave and the distal His potential the activity of a bundle branch. Considering these difficulties of identifying both deflections as coming from the His bundle — as far as man is concerned — it is not surprising that in the clinical literature on split His, comments on this problem are usually avoided. The ideal method of validating both potentials is the stimulation of the proximal and distal recording site. This can be done in a reliable way only in animals [5] or in humans during open heart surgery [15]. As another possibility of validation in man it is recommended that simultaneous recordings of the His potentials from the right and left heart together with a bundle branch activity which should then be situated in the $H_2 - V$ interval be carried out [27].

Apart from the locations of the two deflections the time intervals must also fit together. This guideline assistance by the time intervals is justifiable particularly since the times reported so far from H to V and from the bundle branch potentials (RB and LB) to V have been confirmed in humans by measurements made during open heart surgery [14]. However, since this kind of evidence means an extension of the methodology which often can not be carried out in man for temporal and technical reasons, I would recommend the following procedure: validation of the proximal His deflection (H_1) by means of atrial stimulation with the criteria of lengthening of the $A - H_1$ interval with increasing frequencies; validation of the distal His deflection (H_2) by direct stimulation. However, one must be aware that when the part of the His bundle near the bifurcation is stimulated a QRS complex of bundle branch morphology may appear [15, 20]. This happens especially when high stimulation intensities (more than 10 mA) are used which then create an electrical field which influences the bundle branch. But then it is no longer a pure His stimulation, even if before, with the same catheter position, a good potential was recorded. In such cases a pure His bundle stimulation can be reached by reducing the stimulation intensity [15, 20]. In no case, however, is it correct to validate the distal His potential by means of vagal or atrial stimulation or drugs. These procedures are not suitable for a reliable distinction between a distal His deflection (H_2) and a bundle branch potential since with those procedures both deflections move in the same direction.

In dogs the various degrees of intra-His bundle blocks can be produced by ligation of the anterior septal artery [4–6]. Exact percentages concerning the frequency of intra-His lesions in man do not exist since the literature gives only small numbers of cases [13, 17, 23, 27, 35, 36]. French authors discovered 20% intra-His lesions in patients with acute myocardial

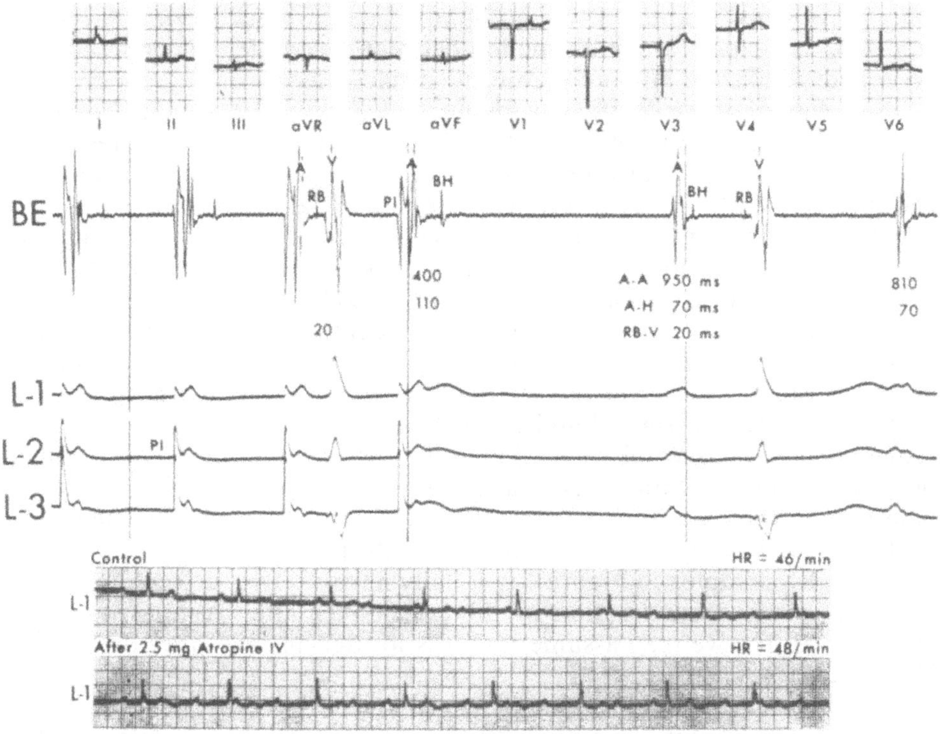

Fig 1. No atropine effect on pacemaker located in the distal part of His bundle in case of complete AV block within His bundle.

infarctions [39] and 18 – 19% in patients with chronic AV blocks [9, 26]. In the German literature reports on these block forms are particularly rare [8, 37]. As in animals, all degrees of intra-His bundle blocks have been described in man. In animals one may speak of a 1st degree His block when a fractioning, notching, and decrease in amplitude together with an increase of duration of the His potential above 20 ms is recorded [4, 6]. With the technique applied to man those findings can not be interpreted with certainty and a 1st degree intra-His block should be diagnosed only when two His deflections appear separated by an isoelectric segment and at the same time a prolonged $H_1 - V$ time and a normal $H_2 - V$ time can be measured.

Concerning the 2nd degree intra-His block both the Wenckebach and the Mobitz type have been described in man [21].

The 3rd degree intra-His block is characterized by the fact that H_1 has a fixed relation to the atrial deflection and H_2 a fixed relation to the QRS complex which is narrow. The frequency of the complete intra-His block is indicated to be 12% [8]. It is important to bear in mind that in the surface electrocardiogram this block form can not be distinguished formally from a complete block in the AV node since in both cases the QRS complex is narrow, provided that there was no bundle branch block before. A certain guideline assistance for the distinction between a complete block in the AV node and within the His bundle in the surface electrocardiogram is given by the behavior of the ventricular frequency following intravenous administration of atropine. In cases of intra-His blocks the ventricular frequency barely increases after atropine [10, 22, 27, 28] (see Figs. 1 and 2). The reason is the lack of vagal influence on the distal His bundle where in these cases the pacemaker is normally located (Fig. 1). However, deviations from this behavior of the pacemaker in the distal His-bundle after atropine or carotid sinus massage have also been observed [35].

In Figure 1 the 12 standard recordings demonstrate the narrow QRS complex. The His bundle electrocardiogram shows that each nonconducted atrium is blocked distal to the His bundle. In front of each narrow QRS complex appears a right bundle potential. The narrow QRS complex proves that the pacemaker is located in the distal part of the bundle proximal to the bifurcation. The surface recordings in the lower part of the figure show that the initial heart frequency of 46/min is increased only negligibly to 48/min after administration of atropine.

The QRS complex in Figure 2 is equally narrow. The surface recordings show the marked acceleration of the pacemaker after administration of atropine, so that we may assume that it is located in the upper part of the His-bundle.

Good correlations of histopathologic and electrophysiologic findings are known when the heart is systemically diseased (amyloid, Lev's disease) [29]. For the His bundle alone such correlations must be interpreted with caution because a correspondence between anatomy (longitudinal separation) [3, 12] and function (evidence of cross connections) [2, 16, 17, 33] does not seem to exist. At this point it should again be mentioned that extracellular recordings do not register lesions in the deeper layers of the structure [19].

If an intra-His bundle block is not discovered, it may lead to misinterpretations concerning the site of block as has been described in animals [4, 32] and in man [7, 18, 35]. By means of time comparisons during open heart surgery [14] we know that with the technique applied to man and with a healthy His bundle the recording normally takes place from the proximal part of the bundle. With a diseased His bundle experience with animals [4, 6] and clinical findings show that it is this same proximal deflection which most often is not recognized, and not least because H_1 may be hidden in the atrial activity [13, 35] and leaves it only after atrial stimulation [35]. Some forms of misinterpretation due to nonrecognition of one or the other component of the split His are the following:

1. If H_1 is not recognized an intra-His bundle lesion may be mistaken for an AV nodal lesion.

2. Likewise, the Mobitz type 2nd degree block within the His bundle can be misinterpreted as a Mobitz type II in the AV node if the proximal His deflection is not recorded. Such a case has been described clinically [18].

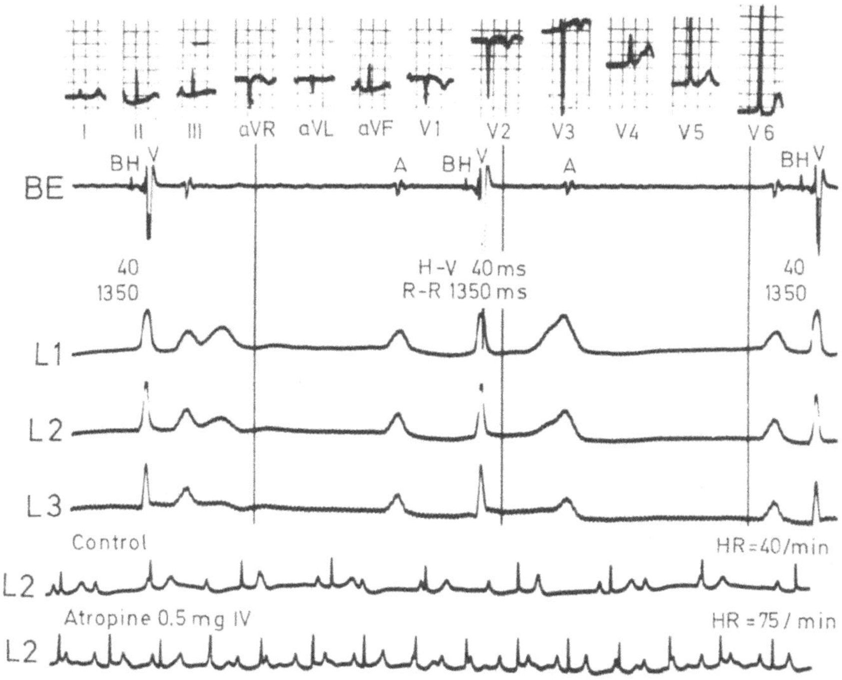

Fig. 2. Positive atropine effect on pacemaker located in proximal His bundle in patient with complete AV block in AV node.

3. If H_1 is not identified it may lead to an erroneous good prognosis in case of an intra-His block combined with a bundle branch block, because a short ("normal") H – V time is measured which in reality is the $H_2 - V$ interval.

4. If on the other hand, with the same constellation as in 3 H_2 is not identified, one might diagnose a bilateral bundle branch block because "H – V" is prolonged.

These examples of possible misinterpretations when missing one or the other deflection of the split His show the significance of a correct recording of double potentials for the prognosis of conduction disturbances. Since for temporal and technical reasons it is not always possible to use several catheters the His bundle area must be explored if an intra-His lesion is suspected [35]. The fact that at least with a diseased His bundle we do not always record the activity of the whole structure and that the potential actually recorded only represents the activity of a part of the His bundle may be evaluated as an indirect confirmation of the findings of Alanis and Scherlag [1, 31]. The following example shows how we can come to the correct diagnosis by exploring the His-bundle area (see Fig. 3) [20].

Figure 3, a – d, shows examples of false measurements of the H – V time and misinterpretations of block localization. Part d shows the correct dia-

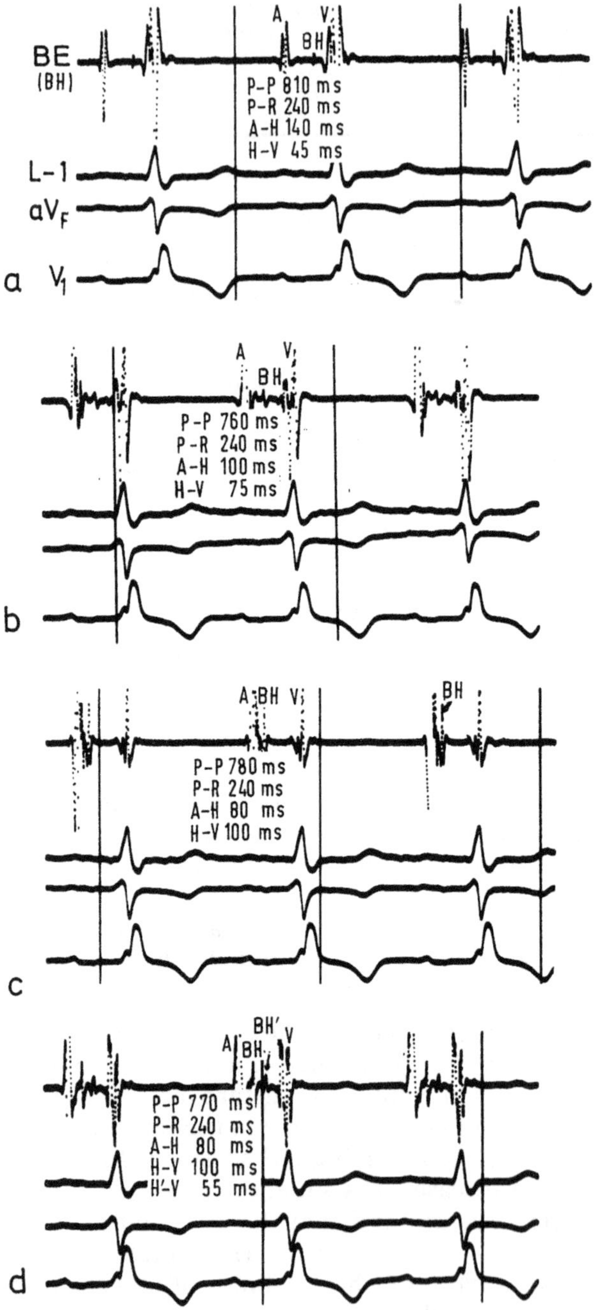

Fig. 3 a – d. (a – c) False measurements of H-V time and mis-interpretations of block localization. (d) Correct diagnoses.

gnoses. In parts a, b, and c, three different H – V intervals are to be seen (45 ms, 75 ms, and 100 ms). Depending on the position of the catheter they comprise the range from normal to pathologic. The correct position of the catheter (d) shows that there is a 1st degree intra-His bundle block.

Summary

The subject requires the discussion of some general questions concerning His bundle recordings in man.

Firstly, is the HB electrogram a unipolar or bipolar recording? Although a bipolar catheter is used, little is known regarding the electrical nature of this recording. Animal studies provide some evidence that in the great majority the HB electrogram is an unipolar proximity recording and represents only occasionally the contribution of both electrodes.

Secondly, to what extent do the surface recordings from the specialized conducting system reflect activity of the underlying tissue? This means especially for the HB electrogram, do the extracellular recordings represent the electrical activity of the entire His bundle or of only a part of it? Do differences exist, regarding this problem, between recordings from a healthy or a diseased His bundle?

Furthermore one of the greatest problems for the clinician is discussed, the validation of the two deflections (HH′ or H_1H_2) in cases of split – His recordings.

This is followed by the description of the various degrees of intra-His bundle lesions; how they can be recognized by the HB electrogram and how this localization can be supposed from the surface ECG. Finally attention is drawn to possible misinterpretations of the site of conduction disorders due to failure of detection of the proximal or the distal deflection in split-His.

References

1. Alanis, J., Gonzales, H., López, E.: The electrical activity of the bundle of His. J. Physiol. **142,** 127 (1958)
2. Bailey, J. C., Spear, J. F., Moore, E. N.: Functional significance of transverse conducting pathways within the canine bundle of His. Amer. J. Cardiol. **34,** 790 (1974)
3. Bharati, S., Lev, M., Wu, D., Denes, P., Dhingra, R., Rosen, K. M.: Pathophysiologic correlations in two cases of split His bundle potentials. Circulation **49,** 615 (1974)
4. El-Sherif, N., Scherlag, B. J., Lazzara, R.: Conduction disorders in the canine proximal His-Purkinjesystem following acute myocardial ischemia. I. The pathophysology of intra-His bundle block. Circulation **49,** 837 (1974)
5. El-Sherif, N., Scherlag, B. J., Lazzara, R., Samet, P.: Pathophysiology of tachycardia- and bradycardia-dependent block in the canine proximal His-Purkinje-system after acute myocardial ischemia. Amer. J. Cardiol. **33,** 529 (1974)
6. El-Sherif, N., Scherlag, B. J., Lazzara, R., Hope, R., Williams, D. O., Samet, P.: The pathophysiology of tachycardia-dependent paroxysmal atrioventricular block after acute myocardial ischemia. Experimental and clinical observations. Circulation **50,** 515 (1974)
7. Fishenfeld, J., Flemig, M. D., Desser, K. B., Benchimol, A.: False localisation of atrioventricular block secondary to failure of "split His" recording. Chest **66,** 288 (1974)

8. Fleischmann, D., Effert, S., Bleifeld, W., Pop, T., Irnich, W.: Lokalisation der Leitungsunterbrechung beim kompletten AV-Block mittels His-Bündel-Elektrographie. – Dtsch. med. Wschr. **100,** 723 (1975)
9. Guerot, C., Valere, P. E., Coste, A., Tricot, R.: Bloc auriculo-ventriculaire localise au tronc du faisceau de His: Le bloc tronculaire. Ann. Cardiol. Angeiol. **21,** 143 (1972)
10. Gupta, P. K., Lichstein, E., Chadda, K.: Electrophysiological features of complete AV-block within the His bundle. Brit. Heart J. **35,** 610 (1973)
11. Hope, R., Berbari, E. J., El-Sherif, N., Williams, D. O., Lazzara, R., Scherlag, B. J.: The His-bundle-electrogram: unipolar or bipolar recording? Clin. Res. **22,** 6 A (1974)
12. James, T. N., Sherf, L.: Fine structure of the His bundle. Circulation **44,** 9 (1971)
13. Krishnaswami, V., Geraci, A. R.: Accelerated A-V conduction associated with complete AV-block. Amer. Heart J. **88,** 463 (1974)
14. Kupersmith, J., Krongrad, E., Waldo, A. L.: Conduction intervals and conduction velocity in the human cardiac conduction system. Studies during open-heart surgery. Circulation **47,** 776 (1973)
15. Kupersmith, J., Krongrad, E., Browman, F. O., Malm, J. R., Waldo, A. L.: Pacing the human cardiac conduction system during open-heart surgery. Circulation **50,** 499 (1974)
16. Lazzara, R.: Conduction pathways within the His bundle and bundle braches – The importance of transverse interconnections. In: His Bundle Electrocardiography and Clinical Physiology. Narula, O. S. (ed.). Philadelphia: F. A. Davis, 1975, p. 37
17. Lazzara, R., Yeh, B. K., Samet, P.: Functional transverse interconnections within the His bundle and bundle branches. Circulat. Res. **32,** 509 (1073)
18. Mandel, W. J., Kermaier, A., Allen, H. N., Hayakawa, H.: An unusual case of second degree AV-block. A study using His bundle electrograms. Chest **61,** 37 (1972)
19. Meyerburg, R. J., Nilson, K., Zoble, R. G.: Relationship of surface electrogram recordings to activity in the underlying specialized conducting tissue. Circulation **45,** 420 (1972)
20. Narula, O. S.: Validation of His bundle recordings. Limitations of the catheter technique. In: His Bundle Electrocardiographie and Clinical Physiology. Narula, O. S. (ed.). Philadelphia: F. A. Davis, 1975, p. 65
21. Narula, O. S., Samet, P.: Wenckebach and Mobitz II AV-block due to block within the His-bundle and bundle branches. Circulation **41,** 947 (1970)
22. Narula, O. S., Samet, P.: Effect of atropine and glucagon on AV-nodal and His bundle pacemakers in man (Abstract). Circulation **44,** Suppl. II, 205 (1971)
23. Narula, O. S., Scherlag, B. J., Samet, P.: His-bundle blocks and His-bundle rhythms. Dis. Chest **56,** (1969)
24. Narula, O. S., Scherlag, B. J., Samet, P.: Pervenous pacing of the specialized conducting system in man: His bundle and A-V nodal stimulation. Circulation **41,** 77 (1970)
25. Narula, O. S., Scherlag, B. J., Samet, P., Javier, R. P.: Atrioventricular block: Localisation and classification by His bundle recordings. Amer. J. Med. **50,** 146 (1971)
26. Puech, P., Grolleau-Raoux, R., Latour, H., Cabasson, J., Robin, J. M., Baissus, C., Gilbert, M.: Diagnostic des blocs tronculaires hisiens par l'enregistrement endocavitaire et la stimulation du faisceau de His. Arch. Mal. Coeur **65,** 315 (1972)
27. Rosen, K. M., Heller, R., Ehsani, A., Rahimtoola, S. H.: Localisation of site of traumatic heart with His Bundle recordings. Electrophysiologic observations regarding the nature of "split" H potentials. Amer. J. Cardiol. **30,** 412 (1972)
28. Rosen, K. M., Mehta, A., Rahimtoola, S. H., Miller, R. A.: Sites of congenital and surgical heart block as defined by His bundle recordings. Circulation **44,** 833 (1971)
29. Rosen, K. M., Rahimtoola, R. M., Gunnar, R. M., Lev, M.: Site of block diagnosed by His bundle recording. Pathological correlations. Circulation **43** and **44** Suppl. II 64; Abstr. 217 (1971)
30. Sano, T., Nakai, M., Suzuki, F.: Nature of His potential in His electrogram. Jap. Heart J. **13,** 521 (1972)
31. Scherlag, B. J., Berbari, E. J.: Techniques for His bundle recordings. In: His Bundle Electrocardiography and Clinical Electrophysiology. Narula, O. S. (ed.). Philadelphia: F. A. Davis, 1975, p. 51
32. Scherlag, B. J., El-Sherif, N., Lazzara, R.: Latent His bundle lesions: Limitations of standard recording techniques. Circulation **48,** Suppl. IV, 102 (1973)

33. Scherlag, B. J., El-Sherif, N., Lazzara, R.: Bundle branch block due to His bundle lesions. Amer. J. Cardiol. **33,** 169 (1974)
34. Scherlag, B. J., Kosowsky, B. D., Damato, A. N: A technique for ventricular pacing from the His bundle of the intact heart. J. appl. Physiol. **22,** 584 (1967)
35. Schuilenburg, R. M., Durrer, D.: Problems in the recognition of conduction disturbances in the His bundle. Circulation **51,** 68 (1975)
36. Schuilenburg, R. M., Durrer, D.: Conduction disturbances located within the His bundle. Circulation **45,** 612 (1972)
37. Seipel, L., Both, A., Loogen, F.: Klinische Bedeutung der His-Bündel-Elektrographie. Klin. Wschr. **53,** 499 (1975)
38. Spach, M. S., Barr, R. C., Sewer, G. A., Kootsey, J. M., Johnson, E. A.: Extracellular potentials related to intracellular action potentials in the dog Purkinje system. Circulat. Res. **30,** 505 (1972)
39. Touboul, P., Clement, C., Porte, J., Magrina, J., Delahaye, J. P.: Étude electrophysiologique des troubles de conduction auriculo-ventriculaire dans l'infarctus myocardique recent. Arch. Mal. Coeur **65,** 1287 (1972)
40. Varghese, P. J., Elizari, M. V., Lau, S. H., Damato, A. N.: His bundle electrograms of dog. Correlation with intracellular recordings. Circulation **48,** 753 (1973)

Atrioventricular (AV) and Ventriculoatrial (VA) Conduction Pattern in Patients with Short P – R Interval and Normal QRS Complex

L. SEIPEL, G. BREITHARDT, and A. BOTH

The electrocardiographic finding of a short P – R interval and a normal QRS complex has been described by several authors [8, 15, 28, 35, 55]. In case of simultaneously occurring arrhythmias, it is usually designated as the LGL [35] or the CLC [15] syndrome.

Most authors assume as the underlying pathophysiologic mechanism a partial or complete bypass of the AV node by an accessory pathway or by the posterior internodal tract (James fiber) [30] with a direct insertion in the bundle of His [8, 12, 21, 22, 32, 37, 43, 48]. The existence of a bypass tract has been anatomically proved in a case with an LGL syndrome [9]. On the basis of clinical findings connections to the right bundle branch have also been discussed [52]. If so, the pattern would constitute a special form of the pre-excitation syndrome. A further explanation would be a functional longitudinal dissociation of the AV node with a rapidly and slowly conducting pathway [11, 12, 37, 42]. An anatomically small AV node may also cause a short conduction time between the atrium and the ventricle [1, 11, 17, 50]. Further explanations would be an isorhythmic dissociation between the atrium and the ventricle [11] as well as delayed excitation of the atrial myocardium ("delayed P") with normal conduction via internodal tracts to the AV node and the ventricle [3, 53]. Both possibilities seem to be hypothetical. In addition, the significance of the internodal tract as a specialized pathway for internodal conduction remains controversial [33]. An inferior left atrial pacemaker with an additional accessory pathway has also been made responsible for the "masked WPW syndrome" [7]. In addition, an increased conduction velocity in the bundle of His or in Mahaim fibers has been discussed [6, 21, 37].

Methods and Results

In 21 patients with the syndrome of short P – R interval ($\leqq$0.12 s) and one patient with a normal P – R interval and widened QRS complex, atrioventricular conduction was analyzed. During His bundle electrography in all cases atrial stimulation was performed. In five patients the right ventricle was stimulated additionally. In each case, high rate atrial stimulation at increasing rates and single premature atrial stimulation (extrastimulus technique) during spontaneous rhythm was done. In 10 cases, the extrastimulus technique was used for estimation of refractory periods during a constant pacemaker-induced rate. In eight cases the procedure was repeated after application of verapamil (0.1 mg/kg i.v.).

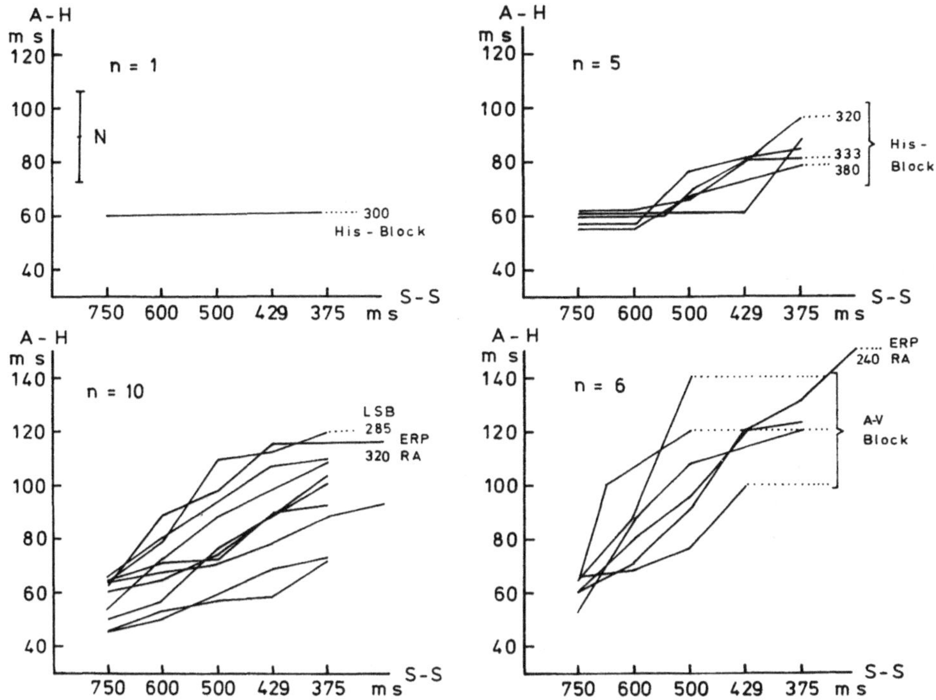

Fig. 1. Behavior of the AH interval during high rate atrial stimulation at increasing rates in 22 patients with LGL-syndrome.
N = normal value of A-H interval.

During rest, His bundle electrography yielded a normal atrial conduction time. The P – A interval was, on an average, 26.1 ± 7.9 ms (normal value of our laboratory: 27 ± 8.2 ms [47]. The A – H interval was significantly shorter (57.4 ± 7.4 ms) compared to normal persons (89 ± 17.2 ms [47]). Nevertheless, in some patients the A – H interval was in the lower range of our normal value. The H – V time was 38.4 ± 7.9 ms which is slightly shorter than the normal value in our laboratory (43 ± 6.9 ms). The HBE of the patient with normal P – R interval and widened QRS complex showed a short A – H time (56 ms) and a prolonged H – V interval (70 ms).

During high rate atrial stimulation the H – V interval did not change. As to the A – H time, different patterns could be observed (Fig. 1). In one patient the A – H time remained constant up to block even during high rate atrial stimulation (group I). In five patients the A – H time did not change up to a distinct stimulation rate, after which it suddenly increased (group II). In both groups the conduction block at high rates usually occurred in the His-Purkinje system. In 16 patients a more or less pronounced continuous prolongation of the A – H interval was observed at increasing rates. Some patients demonstrated a marked increase of the A – H interval with block in the AV node at relatively low stimulation rates. In one of

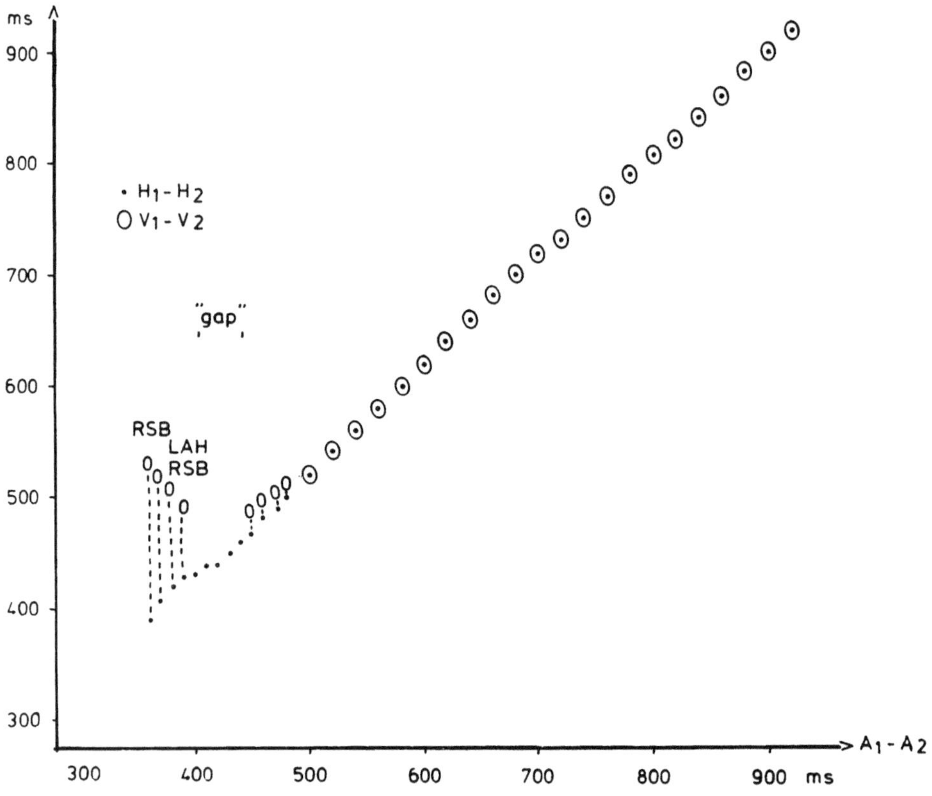

Fig. 2. Gap phenomenon of AV conduction within His-Purkinje system (so-called type II gap) during atrial premature stimulation. The H_1H_2 intervals and the V_1V_2 intervals, respectively, are plotted against the A_1A_2 intervals. As the A-H interval remains nearly constant during premature stimulation, the H_1H_2 intervals lie on a line with an angle of 45°. As soon as the H_1-H_2 intervals reach a critical value, block distal to the His potential occurs (*gap*). At further shortening of the H_1H_2 interval the impulse is again conducted to the ventricle with marked prolongation of the H_2V_2 intervals (therefore H_1H_2 and V_1V_2 intervals no longer lie on the same line).

these cases, there was at first a prolongation of the A – H interval which then remained constant at higher rates until block occurred. In this third group of patients there were also cases with a clinically typical LGL syndrome and recurrent tachycardias.

The effect of premature atrial stimulation (extrastimulus technique) on the A – H interval corresponded principally to the one during high rate test. With increasing prematurity of the stimulus, the A – H interval within the different groups of cases either remained constant or showed a sudden or continuous prolongation. The refractory periods in some of these patients were shorter than in normal persons. However, the small number of patients does not allow statistical conclusions. In patients with short P – R intervals a gap phenomenon (type I and type II) was frequently observed

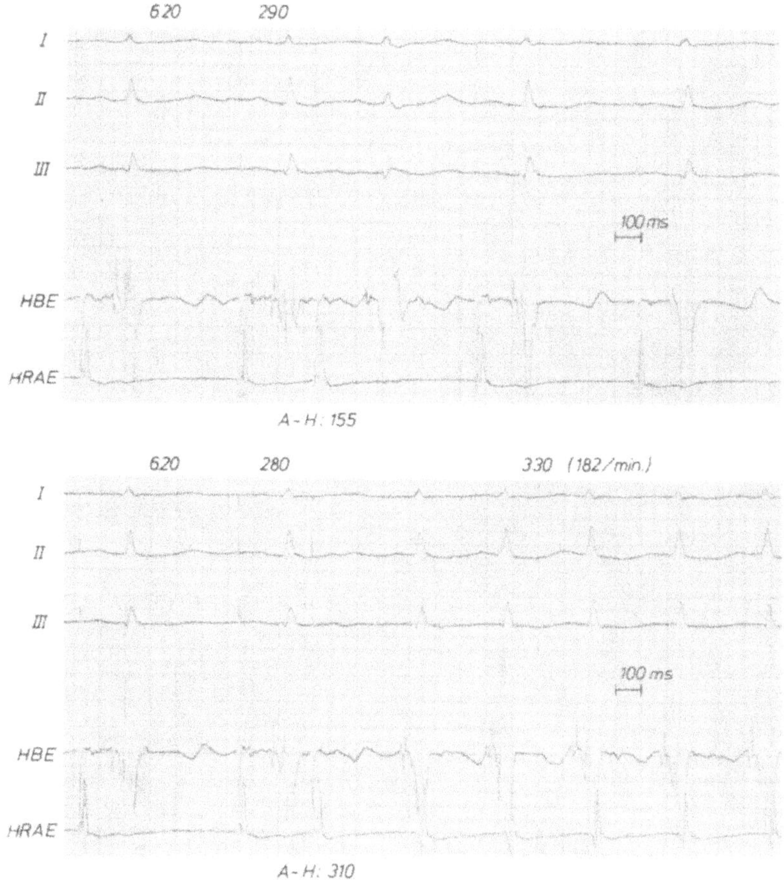

Fig. 3. Initiation of supraventricular tachycardia by atrial premature stimulation. Shortening of coupling interval from 290 to 280 ms leads to sudden prolongation of A-H interval from 155 to 310 ms. This initiates tachycardia, probably due to reentry of AV node.

(Fig. 2). In the cases of group II a sudden prolongation of the A – H interval during single premature stimulation occurred at a distinct prematurity of the stimulus. At this critical coupling interval, supraventricular tachycardias were frequently initiated. During these tachycardias the high atrial potential coincided with the ventricular complex of the preceding beat. The atrial potentials differed from the potentials during spontaneous sinus rhythm and the ventricular complexes were always preceded by a His potential with unchanged H – V intervals (Fig. 3). It is noteworthy that in single cases with very high rates these tachycardias could be interrupted only by high rate stimulation, but not by application of single stimuli.

In two cases a different behavior of ventriculoatrial (VA) conduction in comparison to atrioventricular (AV) conduction was found. In these two patients, the AV conduction time increased progressively during high rate

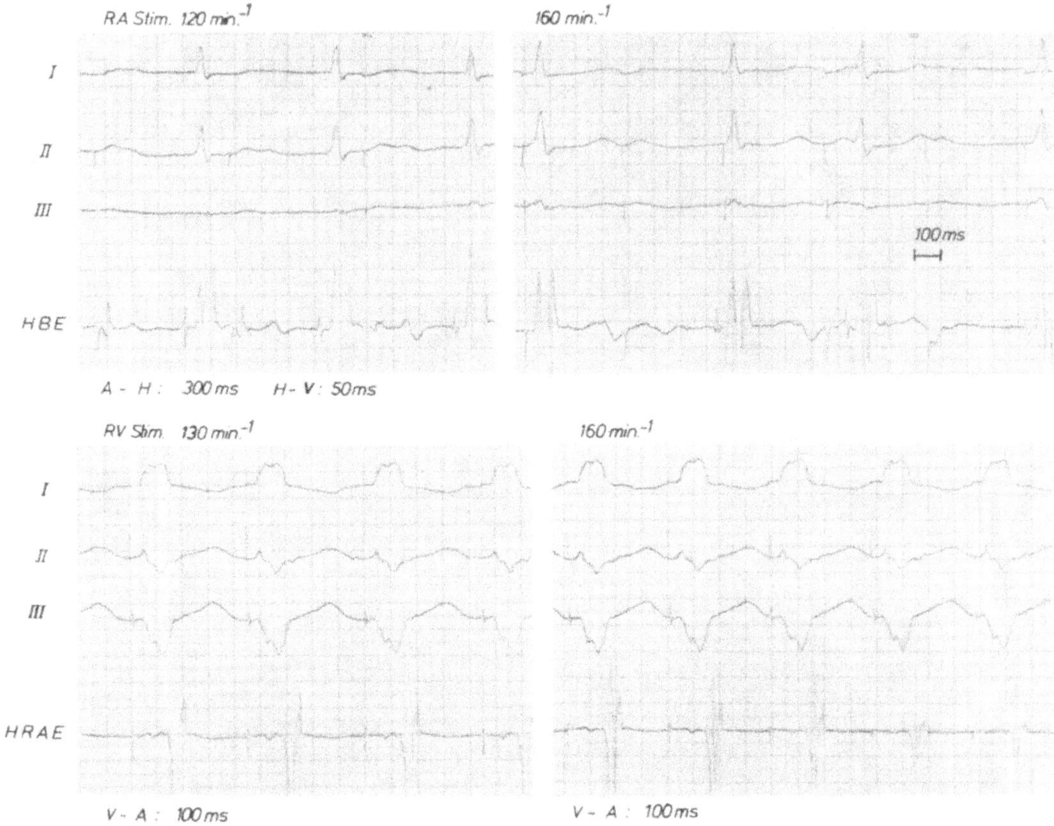

Fig. 4. Different behavior of AV and VA conduction in a patient with a short P-R interval. During high rate atrial stimulation a prolongation of the A-H interval and block within the AV node occurs (*above*). During ventricular stimulation at identical rates 1 : 1 conduction without prolongation of VA interval is documented (*below*).

or single premature atrial stimulation. This prolongation was due to a prolongation of the A – H interval. At shorter cycle lengths a block occurred after the A wave. During ventricular stimulation, however, the retrograde VA conduction time was constant, independent of the frequency or the coupling interval of the stimuli (Fig. 4).

Verapamil was given to eight patients with short P – R interval and abnormal behavior of the A – H interval during control stimulation. There was no, or only a slight, prolongation of the A – H interval compared to the control value. During high rate stimulation, the degree of prolongation of the A – H interval was principally identical to the control stimulation. These results differ from the effects of verapamil in 10 normal cases in whom it caused a marked prolongation of the A – H interval with a more pronounced effect during high rate stimulation. These differences were significant [46].

Discussion

By use of His bundle electrography a further analysis of the short P – R interval in patients with the LGL syndrome is possible [4, 11 – 13, 16, 17, 25, 29, 36, 37, 42, 46]. Atrial depolarization occurs in normal sequence from the high to the low atrium (exclusion of an ectopic focus). The atrial conduction time (P – A interval) is normal which allows exclusion of a delayed excitation of the atrial myocardium. The ventricles are activated via the bundle of His. The most important finding is the short conduction time between the low right atrium and the bundle of His (A – H interval). This indicates an abnormally rapid conduction in the region of the AV node. However, in some cases with LGL syndrome the A – H time may be within the lower range of normal. Thus, in these cases the findings in the HBE during sinus rhythm do not allow a proper separation from normal persons. The H – V time frequently is relatively short. Besides a high conduction velocity in the His-Purkinje system [6, 21, 37], it is also conceivable that a distal insertion of the James fiber to the bundle of His causes a shortening of the H – V interval [19].

In addition to the findings during sinus rhythm, the "dynamical" analysis of AV conduction by use of atrial and ventricular stimulation leads to significantly greater information. The physiologic mechanism responsible for the short P – R interval can be further analyzed. During high rate atrial stimulation, at least three different patterns of AV conduction may be distinguished [4, 12, 16, 29, 37, 42, 46]. A constant conduction time during high rate stimulation until block gives evidence for a complete bypass of the AV node by an accessory tract. This finding is very rare.

A sudden prolongation of the A – H interval at a distinct rate of stimulation is conceivable with either a short circuit of the AV node by a James fiber or a functional dissociation within the AV node. As soon as the refractory period of the rapidly conducting pathway is reached, the conduction occurs via the more slowly conducting pathways with shorter effective refractory period. A continuous prolongation of the A – H interval at increasing rate indicates that the AV node is involved in the AV conduction. The short A – H interval at spontaneous rhythm and the merely slight prolongation during stimulation in some cases might be due to a small AV node. The marked prolongation of the A – H time and the premature block during high rate stimulation in some cases with the LGL syndrome is noteworthy. In these cases, it is probably not possible to imitate the conduction pattern during sinus rhythm by ectopic atrial stimulation [46]. As other authors have shown, different positions of the catheter within the right atrium may cause a change of AV conduction [1, 6, 56]. It should be stressed that the short A – H time does not in each case lead to a short

P – R interval. Single patients with normal or prolonged P – R interval or even with AV block may demonstrate an atypical behavior of the A – H time as in the LGL syndrome [13, 34]. This is exemplified by the case with normal P – R interval and bundle branch block who demonstrated a short A – H interval and a prolonged H – V time.

In several cases the atrial exstrastimulus technique reveals abnormally short refractory periods within the AV node. The present data are not yet sufficient for statistical evaluation. Bisset et al. [5] were able to demonstrate significantly shorter refractory periods within the AV node in patients with short P – R interval compared to normal cases. In our cases a gap phenomenon of the AV conduction is a relatively frequent finding due to the abnormal behavior of the AV node.

A functional dissociation of AV conduction is an important condition for the initiation of tachycardia. In several patients a sudden prolongation of the A – H interval occurs at critical coupling intervals leading to a tachycardia. These tachycardias fulfill the typical criteria for AV node reentry [18, 26, 27, 38, 40, 57, 60]. However, not all supraventricular tachycardias were initiated by a sudden A – H prolongation. In a few cases, it is not possible to interrupt tachycardias by premature atrial stimuli, but only by high rate stimulation. This confirms previous observations [40].

Ventricular stimulation may be able to uncover concealed accessory connections between the atrium and ventricle. These may remain undetected during atrial stimulation as the accessory pathway is blocked antegradely and conducts only retrogradely. In two of our cases, we found such a divergent behavior of antegrade (AV) and retrograde (VA) conduction between atrium and ventricle. The existance of similar "retrograde preexcitation syndromes" has been proved even in cases with normal P – R interval [39, 41, 51, 54, 57]. They may be responsible for reentry tachycardias via the ventricles with antegrade conduction through the normal pathways and retrograde conduction via the accessory pathway.

Verapamil had no, or only, a slight effect on AV conduction in patients with the LGL syndrome. This supports the assumption of abnormal conductivity in the region of the AV node. Verapamil acts exclusively on the AV node. Thus, in patients with the short P – R interval, the AV node must be more or less functionally excluded from atrioventricular conduction.

The study of patients suspected to have the LGL syndrome or of patients with tachycardias and normal P – R interval, is of clinical significance. Besides establishing the diagnosis, the analysis of AV and VA conduction is a prerequisite for effective therapy. In addition, it is important to analyze the tachycardia zone [38]. This examination is even necessary if one has in mind to treat the tachycardias by implantation of an inductively working high rate pacemaker [23, 33 a, 38, 59]. Since high rate atrial stimulation in patients with an accessory pathway may lead to ventricular tachycardia, the effect of high rate atrial stimulation has to be tested before implantation of such a device.

The analysis of AV conduction during high rate pacing and the definition of the refractory periods may also have great prognostic significance. Patients with short refractory periods of the AV conduction system, or with 1 : 1 conduction at high rates of stimulation, are threatened by atrial fibrillation or flutter which may induce ventricular tachycardia. In patients with LGL syndrome, atrial fibrillation is more frequent than in normal cases [6, 16, 35, 45]. Probably in these patients the occurrence of sudden death [13, 35] is due to this mechanism. Furthermore, it is possible that in case of a short refractory period of the AV conduction system, very early premature atrial beats may be conducted to the ventricles initiating ventricular fibrillation by an R on T phenomenon [13]. This has been demonstrated in young mammalians which have a very short refractory period of the AV node [44]. In these cases His bundle electrography should be used to study the effect of antiarrhythmic drugs on the refractory period of the AV conduction system. Before resuming surgical procedures such as interruption of the bundle of His, an exact electrophysiologic study of the patient is necessary [24, 49].

The new diagnostic possibilities of intracardiac recording and stimulation have made the delineation of the LGL syndrome even more complex. A generally acceptable definition of this syndrome can neither be given from the clinical data nor from the results of the electrophysiologic studies. On the one side, the definition of this syndrome by a short P – R interval with normal QRS complex is not sufficient. Electrophysiologic studies have shown, that even patients with normal P – R interval and widened QRS complexes may show abnormal conductivity within the AV node similar to the LGL syndrome. On the other hand, the findings in the HBE are not uniform in patients with a clinically defined LGL syndrome as the A – H interval may lie within the lower range of normal persons. Nor does atrial stimulation give a proper solution to this problem. It seems at least unjustified to include only those cases in the LGL syndrome that present an abnormal pattern of the A – H interval during stimulation. Some patients with a typical LGL syndrome (short P – R interval with tachycardias) may demonstrate during stimulation a completely normal pattern with prolongation of the A – H interval although they had a short A – H interval during sinus rhythm. Nevertheless, these patients cannot be regarded as normal. Therefore it seems difficult to refer to the so-called LGL syndrome as an entity. It remains a semantic question how to define the LGL syndrome [12, 13]. In this situation, the clinical and electrophysiologic findings should be described as exactly as possible.

Summary

In 21 patients with short P–R interval ($\leqq 0.12$ s), normal QRS complex and arrhythmias (LGL or CLC syndrome), His bundle electrography and atrial as well as ventricular stimulation (high rate test, extrastimulus technique) were performed. In addition, one patient with normal P – R interval was included. During sinus rhythm the intra-atrial conduction time (P – A interval) was normal (26.1 ± 7.9 ms). The A – H interval (57.4 ± 7.4 ms) was significantly shorter than our normal value (89 ± 17.2 ms). However, in some patients with the LGL syndrome the A – H interval was in the lower normal range. The mean H – V time was 38.4 ± 7.9 ms (normal range 43 ± 6.9 ms). The patient with the normal P – R interval showed a short A – H time and a prolonged H – V interval.

During rapid atrial stimulation with stepwise increase of frequency, the H – V interval remained unchanged. As to the A – H interval, three different patterns could be observed: (1) The A – H interval remained unchanged up to block within the His-Purkinje system (1 case). (2) A sudden prolongation of the A – H interval at a critical rate (5 cases). (3) A continuous prolongation of the A – H interval according to the driving frequency (16 cases). As far as ventricular stimulation was performed, the VA conduction showed in principle the same behavior with two exceptions. In these two patients the antegrade AV conduction time was prolonged at shorter cycle length whereas the retrograde VA conduction remained unchanged. Typical reentry tachycardias were induced and terminated by atrial stimuli.

In addition, the effect of verapamil (0.1 mg/kg i.v.) was tested. This drug showed little or no effect on the A – H interval in these patients whereas in a control group the A – H time was prolonged significantly after drug application.

The results indicate an abnormal behavior of AV conduction in many patients with short P – R interval. As far as conclusions from the clinical data may be drawn, an accessory pathway completely bypassing the AV node (James fiber) is a rare condition. With respect to these findings it seems to be difficult to refer to the so-called LGL syndrome as an entity.

References

1. Amat y Leon, F., Denes, P., Wu, D., Pietras, R. J., Rosen, K. M.: Effects of atrial pacing site on atrial and atrioventricular nodal function. Brit. Heart J. **37,** 567 (1975)
2. Anderson, R. H., Thaper, M. K., Arnold, R., Jones, R. S.: Study of conducting tissue in a case of ventricular preexcitation. Brit. Heart J. **35,** 566 (1973)
3. Bellet, S., Jedlicka, J.: Sinoventricular conduction and its relation to sino-atrial conduction. Amer. J. Cardiol. **24,** 831 (1969)
4. Bissett, J. K., Thomson, A. J., de Soyza, N., Murphy, M. L.: Atrioventricular conduction in patients with short PR intervals and normal QRS complexes. Brit. Heart J. **35,** 123 (1973)
5. Bisset, J. K., de Soyza, N., Kane, J. J., Murphy, M. L.: Altered refractory periods in patients with short P-R intervals and normal QRS complex. Amer. J. Cardiol. **35,** 487 (1975)
6. Boineau, J. P., Moore, E. N., Spear, J. F., Sealy, W. C.: Basis of clinical-ECG variations in right and left ventricular preexcitation: A unitary concept of WPW. In: Cardiac Arrhythmias. Dreifus, L. S., Likoff, W. (eds.). New York: Grune & Stratton, 1973, p. 421
7. Boineau, J. P., Moore, E. N., Spear, J. F., Sealy, W. C.: Basis of static and dynamic electrocardiographic variations in Wolff-Parkinson-White syndrome. Amer. J. Cardiol. **32,** 32 (1973)

8. Burch, G. E., Kimball, J. L.: Notes on the similarity of QRS complex configurations in the Wolff-Parkinson-White syndrome. Amer. Heart J. **32,** 560 (1946)
9. Brechenmacher, C., Laham, J., Iris, L., Gerbaux, A., Lenègre, J.: Étude histologique des voies anomales de conduction dans un syndrome de Wolff-Parkinson-White et dans un syndrome de Lown-Ganong-Levine. Arch. Mal. Coeur **67,** 507 (1974)
10. Breithardt, G., Seipel, L., Both, A., Gleichmann, U.: Klinische Bedeutung und Diagnostik des LGL-Syndroms. Med. Welt (N. F.) **25,** 117 (1974)
11. Caracta, A. R., Damato, A. N., Gallagher, J. J., Josephson, M. E., Varghese, P. J., Lau, S. H., Westura, E. E.: Electrophysiologic studies in the syndrome of short P-R interval, normal QRS complex. Amer. J. Cardiol. **31,** 245 (1973)
12. Castellanos, A., Castillo, C. A., Agha, A. S., Tessler, M.: His bundle electrograms in patients with short P-R intervals, narrow QRS complexes and paroxysmal tachycardias. Circulation **43,** 667 (1971)
13. Castellanos, A., Vagueiro, M. C., Befeler, B., Myerburg, R. J.: Syndrome of short P-R, narrow QRS and repetitive supraventricular tachyarrhythmias: the possible occurrence of the R-on-T phenomenon and the limits of this syndrome. Europ. J. Cardiol. **2,** 337 (1975)
14. Castellanos, A., Myerburg, R. J.: Repetitive supraventricular tachycardias in context. Amer. Heart J. **90,** 131 (1975)
15. Clerc, A., Lévy, R., Cristesco, C.: A propos du raccourcissement permanent du l'espace P-R de l'electrocardiogramme sans déformation du complexe ventriculaire. Arch. Mal. Coeur **31,** 569 (1938)
16. Coumel, P., Waynberger, M., Slama, R., Bouvrain, Y.: Le syndrome de P-R court, avec complex QRS normal. Particularités électrocardiographiques. Arch. Mal. Coeur **65,** 161 (1972)
17. Damato, A. N., Gallagher, J. J., Lau, S. H.: Applications of His bundle recordings in diagnosing conduction disorders. Progr. Cardiovasc. Dis. **14,** 601 (1972)
18. Denes, P., Wu, D., Dhingra, R. C., Chuquimia, R., Rosen, K. M.: Demonstration of dual A-V nodal pathways in patients with paroxysmal supraventricular tachycardia. Circulation **48,** 549 (1973)
19. Douglas, J. E.: Lown-Ganong-Levine syndrome. Circulation **45,** 1143 (1972)
20. Durrer, D.: Electrical aspects of human cardiac activity: A clinical physiological approach to excitation and stimulation. Cardiovasc. Res. **2,** 1 (1968)
21. Durrer, D., Schuilenburg, R. M., Wellens, H. J. J.: Pre-excitation revisited. Amer. J. Cardiol. **25,** 690 (1970)
22. Ferrer, M. I.: New concepts relating to the preexcitation syndrome. J. Amer. med. Ass. **201,** 162 (1967)
23. Fruehan, C. T., Meyer, J. A., Klie, J. H., Johnson, L. W., Obeid, A. I., Smulyan, H., Eich, R. H.: Refractory paroxysmal supraventricular tachycardia. Treatment with patient controlled permanent radio frequency atrial pacemaker. Amer. Heart J. **87,** 299 (1874)
24. Garcia, R., Arciniegas, E.: Recurrent atrial flutter. Treatment with a surgical induced atrioventricular block and ventricular pacing. Arch. intern. Med. **132,** 754 (1973)
25. Gleichmann, U., Seipel, L., Loogen, F.: His-Bündel Elektrographie beim Präexcitationssyndrom. Verh. dtsch. Ges. Kreisl.-Forsch. **39,** 217 (1973)
26. Goldreyer, B. N., Damato, A. N.: The essential role of atrioventricular conduction delay in the initiation of paroxysmal supraventricular tachycardia. Circulation **43,** 679 (1971)
27. Goldreyer, B. N., Bigger, J. T.: Site of reentry in paroxysmal supraventricular tachycardia in man. Circulation **43,** 15 (1971)
28. Holzmann, M., Scherf, D.: Über Elektrokardiogramme mit verkürzter Vorhof-Kammer-Distanz und positiven P-Zacken. Z. klin. Med. **121,** 404 (1932)
29. Iannone, L. A.: Electrophysiology of atrial pacing in patients with short PR interval, normal QRS complex. Amer. Heart J. **89,** 74 (1975)
30. James, T. N.: The connecting pathways between the sinus node and the av node and between the right and left atrium in the human heart. Amer. Heart J. **66,** 498 (1963)
31. James, T. N.: Morphology of the human atrioventricular node with remarks pertinent to its electrophysiology. Amer. Heart J. **62,** 756 (1961)
32. James, T. N., Sherf, L.: Spezialized tissues and preferential conduction in the atria of the heart. Amer. J. Cardiol. **28,** 414 (1971)

33. Janse, M. J., Anderson, R. H.: Specialized internodal atrial pathways – fact or fiction? Europ. J. Cardiol. **2,** 117 (1974)
33 a. Kahn, A., Citron P.: Patient initiated rapid atrial pacing to manage supraventricular tachycardia. Circulation Suppl. **49 – 50**/III, 58 (1974)
34. Krishnaswami, V., Geraci, A. R.: Accelerated A-V conduction associated with complete A-V block. Amer. Heart J. **88,** 463 (1974)
35. Lown, B., Ganong, W. F., Levine, S. A.: The syndrome of short P-R interval, normal QRS complex and paroxysmal rapid heart action. Circulation **5,** 693 (1952)
36. Luckmann, E., Hossmann, V., Runge, M.: His-Bündel Elektrogramm beim Lown-Ganong-Levine-Syndrom. In: Diagnostik und Therapie von Herzrhythmusstörungen. Haan, D. (ed.). Uelzen: Med. Liter. Verl. Ges., 1973, p. 139
37. Mandel, W. J., Danzig, R., Hayakawa, H.: Lown-Ganong-Levine syndrome. Circulation **44,** 696 (1971)
38. Mandel, W. J., Laks, M. M., Obayashi, K., Bilder, P.: Prolongation of the tachycardia zone: A possible mechanism for medical failure in paroxysmal supraventricular tachycardia. Europ. J. Cardiol. **3,** 117 (1975)
39. Narula, O. S.: Retrograde pre-excitation. Comparison of antegrade and retrograde conduction intervals in man. Circulation **50,** 1129 (1974)
40. Neuss, H., Nowak, F. G.: Supraventrikuläre Tachykardien durch Erregungsumkehr im AV-Knoten. Herz Kreislauf **5,** 340 (1973)
41. Neuss, H., Schlepper, M., Thormann, J.: Analysis of re-entry mechanisms in three patients with concealed Wolff-Parkinson-White syndrome. Circulation **51,** 75 (1975)
42. Nowak, F. G., Neuss, H.: Verhalten der av-Überleitung unter Frequenzbelastung bei Patienten mit kurzer PQ-Zeit. Verh. dtsch. Ges. Kreisl.-Forsch. **40,** 406 (1974)
43. Pick, A., Katz, L. N.: Disturbances of impulse formation and conduction in the pre-excitation (WPW) syndrome. Amer. J. Med. **19,** 759 (1955)
44. Preston, J. B., McFadden, S., Moe, G. K.: Atrioventricular transmission in young mammals. Amer. J. Physiol. **197,** 236 (1959)
45. Reinikainen, M.: Observations on the syndrome with short P-Q interval and normal QRS complex. Ann. Med. intern. Fenn. **50,** 149 (1961)
46. Seipel, L., Both, A., Loggen, F.: Die atrioventrikuläre Erregungsleitung beim Lown-Ganong-Levine-Syndrom. Z. Kardiol. **64,** 20 (1975)
47. Seipel, L., Both, A., Loggen, F.: Klinische Bedeutung der His-Bündel Elektrographie. Klin. Wschr. **53,** 499 (1975)
48. Sherf, L., James, T. N.: A new electrocardiographic concept: Synchronized sinoventricular conduction. Chest **55,** 127 (1969)
49. Slama, R., Coumel, P., Motte, G., Blondeau, P., Aigueperse, J., Piwnica, A., Cachera, J. P., Bouvrain, Y.: Section volontaire di faisceau de His pour troubles du rhythme graves. Arch. Mal. Coeur **64,** 27 (1971)
50. So, C. S., Merkele, F.: Kurze PQ-Zeit unter besonderer Berücksichtigung des Lown-Ganong-Levine Syndroms. Münch. med. Wschr. **117,** 495 (1975)
51. Spurell, R. A. J., Krikler, D. M., Sowton, E.: Concealed bypasses of the atrioventricular node in patients with paroxysmal supraventricular tachycardia revealed by intracardiac stimulation and verapamil. Amer. J. Cardiol. **33,** 590 (1974)
52. Spracklen, F. H. N., Witham, A. C., Beck, W.: Pre-excitation of the right bundle of His. A new electrocardiographic syndrome. S. Afr. med. J. **48,** 1790 (1974)
53. Théry, C., Lékieffre, J., Carré, A., Warembourg, H.: Le syndrome PR court-QRS normal: Forme particulière de bloc sino-auriculaire? (Avec étude anatomique des voies de conduction). Arch. Mal. Coeur **67,** 797 (1974)
54. Tonkin, A. M., Gallagher, J. J., Svenson, R. H., Wallace, A. G., Sealy, W. C.: Antegrade block in accessory pathway conduction in reciprocating tachycardia. Europ. J. Cardiol. **3,** 143 (1975)
55. Wedd, A. M.: Paroxysmal tachycardia. With reference to normotopic tachycardia and the role of extrinsic cardiac nerves. Arch. intern. Med. **27,** 571 (1921)
56. Wellens, H. J. J.: Electrical stimulation of the heart in the study and tratment of tachycardias. Leiden: H. E. S. Kroese, 1971

57. Wellens, J. J., Durrer, D.: The role of an accessory atrioventricular pathway in reciprocal tachycardia. Circulation **52,** 58 (1975)
58. Williams, D. O., Davison, P. H.: Long-term treatment of refractory supraventricular tachycardia by patient-controlled inductive atrial pacing. Brit. Heart J. **36,** 341 (1974)
59. Wise, J. R.: Patient-activated atrial pacing in the treatment of recurrent supraventricular tachycardia. Chest **65,** 212 (1974)
60. Wu, D., Denes, P., Dhingra, R., Pietras, R. J., Rosen, K. M.: New manifestations of dual A-V nodal pathways. Europ. J. Cardiol. **2,** 459 (1975)

The Wolff-Parkinson-White Syndrome

H. J. J. WELLENS

In the patient with the Wolff-Parkinson-White (WPW) syndrome occurrence and severity of cardiac arrhythmias will be influenced by the electrophysiologic properties of the accessory atrioventricular connection.

The introduction of programmed electrical stimulation of the heart [5] made it possible to study these properties directly in the patient suffering from the syndrome. Over the past years this method of investigation has been applied to 125 patients with the WPW syndrome, referred to the University Department of Cardiology in Amsterdam. Results of these studies will be discussed in this article.

Material and Methods

Techniques of programed electrical stimulation have been described elsewhere [18]. One hundred and twenty-five patients were studied. Age varied from 8 to 76 years. There were 82 males and 43 females. Classification according to type of WPW was done by applying Rosenbaum's classification [11] to QRS configuration of the earliest atrial premature beat conducted over the accessory pathway during atrial pacing [19]. Eighty-five patients were classified as type A, and 34 as type B. Six patients could not be classified. The configuration of their QRS complex in lead V_1 fit neither the criteria for type A, nor for type B.

Electrophysiologic Properties of the Accessory Pathway

When the single test stimulus technique was applied during atrial pacing and the shortest value chosen from pacing at three different basic pacing rates, the effective refractory period of the accessory pathway was found to vary from 180 to 800 ms. In 40 patients the length of the effective refractory period of the accessory pathway was 250 ms or less. Table 1 shows age, variation in length, and the mean value of the effective refractory period of the accessory pathway in atrioventricular direction of the 125 patients studied. It has been suggested that the length of the effective refractory period of the accessory pathway increases with age [7]. The mean values shown in Table 1 do not support this supposition in the age group 11 – 60 years. Not enough data are available from patients under 10 and above 60 years of age. Single determinations of the length of the effective refractory period of the accessory pathway in different age groups do not,

Table 1. Relation between age, range, and mean value of effective refractory period of accessory pathway (ERP_{AP})

Age (years)	No Patients	Range ERP_{AP} (ms)	Mean ERP_{AP} (ms)
0 – 10	1		180
11 – 20	21	200 – 800	285
21 – 30	33	200 – 600	310
31 – 40	21	180 – 530	301
41 – 50	21	220 – 700	330
51 – 60	21	200 – 700	310
61 – 70	6	240 – 600	360
> 70	1		410

Table 2. Criteria for differentiation during ventricular pacing between ventriculoatrial conduction over accessory pathway and over His-AV node pathway

A Suggestive for VA conduction over accessory pathway:

1. Absence of increase in VA conduction time following stimuli given with increasing prematurity
2. Activation of low left atrium (in case of a left-sided accessory pathway) or activation of low right atrium (if a lateral right-sided accessory pathway is present) prior to atrial activation in His bundle recording.
3. A time relation between retrograde His bundle activation and retrograde atrial activation not compatible with VA conduction over AV node (either a short interval between His and retrograde atrial activation, or activation of bundle of His synchronous with or following retrograde atrial activation)
4. No change in VA conduction time following administration of atropine

B Suggestive for VA conduction over His-AV node pathway:

1. Gradual increase in VA conduction time with appearance of His bundle electrogram and a pro rata contribution of VA time to increase in VA time following ventricular stimuli given with increasing prematurity
2. Simultaneous activation of low left atrium and atrial activation in His bundle recording
3. Shortening of VA conduction time following administration of atropine

however, give information on the natural history of the electrophysiologic properties of the accessory pathway in the individual patient. Only follow-up studies in the same patient can answer that question.

When conduction over the accessory pathway is stressed by pacing the atrium at increasing pacing rates, block in the accessory pathway characteristically shows a sequence of Mobitz II block, 2 to 1 block, complete block. This is different from the pattern of block developing in the AV node on increasing pacing rate. As known, a Wenckebach type of 2nd degree block precedes 2 to 1 block and complete AV block. During pacing of the ventricle it is possible to study the electrophysiologic properties of the accessory pathway in ventriculoatrial direction. It is important to know how to differentiate between ventriculoatrial conduction over the accessory pathway and over the His-AV node pathway. This is possible by the application of the criteria listed in Table 2. As shown in Table 2 simultaneous registration of atrial activation in the left atrium, the right atrium, and low right atrium at the site of the His bundle recording is essential for determination of VA conduction in patientswith the WPW syndrome [15]. Table 3 shows the results when the criteria proposed in Table 2 were applied to the 125 patients studied. In 20 patients the pathway used during VA conduction could not be decided upon, usually because no left atrial recording was available. It was not possible to predict the properties of the accessory pathway in VA direction from data on the accessory pathway obtained during atrial pacing. In those patients where the length of the refractory period of the accessory pathway could be determined, at identical basic pacing lengths, both in AV and VA direction, the latter was usually found to be shorter [24]. This was recently confirmed by Tonkin et al. [16].

Table 3. Properties of pathway of VA conduction

– Absent	9
– Accessory pathway only or $ERP_{accessory\ pathway} \leqq ERP_{His\text{-}AVN}$	82
– His-AVN only or $ERP_{His\text{-}AVN} < ERP_{accessory\ pathway}$	14
– Unclassifiable	20

Mechanisms of Tachycardia

One hundred and ten of our 125 patients had ECG documentation of tachycardia (Table 4). Six more had a history of tachycardias. During the stimulation study tachycardias with a regular rhythm could be initiated in 98 patients. Site of origin and pathway of tachycardia are listed in Table 5. It was possible in one patient to initiate a ventricular tachycardia by a single atrial premature beat during atrial pacing [27] and in two other patients, an atrial tachycardia by a ventricular premature beat during ventricular pacing. In the majority of patients a tachycardia could be initiated with a tachycardia pathway incorporating the AV node and the accessory pathway. Criteria to differentiate between this type of tachycardia and AV nodal reentrant tachycardia have recently been described [26]. As known, a circusmovement tachycardia incorporating both the AV node and the accessory pathway usually shows AV conduction over the node and VA conduction over the accessory pathway [21]. This type of tachycardia can be initiated by a single atrial premature beat when during atrial pacing the effective refractory period of the accessory pathway is longer than the effective refractory period of the AV node. The same type of tachycardia can be initiated by a ventricular premature beat during ventricular pacing. Then the effective refractory period of the accessory pathway has to be shorter than the effective refractory period of the His-AV node pathway. Since the effective refractory period of the accessory pathway shortens [16, 25], and the effective refractory period of the AV node lengthens, on increasing basic pacing rate, it follows that in order to facilitate initiation of tachycardia during cardiac pacing atrial pacing should be done at the slowest possible pacing rate and ventricular pacing at a fast pacing rate. Termination of a circus-movement tachycardia can be accomplished by creating an area of refractoriness ahead of the circulating impulse [5]. When pacemaker implantation is considered for long-term treatment of

Table 4. Type tachycardia electrocardiographically documented in 125 patients studied

Documented atrial fibrillation	21
Documented supraventricular tachycardia	78
Documented atrial fibrillation + supraventricular tachycardia	11

Table 5. Type tachycardia initiated during electrical stimulation

Atrial tachycardia	2
AV nodal tachycardia	8
CM tachycardia incorporating AP	72
Ventricular tachycardia	1
Undetermined	15

Abbreviations:
AP = Accessory pathway
CM = Circus movement

patients with the WPW syndrome suffering from circus-movement tachycardia it is essential to determine the pathway used during tachycardia to insure proper selection of the stimulation site for the permanently implanted electrode.

The Role of a "Concealed" Accessory Pathway in Tachycardia

As described the properties of the accessory pathway differ when antegrade and retrograde conduction over this structure are compared. As listed in Table 3 nine of 125 patients with intact conduction in AV direction failed to show conduction in VA direction over the accessory pathway. Recently, examples of the reverse situation have been published [3, 9, 12, 25, 26, 30]. In these patients an accessory pathway only conducting in VA direction can be incorporated in the tachycardia circuit. Elucidation of such a situation is of obvious importance not only as far as drug therapy or implantation of a pacemaker is concerned but also when surgical interruption of the tachycardia circuit is considered.

Atrial Fibrillation and the WPW Syndrome

Under normal circumstances the properties of the AV node protect the ventricle against high ventricular rates when atrial fibrillation supervenes. In patients with the WPW syndrome this is not true when the accessory pathway has a short effective refractory period. The development of ventricular fibrillation following onset of atrial fibrillation has been reported in these patients [1, 2, 4, 8, 17]. Thirty-two of our patients had electrocardiographic documentation of atrial fibrillation. Concomitant heart disease, which may have precipitated the occurrence of the arrhythmia, is listed in Table 6. It is of interest that in 17 patients no cardiac abnormality other then the WPW syndrome could be identified. Sixteen of these 17 patients

Table 6. Cardiac abnormalities in patients with WPW syndrome suffering from atrial fibrillation

Rheumatic heart disease	6
Coronary heart disease	3
Sick Sinus	3
Ebstein's anomaly	1
Prolapse mitral valve	2
No abnormality identifiable	17
	32

had type A WPW, 12 were under 40 years of age, and 7 under 30 years of age. This suggests that the presence of an accessory pathway (especially when type A) predisposes to the development of atrial fibrillation. We have found that atrial fibrillation in patients with the WPW syndrome can be initiated by a ventricular premature beat which is conducted over the accessory pathway towards the atrium and also by deterioration of a circus-movement tachycardia into atrial fibrillation.

The dangers of atrial fibrillation for the individual patient with the WPW syndrome can be predicted from the outcome of the stimulation study. A good correlation has been demonstrated between the length of the effective refractory period of the accessory pathway and the mean ventricular rate during atrial fibrillation [16, 25].

Effect of Drugs

The effect of several drugs on the electrophysiologic properties of the accessory pathway and the AV node has been studied (Table 7). During nearly all these investigations the drug was given intravenously over a short period of time. One should realize that these data must be used with caution in predicting the effect after oral drug administration.

Table 7. Effect of drugs on accessory pathway and AV node in patients with the WPW syndrome [7, 10, 13, 14, 20, 22, 23, 29]

	Change in RP AV node	Change in RP AP
Digitalis	+	–
Quinidine	– ← → +	0 ← → +
Procaineamide	0	+
Ajmaline	0	+
Lidocaine	0	0 ← → +
Propranolol	+	0
Verapamil	+	– ← → 0
Atropine	–	0
Disopyramide	0 ← → +	0 ← → +
Amiodarone	+	+
Diphenylhydantoin	– ← → +	0 ← → +

Abbreviations:
AP = accessory pathway;
RP = refractory period;
– = shortening;
+ = lengthening;
0 = no change

Differences in pharmacokinetics following venous versus oral administration may explain why a drug which was found to be useful following venous administration is found to be ineffective when given orally. Stimulation studies correlating the effects following acute (intravenous) and chronic (oral) administration are needed to decide upon the relevance of the results from the acute study for further oral treatment [28].

Indications for Stimulation Studies in the Patient with the WPW Syndrome

Programmed electrical stimulation of the heart should be done in:

1. Patients with documented episodes of atrial flutter or atrial fibrillation with high ventricular rate. The length of the effective refractory period of the accessory pathway should be measured and the drug determined that causes the greatest amount of lengthening of that refractory period. If lengthening of the refractory period of the accessory pathway can not be accomplished by pharmacologic means, surgical interruption of the accessory pathway should be considered.
2. Patients whose tachycardias can not be controlled by drug therapy: In these patients site and mechanism of tachycardia should be studied. Based upon the outcome of these studies the drug that seems most appropriate should be given and its effect evaluated. If drug therapy is unsuccessful the feasibility of therapy by a chronically implanted pacemaker or the necessity of surgical interruption of the tachycardia circuit should be determined.

Preferably all patients with the WPW syndrome should be studied by programmed stimulation. Only by doing this and by repeating the study over the years can the natural history of the properties of the accessory pathway be elucidated. Especially needed is this information for guiding the asymptomatic patient who has a short refractory period of his accessory pathway.

Summary

Data are discussed from programmed electrical stimulation in 125 patients with pre-excitation, with emphasis upon:

1. Classification of pre-excitation.
2. Properties of the accessory pathway in AV and VA direction.
3. Mechanisms of tachycardia.
4. Atrial fibrillation and pre-excitation.
5. Effect of drugs.

References

1. Ahlinger, S., Granath, A., Holmer, S.: Wolff-Parkinson-White syndrom med paroxysmal atrieflimmer overgaende i ventrikelflimmer. Nord méd **70,** 1336 (1963)
2. Castillo-Fenoy, A., Goupil, A., Offenstadt, G.: Syndrome de Wolff-Parkinson-White et mort subite. Ann. Méd. Interne (Paris) **124,** 871 (1973)
3. Coumel, Ph., Attuel, P.: Reciprocating tachycardia in overt and latent pre-excitation. Influence of functional bundle branch block on the rate of the tachycardia. Europ. J. Cardiol. **1,** 423 (1974)
4. Dreifus, L. S., Haiat, R., Watanabe, Y., Truex, R.: Ventricular fibrillation: a possible mechanism of sudden death in patients with the Wolff-Parkinson-White syndrome. Circulation **43,** 520 (1971)
5. Durrer, D., Schoo, L., Schuilenburg, R. M., Wellens, H. J. J.: Role of premature beats in the initiation and the termination of supraventricular tachycardia in the Wolff-Parkinson-White syndrome. Circulation **36,** 644 (1967)
6. Mandel, W. J., Laks, M., Obayashi, K., Clifton, J.: Electrophysiologic features of the W.P.W. syndrome: modification by procaine amide (abstr.) Circulation **48** – IV: 195 (1973)
7. Mandel, W. J., Laks, M. M., Fink, B., Obayashi, K.: Comparative electrophysiologic features of the W.P.W syndrome in the pediatric and adult patient. Amer. J. Cardiol. **33,** 155 (1974)
8. Martin-Noel, P., Denis, B., Grunwald, D.: Deux cas mortels de syndrome de Wolff-Parkinson-White. Arch. Mal. Coeur **63,** 1647 (1970)
9. Neuss, H., Schlepper, M., Thormann, J.: Analysis of re-entry mechanisms in three patients with concealed W.P.W syndrome. Circulation **51,** 75 (1975)
10. Rosen, K. M., Bärwolf, C., Elsani, A., Rahimtoola, S. H.: Effects of lidocaine and propranolol in the normal and anomalous pathways with pre-excitation. Amer. J. Cardiol. **30,** 801 (1972)
11. Rosenbaum, F. F., Hecht, H. H., Wilson, F. N., Johnston, E. D.: Potential variations of the thorax and the esophagus in anomalous atrioventricular excitation (Wolff-Parkinson-White syndrome). Amer. Heart J. **29,** 281 (1945)
12. Spurrell, R. A. J., Krikler, D. M., Sowton, E.: Concealed bypass of the atrioventricular node in patients with paroxysmal supraventricular tachycardia revealed by intracardiac electrical stimulation and verapamil. Amer. J. Cardiol. **33,** 590 (1974)

13. Spurrell, R. A. J., Krikler, D. M., Sowton, E.: Effects of verapamil on electrophysiological properties of anomalous atrioventricular connection in Wolff-Parkinson-White syndrome. Brit. Heart. J. **36**, 256 (1974)
14. Spurrell, R. A. J., Thorburg, C. W., Camm, J., Sowton, E., Deuchar, D. C.: Effects of disopyramide on electrophysiological properties of specialized conduction system in man and on accessory atrioventricular pathway in Wolff-Parkinson-White syndrome. Brit. Heart. J. **37**, 861 (1975)
15. Svenson, R. H., Miller, H. C., Gallagher, J. J., Wallace, A. G.: Electrophysiological evaluation of the Wolff-Parkinson-White syndrome: Problems in assessing antegrade and retrograde conduction over the accessory pathway. Circulation **52**, 552 (1975)
16. Tonkin, A. M., Miller, H. C., Svenson, R. H., Wallace, A. G., Gallagher, J. J.: Refractory period of the accessory pathway in the Wolff-Parkinson-White syndrome. Circulation **52**, 563 (1975)
17. Touche, M., Jouvet, M., Touche, S.: Fibrillation ventriculaire au cours d'un syndrome de Wolff-Parkinson-White. Réduction par choc électrique externe. Arch. Mal. Coeur **59**, 1122 (1966)
18. Wellens, H. J. J.: Electrical Stimulation of the Heart in the Study and treatment of Tachycardias. Baltimore: University Park Press, 1971
19. Wellens, H. J. J.: Contribution of cardiac pacing to our understanding of the Wolff-Parkinson-White syndrome. Brit. Heart J. **37**, 231 (1975)
20. Wellens, H. J. J.: Effect of drugs on Wolff-Parkinson-White syndrome. In: His Bundle Electrography and Clinical Electrophysiology. Narula, O. (ed.) Philadelphia: F. A. Davis, 1975, p. 367
21. Wellens, H. J. J.: The Wolff-Parkinson-White and related syndrome. II The value of cardiac pacing in study and treatment. In: Cardiac Arrhythmias. Krikler, D. M., Goodwin J. F. (eds.) London: W. B. Saunders, 1975, p. 162
22. Wellens, H. J. J., Durrer, D.: Effect of digitalis on atrioventricular conduction and circus-movement tachycardias in patients with Wolff-Parkinson-White syndrome. Circulation **47**, 1229 (1973)
23. Wellens, H. J. J., Durrer, D.: Effect of procaine amide, quinidine and ajmaline in the Wolff-Parkinson-White syndrome. Circulation **50**, 114 (1974)
24. Wellens, H. J. J., Durrer, D.: Patterns of ventriculo-atrial conduction in the Wolff-Parkinson-White syndrome. Circulation **49**, 22 (1974)
25. Wellens, H. J. J., Durrer, D.: Wolff-Parkinson-White syndrome and atrial fibrillation. Amer. J. Cardiol. **34**, 777 (1974)
26. Wellens, H. J. J., Durrer, D.: The role of an accessory A – V pathway in reciprocal tachycardia. Observations in patients with and without the Wolff-Parkinson-White syndrome. Circulation **52**, 58 (1975)
27. Wellens, H. J. J., Lie, K. I., Durrer, D.: Further observations on ventricular tachycardia as studied by electrical stimulation of the heart. Circulation **49**, 647 (1974)
28. Wellens, H. J. J., Liem, K. L., Düren, D. R., Lie, K. I.: Effect of digitalis on A – V nodal tachycardia. Circulation **52**, 779 (1975)
29. Wellens, H. J. J., Lie, K. I., Bär, F., Dohmen, H., Düren, D. R., Durrer, D.: Effect of amiodarone in the Wolff-Parkinson-White syndrome. Amer. J. Cardiol.: in press.
30. Zipes, D. P., De Joseph, R. L., Rothbaum, D. A.: Unusual properties of accessory pathways. Circulation **49**, 1200 (1974)

III. Supraventricular and Ventricular Tachycardias

An in vitro Model of Circulating Excitation in the Absence of an Anatomic Obstacle

M. A. ALLESSIE, F. I. M. BONKE, F. J. G. SCHOPMAN, and W. J. E. P. LAMMERS

The theory of reentry and circus movement of the impulse as a basis for arrhythmias of the heart is very old. Already in 1887, McWilliam described the state of arrhythmic fibrillar contraction (delirium cordis), writing: "The peristaltic contraction travelling along such a structure as the ventricular wall must reach adjacent muscle bundles at different points of time, and since these bundles are connected with one another by anastomosing branches the contraction would naturally be propagated from one contracting fibre to another over which the contraction wave had already passed. Hence the movement would tend to go on until the excitability of the muscular tissue had been lowered, so that it failed to respond with a rapid series of contractions." It is noteworthy that it is not the heart in which circus movement was demonstrated for the first time. The earliest experimental production of circulating excitation was carried out in rings cut from subumbrella tissue of the jellyfish Scyphomedusa [10] (Fig. 1).

It seems questionable whether Mayer himself was fully aware of the importance of this observation with respect to cardiac arrhythmias, emphasizing that: "... isolated circuit-waves, moving constantly in one direction through a circuit, are *not met with* in nature. The heart, or pulsating medusa, contains within itself the means to *prevent* any single pulsation-wave from coursing constantly in one direction through the tissue... such a circuit wave can not take possession of the vertebrate heart." Inspried by these experiments, shortly thereafter, Mines [12] and Garrey [4], independently of each other, extended these experiments to rings of cardiac tissue. They confirmed the results of Mayer and emphasized the important role of circus movement of the impulse in the incidence of arrhythmias in the intact human heart. After reading the paper of Kent [9] in which a right lateral muscular connection between atria and ventricles was described, Mines [13] immediately realized the significance of such an anomalous pathway for the occurrence of tachycardia: Supposing that for some reason an impulse from the atrium reached the main AV bundle but failed to reach this "right lateral" connection. It is possible then that the ventricle would excite the ventricular end of this right lateral connection, not finding it refractory as normally it would at such a time. The wave spreading then to the atrium, might be expected to circulate around the path indicated." Since these early studies, many clinical observations and experimental investigations have provided a large body of evidence that many arrhythmias of the heart are based on a reentrant mechanism [15]. The prediction of Mines [13] about the possibility of circus movement of the impulse from atria → ventricles → atria → ventricles, etc. around the cavity of the heart

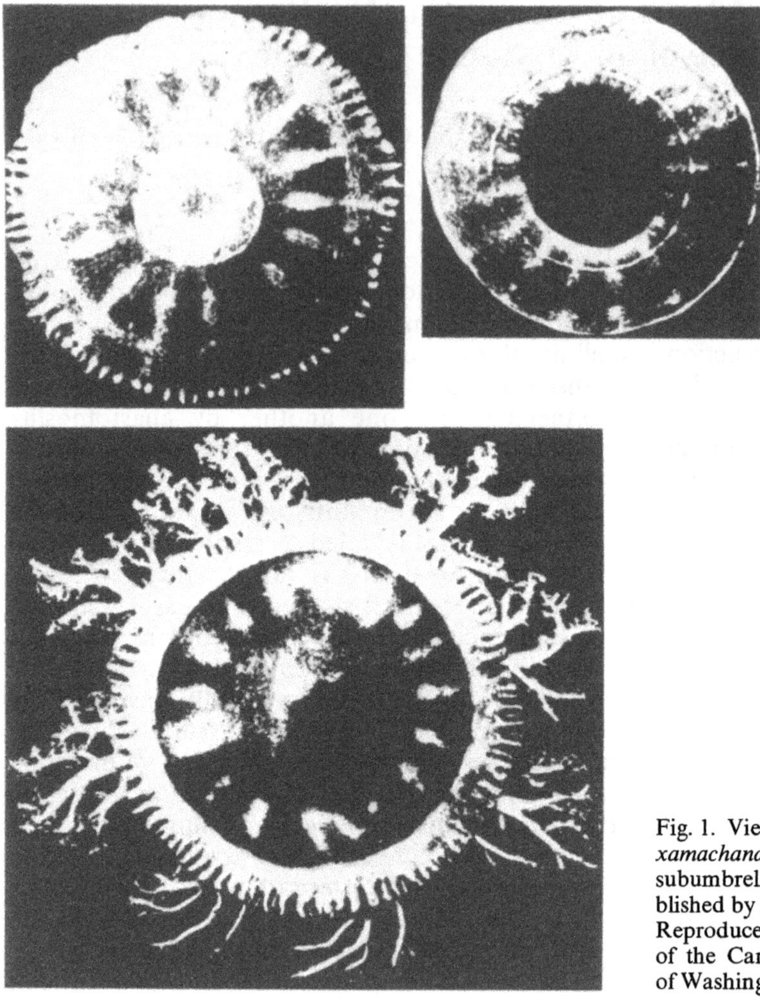

Fig. 1. Views of *Cassiopea xamachana* and the ring of subumbrella tissue, as published by Mayer (1908). Reproduced by permission of the Carnegie Institution of Washington.

has been completely confirmed in patients with the WPW syndrome [3]. Furthermore, evidence has been gathered that some cases of atrial flutter are due to circus movement around the entrances of the caval or pulmonary veins, or around the atrioventricular orifice [16]. Demonstration of circus movement in isolated loops of the Purkinje network offered a possible explanation for some forms of ventricular tachycardia [18].

However, besides this type of circus movement around a gross anatomic obstacle, another form of circus movement can be distinguished in which no central anatomic obstacle is involved [1]. Reentry within the SA node [6] or the AV node [7] might serve as other examples of this latter type of circus movement. Although circus movement in the AV node is described in terms of so-called α and β pathways, the present state of our knowledge does not allow a decision as to whether these pathways have an anatomical substrate or whether they are solely characterized by electrophysiologic differences. Also, on the hypothesis that fibrillation is based on the existence of multiple circulating wavelets [14], the possibility of reentry in small areas of the myocardium is a *conditio sine qua non.*

Circus Movement Within Small Segments of Atrial Muscle

To study the nature and behavior of circus movement in the absence of a central anatomic obstacle, we developed an in vitro model in which circulating excitation can be produced repeatedly by the induction of a single properly timed premature beat. Small segments of atrial muscle were excised from the left atrium of the rabbit. The preparations, measuring about 15×15 mm, consisted of a portion of the atrial appendage and an adjacent part of the body of the atrium. The interatrial band and the part of the atrium containing the entrances of the pulmonary veins were dissected and discarded. Because the preparations did not show any spontaneous activity, they were electrically paced at a regular rate (interval 500 ms). Periods of tachycardia were induced experimentally by the local application of a single properly timed premature stimulus (duration 1 ms, strength 4 times diastolic threshold) after each 20th basic stimulus. In most preparations one or more sites could be found where the induction of a premature impulse evoked "spontaneous" activity, varying from just one

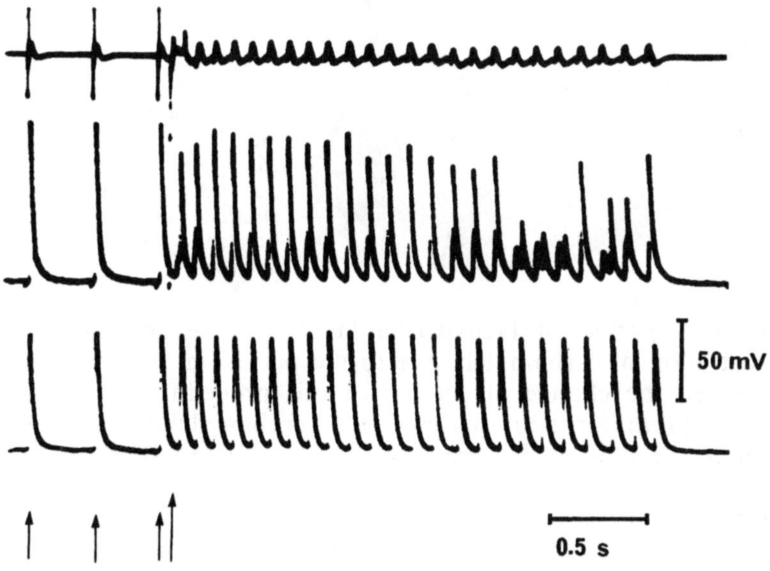

Fig. 2. Electrogram (*top*) and simultaneous intracellular recordings (*bottom*) during initiation of paroxysm of atrial tachycardia by induction of single premature beat. Stimuli are indicated by arrows.

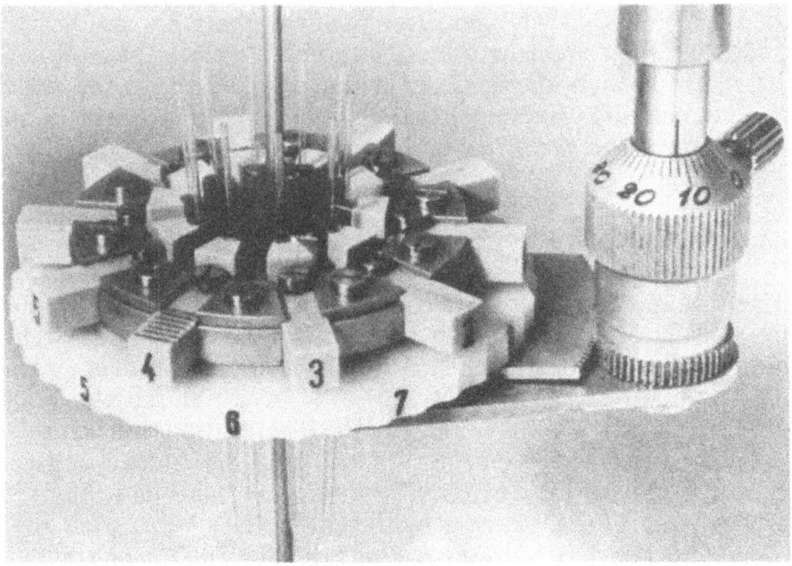

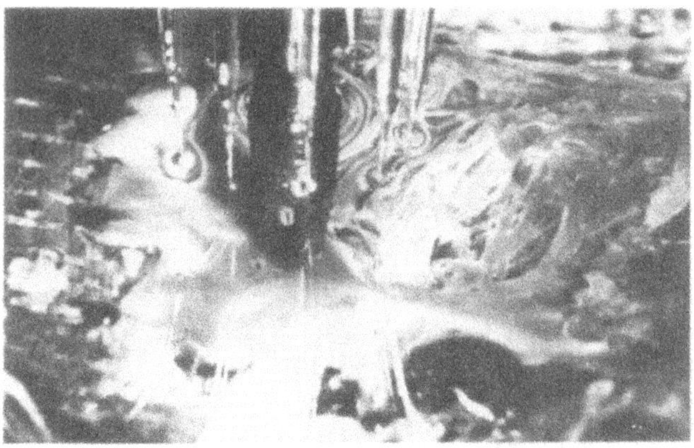

Fig. 3. Apparatus for multiple intracellular recording. Ten microelectrodes are fixed in separate holders mounted on a circle. In the center of the microelectrodes a stimulating electrode is placed. By turning the white wheel, the position of the microelectrodes can be adjusted concentrically. The pinion shown at the right is used to change the position of the electrodes radially over an angle of 36°.
Bottom: Close-up of the electrode arrangement on isolated segment of left atrial muscle.

extra discharge to a period of tachycardia lasting for several minutes (Fig. 2). Administration of carbamylcholine to the perfusion fluid (10^{-6} to 10^{-7} g/ml) enhanced the chance of success of this procedure. Not only was the timing of the premature stimulus less critical, carbamylcholine also increased the number of sites in the preparation where a test stimulus resulted in a paroxysm of tachycardia. Moreover the tachycardias tended to last much longer, in some cases more than 1 h.

To study the sequence of activation during initiation, continuation, and termination of an episode of tachycardia we used a multiple microelectrode technique. Figure 3 shows the apparatus which was developed to manipulate 10 microelectrodes together [17]. Each microelectrode is mounted in a

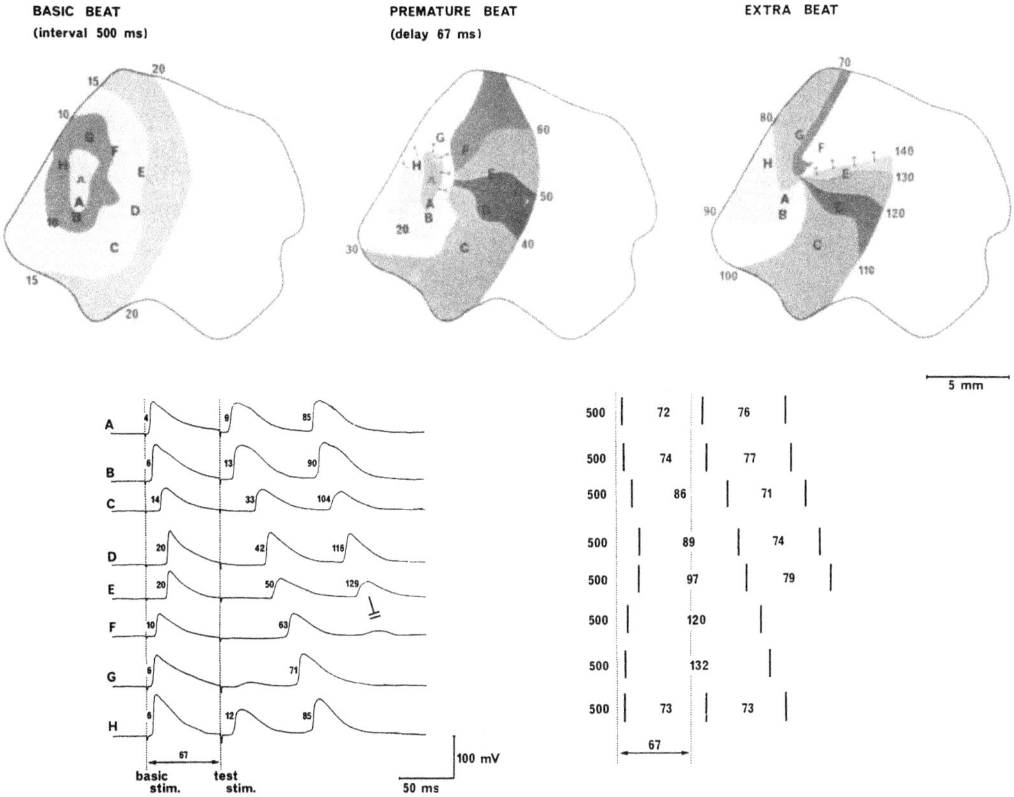

Fig. 4. Maps of spread of activation in a small piece of atrial muscle during regular driving (interval 500 ms), a premature beat (coupling interval 67 ms) and a subsequent "spontaneous" beat. Site of stimulation is indicated on maps by a stimulus symbol (⎍). Double bars indicate conduction block. At bottom the transmembrane potentials of eight fibers (*A*-*H*), as recorded around the site of stimulation, are given together with a ladder diagram of the coupling intervals of the different fibers. Activation times as well as coupling intervals are given in ms. See text for explanation.

separate holder. These holders are fitted on to a large wheel in such a way that by turning the wheel, all microelectrodes are displaced concentrically. With the pinion shown at the right, the position of the microelectrodes can be changed radially over an angle of 36°. With this apparatus attached to a manipulator driven by a stepper motor, and a stimulating electrode placed in the center of the microelectrodes, it is possible to record transmembrane potentials simultaneously at any distance around the site of stimulation. Figures 4 and 5 show the results of an experiment in which the excitation process was mapped with this multiple microelectrode technique. In this experiment a single premature stimulus, elicited 67 ms after the basic stimulus, was followed by two discharges. During basic rhythm, there was a more or less radial spread of the excitation wave from the site of stimulation. This conduction pattern was completely changed during the propagation of the premature impulse. First of all the speed of propagation was diminished considerably. The most striking change, however, was that orthograde conduction was succesful only in one direction (downward in Fig. 4, fibers A, B, and C). In the other directions (the upper and right side of the atrial segment, fibers D, E, F and G) the impulse was conducted only for a short distance before it died out completely. This decremental conduction resulting in local conduction block of the premature impulse is illustrated in Figure 5. In the area of block, the fibers a and b, which were

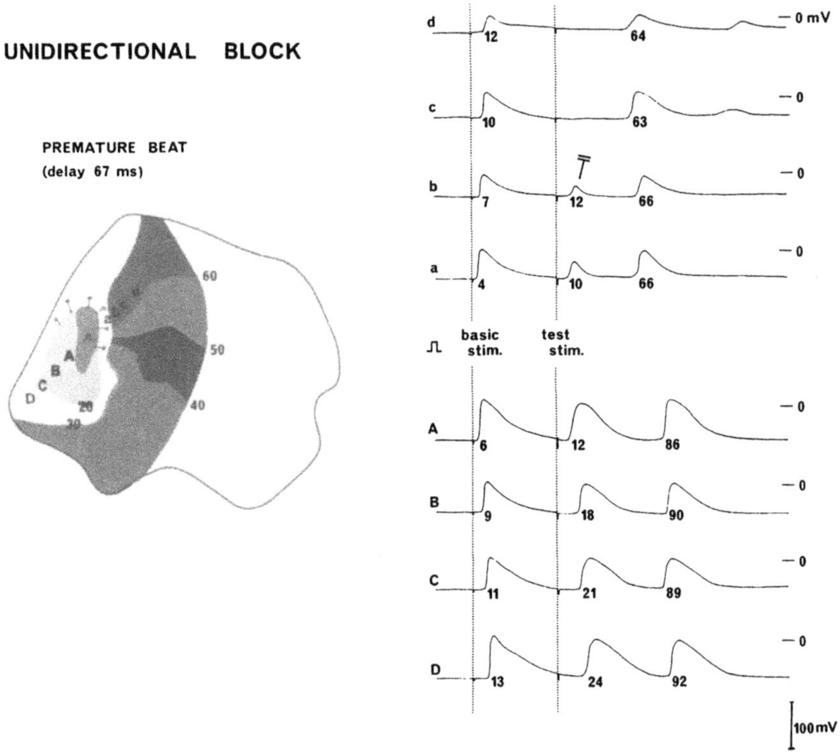

Fig. 5. Map of excitation of atrial segment during premature beat together with action potentials of four fibers on either side of stimulation electrode to demonstrate nature of unidirectional block. Fibers A-D respond with a full blown action potential to the premature stimulus. On the contrary, fibers a and b, at the opposite side of the stimulation electrode, only show a small response which is unable to excite fibers c and d.

rather close to the site of stimulation, still showed a premature response. However, this premature response, being of small amplitude and rate of rise and of short duration, was unable to excite the more remote fibers c and d. The occurrence of unidirectional conduction block forced the premature impulse to turn around the area where orthograde propagation had failed. The resulting sequence of activation can be traced from the maps and the intracellular recordings given in Figure 4.

During the premature beat the impulse was conducted in a roundabout way from fiber A to B to C ... G. As a result of this detour, fiber G was activated with a delay of as much as 71 ms after the premature stimulus. This long delay was sufficient for fiber H and A to restore their excitability after already being activated orthogradely. Consequently the turning excitation wave could re-excite these fibers in a retrograde direction and the impulse was entrapped in a circuitous route. On many occasions the impulse kept circulating for many revolutions, giving rise to longer or shorter periods of tachycardia. In the example shown here, the circulating impulse was already interrupted on its second round trip resulting in just one extra beat. The interruption of the circus movement took place in the area of fibers E and F. There the circulating impulse was conducted with decrement leading the complete extinction of the impulse. The last activity during the extra beat was recorded from fiber E. The relative action potential was of small amplitude and rate of rise. Fiber F only showed an electrotonic hump. This spontaneous interruption of a circus movement may occur when in a part of the circuit recovery of excitability lasts longer than the revolution time of the circulating impulse. As demonstrated earlier [2], the part of the atrium where orthograde conduction of the premature beat is blocked generally exhibits a longer refractory period than the area where direct propagation of the premature impulse is successful. Since in fibers E and F orthograde propagation of the premature impulse failed, it may be assumed that this area showed a relatively slow recovery of excitability. Furthermore, it can be expected that such a disparity in refractory periods along the circular pathway is enhanced after the premature beat. In the diagram next to the action potentials in Figure 4 it is shown that the abrupt change from a radial spread of the activation during basic rhythm into a circuitous propagation during the premature beat leads to great local differences in coupling interval between the basic action potential and the premature response. In this example the time interval between the depolarizations during the basic beat and the premature beat ranged from 72 ms in fiber A to 132 ms in fiber G. Since the rate of recovery of excitability depends on the duration of the preceding cycle length [5, 8], it may be expected that the refractory period after the premature beat will be progressively longer going from A to G. Consequently, on its second round trip the impulse will encounter tissue in a progressively less advanced state of excitability, which may result readily in extinction of the circulating impulse.

Theoretical Considerations on the Differences Between Circus Movement With and Without the Involvement of a Central Anatomical Obstacle

In the presence of a central anatomic obstacle, the length of a circular pathway is defined by the perimeter of the obstacle. Provided the perimeter of the obstacle is long enough with respect to the conduction velocity of the impulse and the refractory period of the tissue, the impulse will, on its circuitous route, find the tissue ahead recovered from the preceding excitation, and the process can sustain itself indefinitely. In such a circuit there is an "excitable gap" between the head and the tail of the circulating wave, i.e. the "wavelength" (the product of the refractory period and conduction velocity) is shorter than the length of the circuit. On the other hand, when an anatomic obstacle is not involved, the dimensions of a reentrant pathway will be determined by the shortest possible route in which the impulse can continue to circulate. Such a smallest possible circuit is characterized by the fact that the "stimulating efficacy" of the circulating wavefront is just enough to excite the tissue ahead which still is in its relative refractory phase. In such a circuit there is no excitable gap. The wave front is moving at submaximal speed through relatively refractory tissue. The wavelength of the circulating impulse is a "tight fit" with the length of the circuit. This implies that neither the dimensions nor the position of this type of circus movement are fixed. A change in the wavelength of the circulating excitation must lead to changes in position and length of the reentrant pathway. Thus it can be expected that a shortening of the refractory period or a depression of conduction velocity will result in a reduction of the proportions of the circus movement. On the other hand, prolongation of the refractory period or acceleration of the conduction will enlarge the minimal mass of cardiac tissue which is required for circus movement.

From the foregoing it may be expected that the two different models of circus movement will respond differently to variations in electrophysiologic properties of the fibers composing the circuit. Changes in conduction velocity or refractory period, occurring spontaneously or induced by cardiac drugs, might have a quite distinct effect on the frequency of both types of circus movement tachycardia. For instance, if the refractory period in atrial muscle is abbreviated by vagal stimulation or cholinergic drugs, the revolution time of circus movement around a gross obstacle will be only slightly influenced. As the length of the circular pathway is fixed, the main effect will be an enlargement of the excitable gap. The small acceleration of the conduction velocity in the myocardium which is associated with vagal stimulation will eventually result in a slight acceleration of the tachycardia. On the contrary, in the case of circus movement without a central obstacle, abbreviation of the refractory period will enable the impulse to circulate in a smaller circuit. This shortening of the path length, resulting in a marked decrease of the revolution time, may lead to a considerable acceleration of the tachycardia, or, as is often observed in clinical cases, the atria may be thrown into fibrillation.

Thus far, we have done only some preliminary experiments to test the validity of the models. We compared the effect of carbamylcholine (10^{-7} M) on the frequency of long-lasting tachycardias in rings of atrial muscle with the effect on tachycardias in intact segments of atrial myocardium. It was found that in the ring-shaped preparations, carbamylcholine had only a slight accelerating effect. Interruption of the tachycardia was never observed. In contrast, the rate of tachycardia in the intact preparations was increased considerably under the influence of carbamylcholine. In some cases the tachycardia was suddenly interrupted. Conversion of tachycardia into fibrillation did not occur, probably because the isolated pieces of myocardium were too small to accomodate more than one circulating impulse. These observations are in good agreement with the hypothesis of the two types of circus movement, pointing out that a circus-movement tachycardia may respond differently to changes in electrophysiologic properties of the heart, depending on the involvement of an anatomic obstacle. This might have important consequences for the treatment of tachyarrhythmias.

Summary

For the explanation of tachycardia and fibrillation two alternative mechanisms are available: that of ectopic rapid impulse formation and that of circus movement of the cardiac impulse. The concept of circulating excitation as proposed by Mines in 1913, is based on experiments with ring-shaped preparations cut from cardiac tissue. Since then, also in the intact heart, some cases of tachycardia have been found which are based on circus movement of the impulse around a gross anatomic obstacle like the entrance of the caval veins (atrial flutter) or the cavity of the heart (tachycardia associated with the WPW syndrome). Demonstration of circus movement around loops formed by the Purkinje network offered a possible explanation for ventricular tachycardia.

However, there is also evidence that reentry and circus movement can take place without the involvement of a large anatomic obstacle (reentrant tachycardias arising in the area of the AV or SA node). Furthermore, in the theory that fibrillation is based on the existence of multiple circulating wavelets, the possibilities of reentry in small areas of the myocardium is a "conditio sine qua non."

The authors studied the mechanism of tachycardias which can be evoked experimentally in small isolated segments of the left atrium of the rabbit by induction of a single properly timed premature beat. By means of multiple microelectrode recordings the excitation of the preparation during the initiation of tachycardia could be traced accurately. It could be demonstrated that the tachycardias were based on a circus movement of the impulse through a relatively small part of the myocardium. Circus movement was initiated because the impulse of the premature beat was conducted only in one direction, while in the other directions conduction occurred with decrement resulting in an antegrade conduction block. It turned out that the occurrence of unidirectional conduction block was caused by a considerable spatial dispersion in refractory periods.

Intracellular recordings from the center of the circulating excitation showed that this area was continuously invaded by centripetal wavelets. These observations resulted in a new model of circus movement (the "leading circle" concept) applicable to those cases of circulating excitation in which no central anatomic obstacle is involved.

References

1. Allessie, M. A., Bonke, F. I. M., Schopman, F. J. G.: Circus movement in rabbit atrial muscle as a mechanism of tachycardia. Circulat. Res. **33**, 54 – 62 (1973).
2. Allessie, M. A., Bonke, F. I. M., Schopman, F. J. G.: Circus movement in rabbit atrial muscle as a mechanism of tachycardia. II. The role of nonuniform recovery of excitability in the occurrence of unidirectional block, as studied with multiple microelectrodes. Circulat. Res. In press, 1976.
3. Durrer, D., Wellens, H. J. J.: The Wolff-Parkinson-White syndrome anno 1973. Europ. J. Cardiol. **1/4**, 347 – 367 (1974)
4. Garrey, W. E.: Nature of fibrillary contraction of the heart: its relation to tissue mass and form. Amer. J. Physiol. **33**, 397 – 414 (1914)
5. Han, J., Moe, G. K.: Nonuniform recovery of excitability in ventricular muscle. Circulat. Res. **14**, 44 – 60 (1964)
6. Han, J., Malozzi, A. M., Moe, G. K.: Sino-atrial reciprocation in the isolated rabbit heart. Circulat. Res. **22**, 355 – 362 (1968)
7. Janse, M. J., van Capelle, F. J. L., Freud, G. E., Durrer, D.: Circus movement within the AV node as a basis for supraventricular tachycardia as shown by multiple microelectrode recording in the isolated rabbit heart. Circulat. Res. **28**, 403 – 414 (1971)
8. Janse, M. J., Van der Steen, A. B. M., van Dam, R. Th., Durrer, D.: Refractory period of the dog's ventricular myocardium following sudden changes in frequency. Circulat. Res. **24**, 251– 261 (1969)
9. Kent, S. A. F.: Observations on the auriculo-ventricular junction of the mammalian heart. Quart. J. Physiol. **7**, 193 – 195 (1913)
10. Mayer, A. G.: Rhythmical pulsation in scyphomedusae: Part II. Papers Tortugas Lab Carnegie Institution of Washington **1**, 115 – 131 (1908)
11. McWilliam, J. A.: Fibrillar contraction of the heart. J. Physiol. (Lond.) **8**, 296 – 310 (1887)
12. Mines, G. R.: On dynamic equilibrium in the heart. J. Physiol. (Lond.) **46**, 349 – 383 (1913)
13. Mines, G. R.: On circulating excitations in heart muscles and their possible relation to tachycardia and fibrillation. Trans. Roy. Soc. Can. **4**, 43 – 53 (1914)
14. Moe, G. K.: On the multiple wavelet hypothesis of atrial fibrillation. Arch. int. Pharmacodyn. **140**, 183 – 188 (1962)
15. Moe, G. K.: Evidence for reentry as a mechanism of cardiac arrhythmias, Rev. Physiol. Biochem. Pharmac. **72**, 56 – 81 (1975)
16. Rytand, D. A.: Circus movement (entrapped circuit wave) hypothesis and atrial flutter. Ann. intern. Med. **65**, 125 – 159 (1966)
17. Schreurs, A. W., Selij, A. P. L., Allessie, M. A., Bonke, F. I. M.: A concentrically and radially adjustable holder for ten microelectrodes. Pflügers Arch. ges. Physiol. **346**, 167 – 170 (1974)
18. Wit, A. L., Cranefield, P. F., Hoffman, B. F.: Slow conduction and reentry in the ventricular conducting system. II. Single and sustained circus movement in networks of canine and bovine Purkinje fibers. Cirulat. Res. **30**, 11 – 22 (1972)

Clinical and Electrocardiographic Features of Supraventricular and Ventricular Tachycardias

D. M. Krikler

Introduction

One can make few useful generalizations about the clinical features of tachyarrhythmias, but the basic clinical tool used in their elucidation is the electrocardiogram; and, as we have heard during previous presentations, this is by no means the final diagnostic tool. Nevertheless it is the one that we most often use, and provided we have the necessary reservations about interpretation, it is a highly practical and indeed essential instrument. What we are here concerned with today are *tachyarrhythmias,* which can be irregular or regular, and which can be associated with two consequential features that may influence the clinical findings: atrioventricular block in the case of some supraventricular tachycardias, and atrioventricular dissociation as the hallmark, if not the invariable one, of ventricular tachycardias. Atrioventricular dissociation can of course occur in its own right under certain circumstances where the pulse rate is fast, but AV block in the presence of a normal sinus rate will require no further consideration because it will present as bradycardia.

Complicating AV block in the presence of supraventricular, and here we mean atrial, tachycardias, implies that the pulse rate, whether measured at the cardiac apex or one of the peripheral pulses, is lower than that of the pacemaker that dominates the heart. We might thus see evidence of rapid and often irregular pulsation in the neck veins, due to the fact that there will often be contraction of the rapidly beating atria against the closed atrioventricular valves. In the presence of AV dissociation such as may be seen with ventricular tachycardia, any atrial activity reflected in the neck veins will have the opposite characteristic: more slowly beating atria will contract intermittently against closed AV valves, producing slow irregular neck vein pulsations of varying intensity. Where the atria fail to contract in a meaningful fashion, e.g., atrial fibrillation, we have a combination of rapidly beating proximal chambers with a relative degree of block in the sense that the distal chambers are beating more slowly, yet without neck vein pulsation. So what we have is a spectrum of some use pointing towards the mechanism, but not always of absolute diagnostic importance.

A few other truisms should be taken into consideration. Ventricular tachycardias more usually complicate more serious cardiac disorders and are more often accompanied by hypotension and cardiac insufficiency, just as much due to the fact that cardiac action is less efficient in their presence. One does, however, see ventricular tachycardia relatively well tolerated, especially if of the uncommon benign variety, and very rapid supraventricular tachycardias extremely poorly tolerated especially if they complicate significant disorders, e.g., myocardial infarction, but on some occasions when unassociated with cardiac disease as such, in, for example, some reciprocating AV nodal tachycardias in which the heart rate is high.

In electrocardiographic diagnosis, one extends the clinical definitions and has the opportunity to see the relationship of atrial and ventricular contractions to each other in the vast majority of cases of tachyarrhythmias. Some of the aspects of the levels at which tachyarrhythmias and bradyarrhythmias are respectively diagnosed, and the mechanisms concerned, are not only reviewed elsewhere in this volume, but the features have been summarized elsewhere [3]. In broad terms rates above 100, in an adult, merit attention. There are two important qualifications; a rapid atrial rate with high-degree atrioventricular block may seem clinically normal, and enhancement of the rate of normal subsidiary pacemaking tissue may produce an arrhythmia within the "normal rate," e.g., atrioventricular dissociation or idioventricular tachycardia.

The occurrence of rapid heart rate may be due to enhancement of the automaticity of the SA node or of other automatic or potentially automatic tissues elsewhere in the heart, or the development of reciprocating mechanisms. When considering enhanced automaticity, one must be concerned not only with ectopic foci that discharge rapidly, but the possibility that the underlying situation is one of parasystolic tachycardia, and this may be seen if there is a varying degree of exit block complicating the tachycardia [2].

Paroxysmal Supraventricular Tachycardia

I. Sinus Tachycardia

Sinus tachycardia is usually due to an exaggeration of the physiologic mechanisms involved in the discharge of the SA node, and is recognized as much for the underlying factors that may produce it as for its electrocardiographic appearances which consist really of no more than sinus rhythm occurring more rapidly. Fever, anxiety, thyrotoxicosis, significant underlying disorders like myocardial infarction – all these factors are well known and require no specific elaboration, but careful clinical examination to define or exclude their presence is clearly of the utmost importance. However, we have recently learnt of the importance of *paroxysmal reciprocating sinus tachycardia.* It has long been suspected that reentry could involve the SA node, occurring as it does in the midst of atrial musculature, the interphase between the node and the neighboring tissues providing a theoretically feasible situation whereby this could occur. Others have noted isolated cases of sinus node reentry [5], with poorly sustained runs of beats. Our experience, based on the clinical detection of cases in which we suspected this disorder some 5 or 6 years ago, has enabled us to confirm with electrophysiologic techniques its existence in at least eight cases [1] and the electrocardiographic features of just such a patient are shown in Figure 1. As can be seen, the P waves in sinus tachycardia are virtually identical to those in sinus rhythm, and the sinus tachycardia is abruptly stopped by the application of carotid sinus pressure with resumption of sinus rhythm at a regular steady rate. Electrophysiologically we have been able to initiate and terminate attacks by suitably timed premature beats injected in the high right atrium close to the SA node. Sometimes there is an alteration in the P wave morphology due we think to

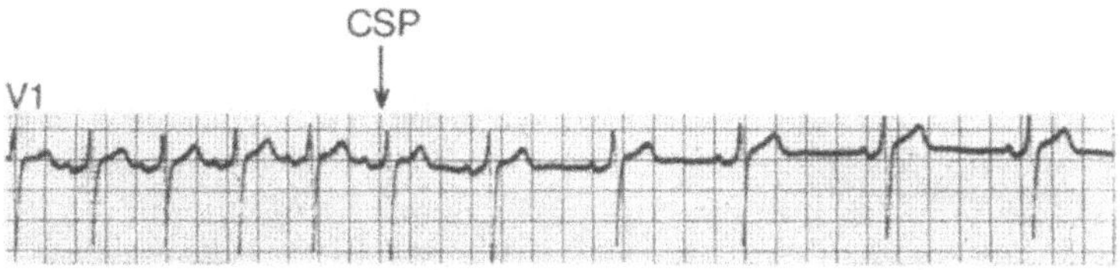

Fig. 1. Paroxysmal reciprocating sinus tachycardia (125 beats a minute) converted to normal sinus rhythm (67 beats a minute) by carotid sinus pressure.

intra-atrial conduction disturbance consequent upon the arrhythmia, but the direction of atrial activation is identical in our cases of paroxysmal reciprocating sinus tachycardia to that in sinus rhythm. The rate tends to be relatively slow, ranging between 90 – 140 beats a minute, though we have had patients in whom there have been much faster runs. Very often these patients have unjustifiably been diagnosed as suffering from anxiety states, and the correct identification of the mechanism has been of great clinical value to them, even if long-term therapy has not really been needed. Agents tending further to slow conduction, and perhaps preventing the establishment of the reentry circuit, e.g., verapamil and beta blockers, have proved most useful in our hands.

II. Reciprocating AV Tachycardia

Attacks with a regular rapid heart rate, with narrow QRS complexes, sudden in onset, and often with a previous history of self-limited episodes, are usually due to this cause. One deduces the presence of a reciprocating mechanism within the AV node, and a consequent regular 1 : 1 AV response. Whether the QRS complexes are preceded or followed by P waves, or whether the latter are hidden in the ventricular activity, is determined by the relative speeds of retrograde and anterograde conduction. Sometimes the QRS complexes are widened because of aberrant ventricular conduction, usually showing a right bundle branch block pattern but occasionally a left, or there may be concealed retrograde penetration of the impulse from one bundle branch into the other. Such tachycardias can often be stopped by vagotonic measures or by pharmacologic agents with similar properties, which, by interfering with conduction within the AV node, lengthen the reciprocating circuit until it can no longer support the continual reentry mechanism.

The above mechanism applies equally well to patients with the Wolff-Parkinson-White or other syndromes associated with anomalous extranodal pathways. During tachycardia the QRS complex will be narrow if the conduction is down the AV node and bundle of His, as it usually is, unless there is also rate-related or other aberration [4].

III. Atrial Tachycardia

Whether due to enhanced activity of atrial myocardial cells that now are able to discharge, or whether there is localized reentry, will be impossible to deduce from the ECG in a patient with paroxysmal atrial tachycardia. Abnormal P waves will be seen and there will be varying degrees of AV block in that the AV node may be unable to conduct the ectopic atrial stimuli in a 1 : 1 relationship either spontaneously or under the influence of vagotonic measures that fail to interrupt the tachycardia itself. The various possibilities are shown in Figure 2: one may get a regular atrial tachycardia with 1 : 1 conduction or with a fixed rate of AV block, or there may be a varying degree of block, sometimes seen as a chaotic atrial rhythm.

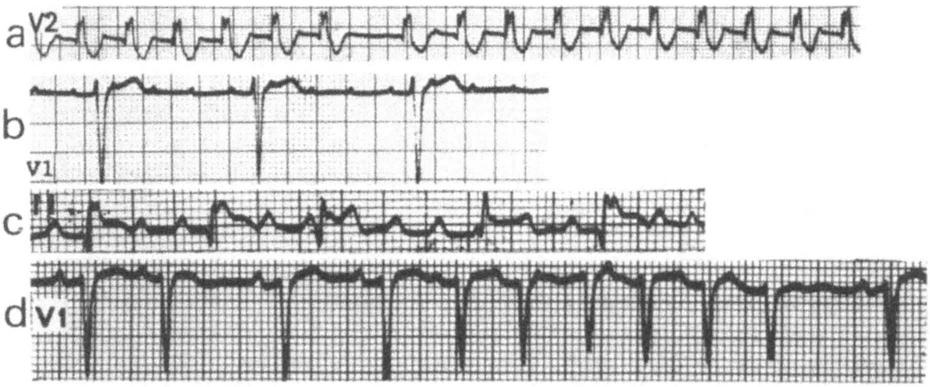

Fig. 2 a – d. Ectopic atrial tachycardia. (a) Atrial tachycardia with 1 : 1 atrioventricular relationship; paroxysm ends with sixth beat, another starts with eighth; seventh beat is of sinus origin. (b) 4 : 1 AV response. (c) Varying AV block. (d) Multifocal atrial tachycardia or so-called chaotic atrial rhythm. [3]

IV. Atrial Flutter and Fibrillation

These rhythms do not strictly fall within the definition of supraventricular tachycardias, but atrial flutter usually presents as a regular tachycardia with 2 : 1 AV response, and sometimes there may be difficulty clinically in making the diagnosis, and in distinguishing the disorder from a reciprocating AV nodal tachycardia or, more usually, from sinus tachycardia. Careful scrutiny of the tracings will usually reveal the nature of the disorder but this may not always be so in the uncommon form of atrial flutter [7]. The response to carotid sinus pressure is often helpful by inducing a high degree of AV block and allowing the underlying flutter waves to be seen more distinctly. The flutter waves are, where seen, always regular, and must be distinguished from the somewhat inconstant fluctuation sometimes encountered in atrial fibrillation; this can be quite coarse at times, but it is never consistently regular to the same extent as in flutter.

Paroxysmal Ventricular Tachycardia

It is becoming more and more apparent that many cases of ventricular tachycardia are due to reentry mechanisms and not enhanced focal activity, and this applies particularly in cardiac ischemia [9]. In the electrocardiographic diagnosis of ventricular tachycardia it is important to remember that wide QRS complexes may reflect aberrant conduction of supraventricular stimuli, and not necessarily indicate a ventricular mechanism. There are a number of types of ventricular tachycardia, illustrated in Figure 3, from which the important aspects of the electrocardiographic diagnosis can also be seen. While the tachycardia is usually regular, this is not always quite precise. Often this degree of irregularity will reflect the fact that the atria are beating at their inherent rate, dissociated from ventricular activity, and suitably timed sinus beats may be able to capture the ventricles either entirely or partially. When the ventricles are captured, the consequent QRS complex will resemble that seen in sinus rhythm; the intermediate situation, where QRS activity reflects both the abnormal ventricular beat and a degree of influence from the atrium, is a fusion complex. Sometimes, however, there is regular 1 : 1 ventriculo-atrial conduction, which can be seen on the ECG as an inverted P wave following each QRS, and here again distinction from supraventricular tachycardia with aberration becomes important. The electrocardiogram may be insufficient, and intracardiac recordings essential.

When ventricular tachycardia is initiated by an extrasystole falling on the T wave of the preceding sinus beat, the subsequent tachycardia complexes may be different, indicating localized reentry, as in Figure 3 b. On the other hand, the more classic appearances of ventricular tachycardia with capture and fusion are best seen when there is a slowly discharging idioventricular tachycardia (Fig. 3 c); this paradoxical situation is sometimes known by other names, e.g., slow ventricular tachycardia. It very often reflects the presence of a discharging focus situated fairly high in the intraventricular conduction system.

The atypical ventricular tachycardia called torsade de pointes is illustrated in Figure 3 d and further discussed elsewhere [3]. A relatively late ventricular extrasystole initiates an undulating series of QRS complexes, with spontaneous termination. Here the ECG appearances are all important as compared with intracardiac studies; and the underlying situations seen in the basic ECG tracing may be essential in order to define the situation. Thus evidence of QT prolongation, sinoatrial or atrioventricular block, or clinical knowledge of the possibility of hypokalaemia or the ingestion of cardiodepressive drugs like quinidine and phenothiazines will all help in the differential diagnosis.

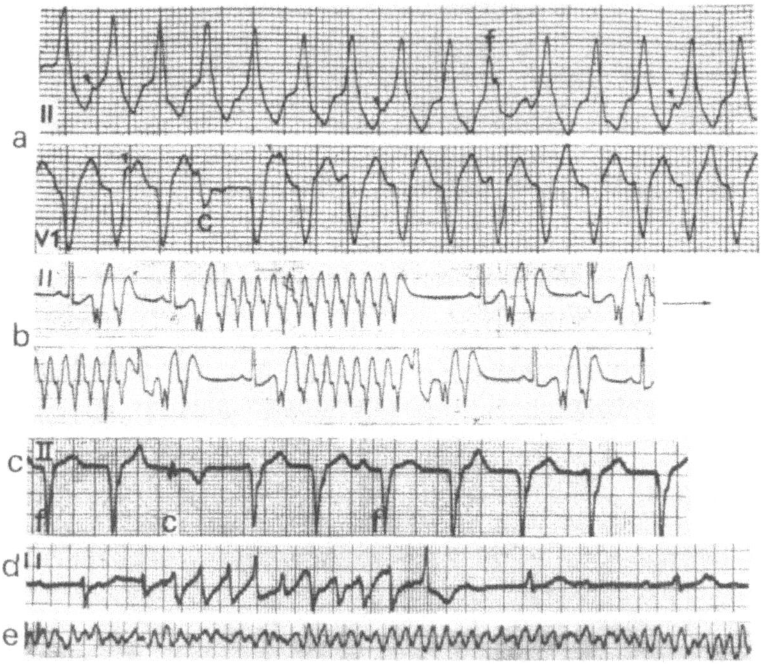

Fig. 3 a – e. Ventricular tachyarrhythmias. (a) Ventricular tachycardia with independent atrial acitivity (some P waves indicates by arrows) and AV dissociation; note fusion *f* and capture *c* beats. (b) Rapid ventricular tachycardia (300 a minute) ("ventricular flutter"), initiated by ventricular extrasystoles coinciding with T waves of sinus beats. Appearances suggest local ventricular reentry. (c) Idioventricular ("slow") ventricular tachycardia with fusion *f* and capture *c* beats. (d) Torsade de pointes complicating complete heart block. (e) Ventricular fibrillation. [3]

Some ventricular tachycardias are benign [6] and not all complicate serious organic cardiac disease. Here the clinical presentation is of the utmost importance and knowledge of a long history and absence of other illness or symptoms will provide useful information in helping define a good prognosis.

Ventricular fibrillation is of course the terminal end stage which is usually diagnosed as "cardiac arrest"; occasionally one sees it in a preterminal ECG (Fig. 3 e).

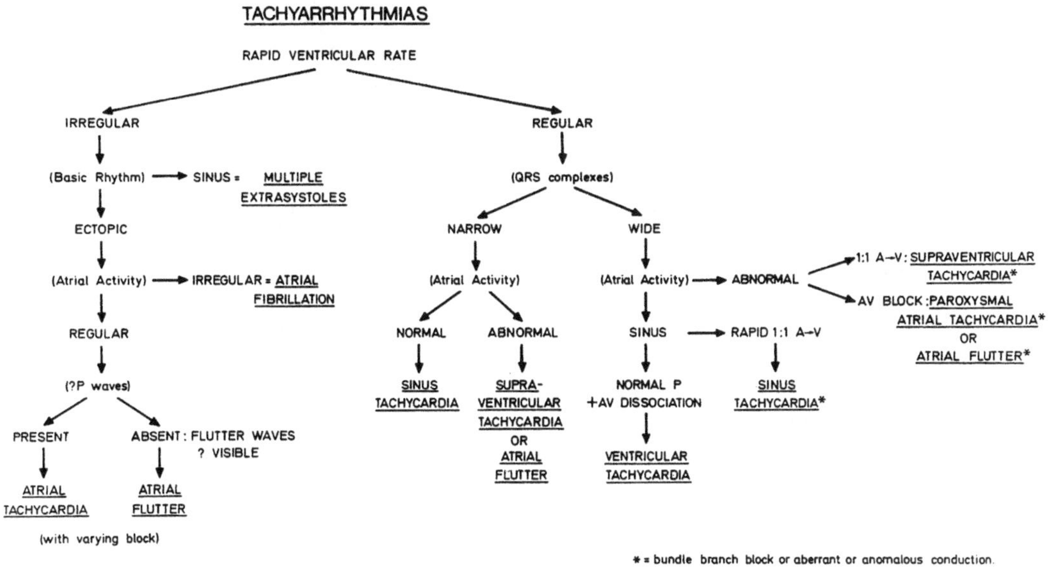

Fig. 4. Flow diagram showing ECG diagnostic approach to tachyarrhythmias. After each situation is recognized (block capitals), statement in parentheses provides next question. [3]

Electrocardiographic Diagnosis

In order to analyse rhythms meaningfully, one needs to approach the ECG in a logical manner. This can be helped by the use of a flow diagram (Fig. 4), in which tachyarrhythmias are subdivided according to whether or not a ventricular response is regular or irregular. Thereafter specific factors can be considered. Clearly the more complex and less common arrhythmias will require separate attention, and here one refers in particular to those complicated by AV dissociation. The important aspects to seek are the P waves and their relationship to the QRS complex, and analysis of the QRS morphology. Sandler and Marriott [8] have usefully distinguished between aberrant ventricular conduction and ventricular tachycardia as regards the different QRS morphologies produced, and as a general rule their comments are highly acceptable. Where typical right bundle branch block patterns are seen, where the QRS complexes all point in the same direction in the chest leads, where the QRS initial vector is the same in tachycardia as in the arrhythmia – under all these circumstances the evidence points towards aberration complicating supraventricular tachycardia.

When examining atrial activity, one must see whether the P waves have retained their normal shape, and note their relationship to the QRS complexes: Do they precede or follow them or are they buried within them, or is their morphology different in tachycardia from that in sinus rhythm? If atrioventricular dissociation can be identified, this can help distinguish supraventricular from ventricular tachycardias. The usefulness of carotid sinus pressure should not be forgotten; it tends to be particularly effective in reciprocating arrhythmias involving the AV node in one or both directions, and perhaps also in the reciprocating tachycardias that affect the SA node, its influence in ectopic atrial tachycardias being generally no more than to increase the degree of any AV block that is present or to induce this if it was absent.

Sometimes, of course, the clinical history gives useful information, and the physical signs of AV dissociation may be a helpful pointer to what will be found on the ECG. Having said all this, and having extracted the maximum of information from the ECG, one must concede that there are a number of cases in which a reliable diagnosis can only be achieved with the use of intracardiac electrography, and it may well be that programmed electric stimulation of the heart will also be needed in order to confirm the nature of the arrhythmia.

Summary

Provided electrocardiographic tracings are carefully examined, and read in conjunction with the clinical setting, it is usually possible to differentiate between supraventricular and ventricular tachycardias and to draw useful conclusions about the underlying mechanisms. There is usually little problem when tachycardias have narrow QRS complexes, when distinction between an atrial origin and reciprocation involving the AV node and/or an anomalous bypass is necessary. In the former case, the tachycardia usually persists under the influence of carotid sinus pressure though AV nodal block may be transiently produced, whereas the latter group either show no response at all or correction to sinus rhythm. An important additional group are the paroxysmal sinus tachycardias, which tend to be relatively slow, and in whom the P waves tend to resemble those seen in sinus rhythm.

The differential diagnosis of regular tachycardias with broad QRS complexes can be difficult. If AV dissociation with capture and fusion beats are seen, ventricular tachycardia can be diagnosed, but there are many reasons why intracardiac electrography may be required for confident distinction between supraventricular tachycardias with aberration on the one hand and ventricular tachycardia on the other. Some variant tachycardias including torsade de pointes have specific features, the diagnosis often being aided when tracings are available that show the previous rhythm and conduction patterns. Intracardiac recordings with programmed electric stimulation can be of diagnostic value in difficult cases and have helped greatly in the elucidation of mechanisms.

Acknowledgments

The work leading to this publication was supported in part by a grant from the British Heart Foundation. Figures 2, 3 and 4 are reproduced by permission of The Lancet.

References

1. Curry, P. V. L., Callowhill, E., Krikler, D. M.: Paroxysmal re-entry sinus tachycardia. Brit. Heart J. **38,** 311 (1976)
2. Friedberg, H. D.: Extrasystoles and parasystole. Brit. J. of hosp. Med. **5,** 148 – 163 (1971)
3. Krikler, D. M.: A fresh look at cardiac arrhythmias, Lancet **1,** 851 – 854, 913 – 918, 974 – 976, 1034 – 1037 (1974)
4. Krikler, D. M.: The Wolff-Parkinson-White and related syndromes. Part I: Presentations and implications. In: Cardiac Arrhythmias: The Modern Electrophysiological Approach. Krikler, D. M., Goodwin, J. F. (eds.), London-Philadelphia-Toronto: W. B. Saunders, 1975, pp. 144 – 161
5. Narula, O. S.: Sinus node re-entry. A mechanism for supraventricular tachycardia. Circulation **50,** 1114 – 1128 (1974)
6. Parkinson, J., Papp, C.: Repetitive paroxysmal tachycardia. Brit. Heart **8,** 241 – 262 (1947)
7. Puech, P., Latour, H., Grolleau, R.: Le flutter et ses limites. Arch. Mal. Coeur **63,** 116 – 144 (1970)
8. Sandler, I. A., Marriott, H. J. L.: The differential morphology of anomalous ventricular complexes of RBBB type in lead VI. Ventricular ectopy versus aberration. Circulation **31,** 551 – 556 (1965)
9. Wellens, H. J. J., Lie, K. I.: Ventricular tachycardia: the value of programmed electrical stimulation. In: Cardiac Arrhythmias: The Modern Electrophysiological Approach. Krikler, D. M. and Goodwin, J. F. (eds.), London-Philadelphia-Toronto: W. B. Saunders, 1975, pp. 182 – 194

Reentry Mechanism Within the His-Purkinje System in Man During Extrasystolic Stimulation of the Right Ventricle *

D. FLEISCHMANN, T. POP, and J. M. T. DEBAKKER

An electrical stimulus elicited during the early recovery phase of the ventricular myocardium may lead to spontaneous ventricular extrasystoles or trains of premature beats. This has been shown by animal studies [2–4, 15–17, 24, 34, 37, 46, 47] especially by the work of Wiggers and Wegria [45, 46]. Wiggers and Wegria [46] defined the short period within the cardiac cycle during which an increased tendency to repetitive firing can be observed as the vulnerable period of the myocardium. Reentry [2, 4, 15, 24, 26, 36, 38, 48, 49] resulting from dissociation in the propagation of the prematurely initiated impulse is suggested as the basic mechanism responsible for the occurrence of the spontaneous beats. However, it still remains controversial whether the conduction disturbance and by this way the reentry pathway are confined to the network of myocardial fibers or include fibers of the His-Purkinje system.

Several reports [5, 6, 29, 32, 33, 36, 39] have been published showing that a vulnerable period of the ventricular myocardium exists also in the human heart. Systematic studies utilizing increasing energy levels are impossible in man. Experience gathered by working with an exactly programable stimulator and electrical stimuli of double diastolic threshold showed that the spontaneous ventricular beats were restricted to one or two extrasystoles. By this method we obtained information not only about the tendency of the human heart to exhibit vulnerability but also about the conduction of prematurely elicited ventricular beats [1]. We think that our results contribute to the understanding of the basic mechanism underlying the origin of echo beats in the chambers of the human heart.

Materials and Methods

For the evaluation of various rhythm disorders intracardial potential recordings combined with stimulation studies were performed in 46 patients. Thirty-six of these patients had a normal QRS complex, 10 cases showed a bundle branch block pattern in the control electrocardiogram; five cases had a right bundle branch block; in two cases the right bundle branch block was combined with a left axis deviation (left anterior fascicular block); a left bundle branch block was present in three cases. Patients with an acute myocardial infarction were excluded from the study.

*This work was supported by the Deutsche Forschungsgemeinschaft SFB 109.

The following parameters were determined for three different basic driving rates — 80/min, 100/min, 120/min — utilizing the extrastimulus method: the refractory periods of the right atrium, the right ventricle, and parts of the atrioventricular conduction system for antegrade and retrograde conduction. This was possible by the simultaneous recording of a bipolar electrogram of the bundle of His [10] according to the method of Scherlag et al. [31], a bipolar electrogram of the right atrium, and several surface electrocardiograms. To stimulate the right ventricle a bipolar electrode catheter was advanced to the right ventricular apex. The right atrium was stimulated by a catheter with four electrodes. The catheter was positioned against the high lateral wall of the right atrium. The two distal electrodes were used for stimulation, the proximal ones for recording the atrial electrogram. The interelectrode distance measured always 10 mm. The stimulation studies were carried out by rectangular pulses of 1 ms duration and double diastolic threshold. The mean diastolic threshold for the right ventricle was 0.48 V ± 0.17 V. We will focus our report on the results of the ventricular stimulation studies; 93 single studies in 46 patients will be considered. The beginning of the relative refractory period of the His-Purkinje system for retrograde AV conduction was defined as follows: the longest premature ventricular beat interval S_1S_2 at which a retrograde H potential became visible and could be delineated from the ventricular potential in the His bundle lead. We realize that the time values obtained are shorter than the actual values because the H potential is obscured in the ventricular potential at the earliest prolongation of the retrograde conduction time. The values for the relative refractory period of the right bundle branch for antegrade AV conduction which are referred to in the discussion have been collected from cases with a functional bundle branch block [11]. The beginning of the relative refractory period of the right bundle branch was defined as the longest H_1H_2 interval at which an incomplete or complete right bundle branch block became manifest in the electrocardiogram.

Results

The Vulnerability of the Ventricular Myocardium

Spontaneous ventricular extrasystoles following a prematurely initiated ventricular test impulse were observed in 27 of 46 cases. This corresponds to a frequency of 59%. In the majority of cases there was only one spontaneous beat after the test impulse, in two cases three or four repetitive beats were seen which ceased spontaneously. Ventricular tachycardias or ventricular fibrillation never occurred although the premature beat interval was shortened in each case until the effective refractory period of the right ventricle was reached. An analysis of the 93 single studies according to the vulnerability, observed at the three different basic driving rates, revealed no statistically significant difference among the three groups (Fig. 1). As can be seen from the Figure 1, however, the number of cases with vulnerability exceeded those without vulnerability at a rate of 80/min whereas this relation was reversed at a rate of 120/min.

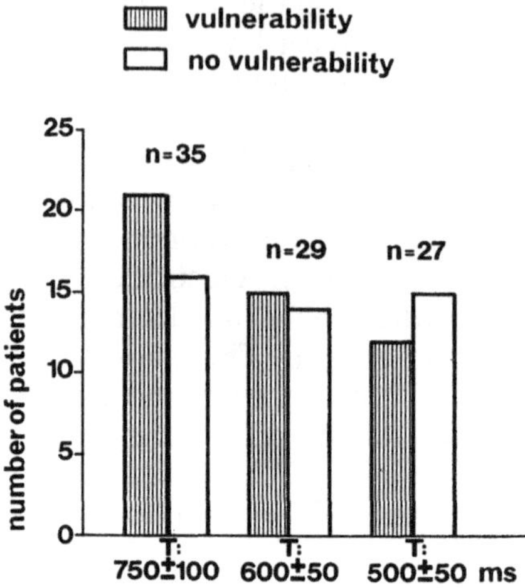

Fig. 1. Vulnerability of right ventricle during extrasystolic stimulation as related to basic driving rate. Abscissa: cycle length T of basic driving rate in ms.

Of the 46 cases 36 had a normal QRS complex in the control electrocardiogram, 10 cases showed a bundle branch block pattern. Spontaneous extrasystoles could be elicited in 24 of the 34 cases with normal intraventricular conduction; only three of the 10 cases with a bundle branch block demonstrated vulnerability to premature stimulation. The morphology of the spontaneous extrasystoles showed a left bundle branch pattern in cases with a normal QRS complex and in one case with an incomplete left bundle branch block suggesting that the extrasystoles originated in the right ventricle. The spontaneous ventricular extrasystoles of two cases with a right bundle branch block, however, had a right bundle branch block pattern. They probably originated in the left ventricular chamber.

The Pattern of Retrograde Intraventricular Conduction During Premature Ventricular Stimulation

When the coupling interval of the premature ventricular test impulse — S_1S_2 interval — was shortened by 10 ms after every tenth beat of a constant ventricular driving frequency, the retrograde His potential could finally be delineated from the ventricular potential in the His bundle electrogram. This occurred at coupling intervals between 300 and 400 ms. The retrograde intraventricular conduction time from the site of stimulation in the right ventricle along the bundle branches to the bundle of His increased constantly with decreasing S_1S_2 intervals. Conduction times measured were in the range between 100 and 350 ms. The longest retrograde conduction time did not coincide in all cases with the values measured shortly before the effective refractory period of the right ventricle. In some

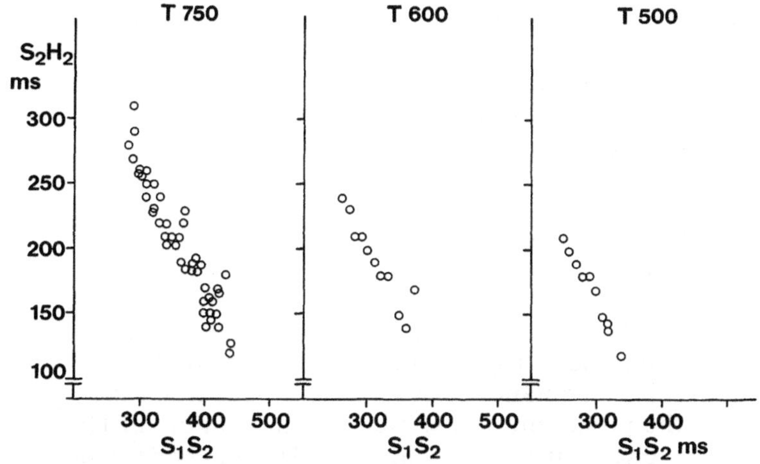

Fig. 2. Retrograde intraventricular conduction time from site of right ventricular stimulation to bundle of His (S_2H_2 interval) vs. basic driving rate. Cycle length T of basic freqency, the S_2H_2 interval (ordinate) and coupling interval S_1S_2 (abscissa) during premature stimulation are given in ms. Decrease in cycle length T leads to shorter retrograde conduction time at same coupling interval; curves are shifted downwards and to the left.

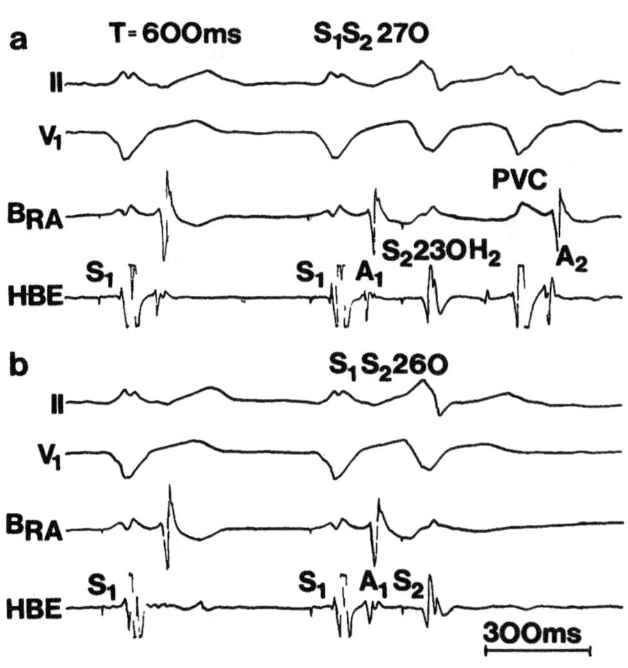

Fig. 3 a and b. Spontaneous ventricular extrasystole occurring after premature electrical stimulation of the right ventricle. In part a and b from above: lead II, V_1, a bipolar atrial (*BRA*) and His bundle (*HBE*) electrogram. Basic rate 100/min corresponding to T=600 ms.Time in ms.(a): Premature ventricular beat S_2 elicited 270 ms after S_1 is slowly conducted to bundle of His H_2. After bundle has been activated spontaneous ventricular extrasystole (*PVC*) occurs (b): Stimulated beat S_2 is elicited only 10 ms earlier (S_1S_2 interval 260 ms). Retrograde conduction to bundle of His is blocked; no H_2 potential can be identified. Spontaneous extra beat does not occur.

cases there were considerable variations in the retrograde conduction times at the same S_1S_2 interval. The retrograde intraventricular conduction time was clearly rate-dependent. An increase of the basic driving rate was followed by shorter conduction times at the same coupling interval of the premature test impulse S_2 (Fig. 2).

Retrograde Intraventricular Conduction Time and Spontaneous Ventricular Beats

The spontaneous ventricular extrasystoles after premature ventricular stimulation occurred only when the retrograde intraventricular conduction time was critically delayed. The spontaneous beats were absent when the retrograde conduction of the premature test stimulus to the bundle of His was blocked (Fig. 3). The phase of vulnerability was less dependent on the timing of the premature impulse within the relative refractory period of the ventricular myocardium than on the delayed retrograde conduction of the premature impulse within the His-Purkinje system (Fig. 4). Tested for a number of cases there was a positive correlation between the retrograde conduction delay within the His-Purkinje system and the frequency of spontaneous extra beats occurring at a certain delayed conduction time.

Discussion

The datas presented show that also in the human in the majority of cases ventricular vulnerability will occur as a result of electrical stimulation during the so-called vulnerable period. There is — according to Wiggers

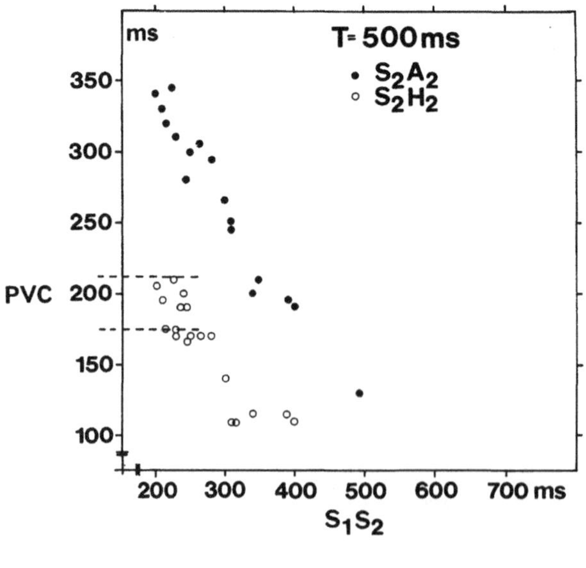

Fig. 4. Occurrence of spontaneous extrasystoles (*PVC*) as related to critically delayed retrograde conduction time. Abscissa: Coupling interval S_1S_2 at basic rate of 120/min (T=500 ms), ordinate: retrograde conduction time to bundle of His (S_2H_2 interval) and retrograde conduction time to atrium (S_2A_2 interval). Time in ms. Spontaneous beats (*PVC*) occurred only when retrograde conduction time to bundle reached 175 ms.

[45] — a strong correlation between impulse strength and the number of spontaneously following extrasystoles. A strong impulse may lead to ventricular fibrillation whereas a weak electrical stimulus provokes only a single artificial beat. We stimulated with impulses of 1 ms duration and double diastolic threshold. The mean impulse strength was in the range of 0.96 V, which corresponds to values used clinically during temporary or permanent electrostimulation. The clinician should therefore be prepared for the occurrence of spontaneous extrasystoles during pacemaker malfunction as the electrical stimuli fall in the early recovery phase of the ventricular myocardium. In only two of 27 cases with vulnerability did we observe trains

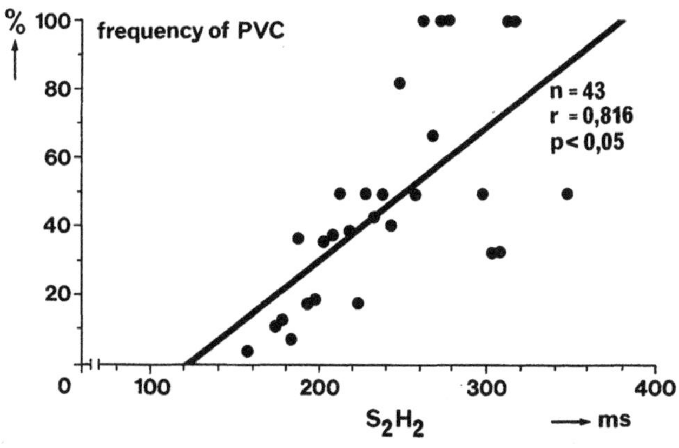

Fig. 5. Correlation between ventricular vulnerability and delayed retrograde conduction to bundle of His (S_2H_2 interval, abscissa) after extrasystolic stimulation of right ventricle.

of extrasystoles. In the other cases one spontaneous extrabeat was seen following the premature test beat. Akhtar et al. [1] reporting a similar study found ventricular vulnerability in 15 of 24 cases; this is in accordance with the frequency described here. The duration of the test impulse used by Akhtar et al. [1] was 1.5 ms; the impulse strength was not stated in detail. Han et al. [16] and Janse [21] used an impulse of 1.5 times diastolic threshold in the dog heart in situ. Both authors found no ventricular vulnerability during premature ventricular stimulation. This result is surprising; as an explanation for the different response upon electrical stimulation between the human and canine heart, other factors besides the relatively low impulse strength have to be considered: different heart size, different anatomy of the intraventricular conduction system, and the young age of the animals. Concerning age, we found, as did Akhtar et al. [1], ventricular vulnerability in young patients without overt heart disease.

De Boer [4] in 1920 reported experiments on ventricular vulnerability of the bled frog heart. According to his theory an electrical impulse given shortly after the recovery phase of the myocardium will lead to spontaneous beats because of delayed conduction and shortening of the refractory period [30] of the premature impulse. De Boer postulated a reentry mechanism causing spontaneous ventricular extrasystoles. The exact mechanism

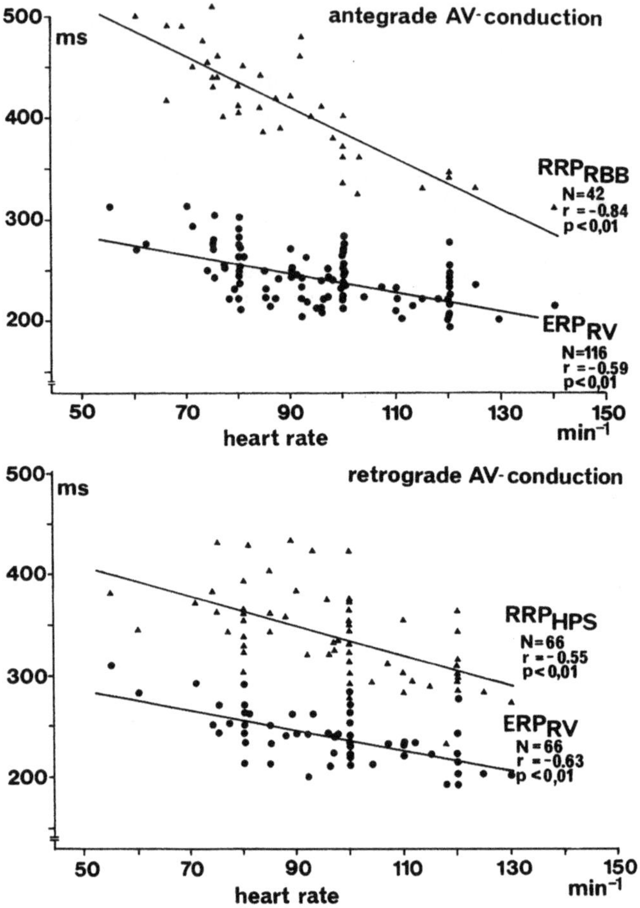

Fig. 6. Refractory periods of human intraventricular conduction system Abscissa: heart rate in beats/min; ordinate: refractory periods in ms.
Upper panel: during antegrade AV conduction: relative refractory period of right bundle branch (RRP_{RBB}) and effective refractory period of right ventricle (ERP_{RV}).
Lower panel: retrograde AV conduction: relative refractory period of His-Purkinje system (RRP_{HPS}) and effective refractory period of right ventricle (ERP_{RV}). Both refractory periods differ for antegrade as well as for retrograde conduction. Refractory periods decrease with increasing heart rate.

underlying the vulnerability to electrical stimulation of the human heart has not been clarified to date [36, 38, 41]. Recording surface potentials of the bundle of His in the human heart [31] during stimulation studies makes it possible, however, to explore more precisely the location and duration of the delayed conduction pathway through the ventricular chamber [1, 12, 13]. The results here reveal a strong correlation between the prematurity of the ventricular test impulse and the retrograde conduction time from the site of stimulation in the right ventricle over the bundle branches to the bundle of His [8]. The retrograde conduction time was at times prolonged above values of 350 ms. We think that the maximal conduction delay during conduction of a prematurely elicited ventricular response is not the ventricular myocardium but either the junction of ventricular to Purkinje fibers or the His-Purkinje system with the longest action potential duration [14, 27, 28].

Figure 6 shows that in the human heart the beginning of the relative refractory period of the right bundle branch for antegrade AV conduction as well as the beginning of the relative refractory period of the His-Purkinje system for retrograde AV conduction are longer than the effective refractory period of the right ventricle. The difference in refractory periods [8, 25, 40, 42] explains the prominent retrograde conduction delay within the His-Purkinje system following a premature ventricular beat and can be regarded as the physiologic basis for the dissociation of conduction within the ventricular myocardium and the His-Purkinje system. A local reentry mechanism [23] is possible when the conduction of a very early elicited ventricular beat is blocked within single Purkinje fibers [22, 48, 49]. A so-called macroreentry [1, 9, 12, 20, 35, 43, 50] including the bundle branches can be conceived during a functional or unidirectional block of the whole fiber system of the right bundle branch for retrograde conduction of a right ventricular impulse which finally transverses the ventricular septum and retrogradly invades the left bundle branch. The dependence of spontaneous beats on a critically delayed retrograde conduction of the test impulse to the bundle of His, the low tendency to ventricular vulnerability in cases with impaired intraventricular conduction as well as the nonoccurrence of spontaneous ventricular beats during retrograde conduction block to the bundle of His are interpreted as favoring the hypothesis of Hoffman [18] concerning the mechanism underlying vulnerability. Hoffman [18], Hoffman and Cranefield [19], Janse [21], Meyerburg et al. [27, 28], and Wit et al. [48, 49] called attention to the difference in refractory periods between the His-Purkinje system and myocardial fibers and indicated a possible reentrant mechanism at the junction of both structures.

Han and Moe [16, 17], Surawicz et al. [37] and Spear et al. [34] locate the maximal conduction delay within the structure of the myocardium. According to their experiments dispersion in recovery of the myocardial fibers following a premature test impulse will lead to delayed conduction within the myocardium. Their theory of a local reentry within the syncytial structure of the myocardium [7, 26], however, cannot satifactorily explain our results.

Summary

Stimulation studies combined with intracardiac potential recording (His bundle electrogram, atrial electrogram) were performed in 46 patients. A phase of ventricular vulnerability could be demonstrated in 27 cases during extrasystolic stimulation of the right ventricle using pulses of 1 ms duration and double diastolic threshold.

The occurrence of the spontaneous premature ventricular beats (PVC) depended on a critically delayed retrograde conduction time within the His-Purkinje system rather than on the timing of premature stimulation within the relative refractory period of the right ventricle.

The difference in refractory periods between the His-Purkinje system and ventricular myocardium is the electrophysiologic basis for the prominent retrograde conduction delay. Spontaneous PVCs were seen in only three out of 10 cases with intraventricular conduction defects. A local reentry at the junction of Purkinje fibers with ventricular myocardium and a macroreentry including the bundle branches are discussed as possible mechanisms for the observed form of vulnerability after extrasystolic ventricular stimulation.

References

1. Akhtar, M., Damato, A. N., Batsford, W. P., Ruskin, J. N., Ogunkelu, J. B., Vargas, G.: Demonstration of reentry within the His-Purkinje-system in man. Circulation **50,** 1150 (1974)
2. Antoni, H.: Physiologische Grundlagen bei der Erzeugung und Unterbrechung von Vorhof- und Kammerflimmern des Herzens durch den elektrischen Strom. Herz/Kreisl. **4,** 324 (1972)
3. Antoni, H., Tägtmeyer, H.: Die Wirkung starker Ströme auf Erregungsablauf und Kontraktion des Herzmuskels. In: Beiträge z. Ersten Hilfe und Behandlung v. Unfällen durch elektr. Strom, Frankfurt: Verlags- und Wirtschaftsges. d. Elektrizitätswerke mbH, 1965
4. De Boer, S.: Eine neue Theorie über das Entstehen von Kammerwühlen. Pflügers Arch. ges. Physiol. **178,** 1 (1920)
5. Büchner, M., Effert, S.: Auslösung tachykarder Arrhythmien durch Extrasystolen. Dtsche med. Wschr. **92,** 2097 (1967)
6. Büchner, M., Effert, S.: Extrasystolie und Herzflimmern. Verh. dtsch. Ges. Kreislforsch. **57,** 18 (1968)
7. Castellanos, A., Jr., Castillo, C. A., Agha, A. S., Myerburg, R. J., Tessler, M. S.: Mechanisms of ventricular tachycardia. In: Cardiac Arrhythmias. Dreifus, L. S., Likoff, W. (eds.), New York: Grune and Stratton, 1973
8. Dam, R. T. v., Hoffman, B. F., Stuckey, J. H.: Recovery of excitability and of impulse propagation in the in situ canine conduction system. Amer. J. Cardiol. **14,** 184 (1964)
9. Durrer, D., Wellens, H. J.: The Wolff-Parkinson-White syndrome anno 1973. Europ. J. Cardiol. **1,** 347 (1974)
10. Fleischmann, D., Mathey, D., Bleifeld, W., Irnich, W., Effert, S.: His-Bündel-Elektrographie bei Patienten mit intraventrikulären Leistungsstörungen. Klin. Wschr. **51,** 1066 (1973)
11. Fleischmann, D., Pop, T.: Unpublished results
12. Fleischmann, D., Pop, T., deBakker, J. M. T.: Zur Frage der Entstehung ventrikulärer Extrasystolen. Kreiserregung im intraventrikulären Leitungssystem. Herz/Kreisl. **7,** 82 (1975)
13. Fleischmann, D., Pop, T., deBakker, J. M. T.: Demonstration of reentry within the His-Purkinje-system in man. Pflügers Arch., Europ. J. Physiol. 359, suppl-R 22 (1975)
14. Gallagher, J. J., Damato, A. N., Varghese, J., Lau, S. H.: Localization of an area of maximum refractoriness or „gate" in the ventricular spezialized conduction system in man. Amer. Heart J. **84,** 310 (1972)
15. Garrey, W. E.: The nature of fibrillatory contraction of the heart; its relation to tissue mass and form. Amer. J. Physiol. **33,** 397 (1914)
16. Han, J., Millet, D., Chizzonitti, B., Moe, G. K.: Temporal dispersion of recovery of excitability in atrium and ventricle as a function of heart rate. Amer. Heart J. **71,** 481 (1966)
17. Han, J., Moe, G.: Nonuniform recovery of excitability in ventricular muscle. Circulation Res.: **14,** 44 (1964)
18. Hoffman, B. F.: Hypothermia and vulnerability. Ann. Acad. Sci.: **80,** 348 (1959)
19. Hoffman B. F., Cranefield, P. F.: Electrophysiology of the Heart. New York: McGraw-Hill, 1960
20. Jahrmärker, H., Theisen, K.: Kammerflattern und Kammerflimmern. In: Herzrhythmusstörungen. Antoni, H., Effert, S. (eds.), Stuttgart: F. K. Schattauer, 1974
21. Janse, M. J.: The effect of changes in heart rate on the refractory period of the heart. Thesis, Amsterdam: Mondeel-Offsetdruckerij, 1971
22. Kao, C. Y., Hoffman, B. F.: Graded and decremental response in heart muscle fibers. Amer. J. Physiol. **194,** 187 (1958)

23. Lüderitz, B., Zacouto, F., Guize, L., Steinbeck, G., Riecker, G.: Ein neues Schrittmacherprinzip zur Suppression ventrikulärer Tachykardien. Verh. dtsch. Ges. Kreisl.-Forsch. **39,** 319 (1973)
24. Mines, G. R.: On circulating excitation in the heart muscle and their possible relation to tachycardia and fibrillation. Trans. roy. Soc. Can. Ser. 3 Vol. **8,** Sect. IV, Geol. and Biol. Sciences 1914
25. Moore, E. N., Preston, J. B., Moe, G. K.: Durations of transmembrane action potentials and functional refraectory periods of canine false tendon and ventricular myocardium. Circulat. Res. **17,** 259 (1965)
26. Moore, E. N., Spear, J. F.: Ventricular fibrillation threshold. Its physiological and pharmacological importance. Arch. int. Med. **135,** 446 (1975)
27. Myerburg, R. J., Gelband, H., Hoffman, B. F.: Confinement of premature impulses in functional compartments of regions of the a-v conducting system. Cardiovasc. Res. **7,** 69 (1973)
28. Myerburg, R. J., Stewart, J. W., Hoffman, B. F.: Electrophysiological properties of the canine peripheral A-V conducting system. Circulat. Res. **26,** 361 (1970)
29. Pick, A.: Manifestation of a vulnerable phase in the human heart. In: Symposion on Sudden Cardiac Death. Surawicz, B., Pellegrino, E. D. (eds.), New York: 1964
30. Sasyniuk, B. J., Mendez, C.: A mechanism for reentry in canine ventricular tissue. Circulat. Res. **28,** 3 (1971)
31. Scherlag, B. J., Lau, S. H., Helfant, R. H., Berkowitz, W. D., Stein, E., Damato, A. N.: Catheter technique for recording His bundle activity in man. Circulation **39,** 13 (1969)
32. Smirk, F. H.: R waves interrupting T waves. Brit. Heart J. **11,** 23 (1949)
33. Smirk, F. H., Palmer, D. G.: A myocardial syndrome with particular reference to the occurance of sudden death and of premature systoles interrupting antecedent T waves. Amer. J. Cardiol. **6,** 620 (1960)
34. Spear, J. F., Moore, E. N., Horowitz, C. N.: Effect of current pulses delivered during the ventricular vulnerable period upon the ventricular fibrillation threshold. Amer. J. Cardiol. **32,** 814 (1973)
35. Spurrell, R. A. J., Sowton, E., Denchar, D. C.: Ventricular tachycardia in 4 patients: evaluated by programmed electrical stimulation of heart and treated in 2 patients by surgical division of anteror radiation of left bundle branch. Brit. Heart J. **35,** 1014 (1973)
36. Surawicz, B.: Ventricular fibrillation. Amer. J. Cardiol. **28,** 268 (1971)
37. Surawicz, B., Gettes, L. S., Ponce-Zumino, A.: Relation of vulnerability to ECG and action potential characteristics of premature beats. Amer. J. Physiol. **212,** 1519 (1967)
38. Surawicz, B., Zumino, A. P.: The vulnerable period of ventricular excitation. In: Mechanisms and Therapy of Cardiac Arrhythmias. Dreifus, L. S., Likoff, W. (eds.), New York: Grune and Stratton 1966
39. Tavel, M. E., Fisch, C.: Repetitive ventricular arrhythmia resulting from artificial internal pacemaker. Circulation **30,** 493 (1964)
40. Trautwein, W.: Elektrophysiologie der Herzmuskelfaser. Ergebn. Physiol. **51,** 131 (1961)
41. Trautwein, W.: Mechanisms of tachyarrhythmias and extrasystoles. In: Symposion on Cardiac Arrhythmias, Sandoe, E., Flensted-Jansen, E., Olesen, K. H. (eds.), Södertälje: AB Astra, 1970
42. Trautwein, W., Dudel, J.: Aktionspotential und Mechanogramm des Warmblüterherzmuskels als Funktion der Schlagfrequenz. Pflügers Arch. ges. Physiol. **260,** 24 (1954)
43. Varghese, P. J., Damato, A. N., Caracta, A. R., Gallagher, J. J., Josephson, M. E., Lau, S. H.: Intraventricular conduction delay as a determinant of atrial echo beats. Circulation **49,** 805 (1974)
44. Wellens, H. J. J., Lie, K. J., Durrer, D.: Further observations on ventricular tachycardia studied by electrical stimulation of the heart. Chronic recurrent ventricular tachycardia and ventricular tachycardia during acute myocardial infarction. Circulation **49,** 647 (1974)
45. Wiggers, C. J.: The mechanism and nature of ventricular fibrillation. Amer. Heart J. **20,** 399 (1940)
46. Wiggers, C. J., Wegria, R.: Ventricular fibrillation due to single, localized induction and condenser shocks applied during the vulnerable phase of ventricular systole. Amer. J. Physiol. **128,** 500 (1939)

47. Mc William, J. A.: Fibrillar contraction of the heart, J. Physiol. (Lond.) **8,** 296 (1887)
48. Wit, A. C., Cranefield, P. F., Hoffman, B. F.: Slow conduction and reentry in the ventricular conducting system II Single and sustained circus movement in networks of canine and bovine fibers. Circulat. Res. **30,** 11 (1972)
49. Wit, A. C., Hoffman, B. F., Cranefield, P. F.: Slow conduction and reentry in the ventricular conducting system I Return extrasystole in canine Purkinje fibers. Circulat. Res. **30,** 1 (1972)
50. Zipes, D. P., De Joseph, R. L., Rothbaum, D. A.: Unusual properties of accessory pathways. Circulation, **49,** 1200 (1974)

Patient Initiated Rapid Atrial Pacing to Manage Supraventricular Tachycardia

A. R. KAHN and P. CITRON

Transient episodes of supraventricular tachycardia (SVT) are usually well tolerated and relatively easily managed in apparently healthy individuals. Four management modalities are presently employed in symptomatic patients. They are:

1. *Drug therapy:* including sedatives, digitalis, quinidine, procainamide, lidocaine, propranolol
2. *Manual neural stimulation:* carotid sinus massage; vagal stimulation such as the Valsalva maneuver [1]
3. *Surgical intervention:* surgical interruption of atrioventricular conduction pathways [10]
4. *Electrical stimulation:* DC cardioversion; temporary external, rapid pacing [7]; artificial pacemakers [12, 13]; carotid sinus nerve stimulation [6].

These tachycardias may, however, result in apprehension, emotional aberrancy, angina, syncope, or congestive heart failure in patients with protracted, recurrent episodes where conventional therapies are not effective or in cases where other underlying cardiovascular diseases exist [3].

This paper reports the results observed in 18 patients who received artificial patient-controlled pacemakers to manage their recurrent episodes of SVT.

Materials and Methods

The pacemaker system used in this study consists of an implanted receiver/lead and an externally worn, patient activated transmitter/antenna [1] (Fig. 1). Energy transmission between the transmitter and receiver is accomplished through radiofrequency (R – F) coupling. Stimulator pulse frequency is controllable at the transmitter between 50 and 300 pulses per minute (ppm). The pulses are conducted via bipolar leads to the right atrium. In 14 patients, myocardial leads were sutured to the right atrial myocardium. Four patients received endocardial atrial leads. Three of these patients had leads placed in the coronary sinus; the fourth received a J-type lead positioned in the right atrial appendage. The radiofrequency receiver used in this pacing system is powered by the transmitted signal and, therefore, contains no batteries.

[1] Specially designed by Medtronic, Inc., Minneapolis, Minnesota, USA.

Each prospective recipient of the described pacing system was thoroughly prescreened to verify an accompanying morbidity to justify evaluation of this management technique. The selection criteria required: (1) that the patients have a history of frequent episodes; (2) that these episodes be drug-refractory; and (3) that temporary external rapid pacing [6] be used to verify the ability to successfully terminate an episode of SVT,

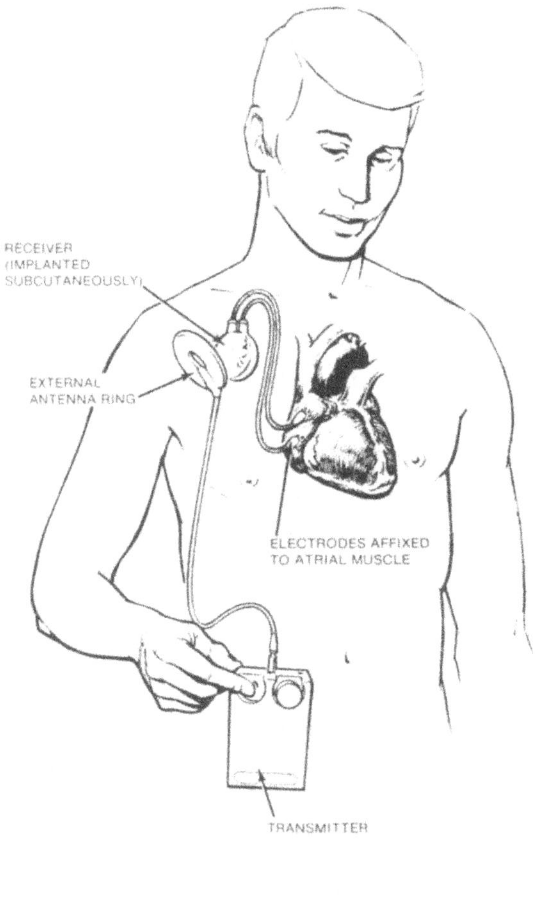

Fig. 1. Schematic representation of radiofrequency pacemaker used in this study.

and concurrently verify that rapid pacing rates were not conducted to the ventricles via anomalous conduction pathways.

Most patients receiving the pacemaker experienced episodes of SVT during the postsurgical hospitalization with these episodes managed using the described system. Figure 2 shows a recording of a tachycardia at a rate of 150 bpm terminated by a brief burst of patient-initiated rapid atrial pacing at a rate of 250 ppm with a subsequent return to normal sinus rhythm.

During a bout of SVT, the patient was required to adjust the pacing rate to the value which had been found effective in reverting the tachycardia during the screening and evaluation process and then activate the transmitter by depressing the ON/OFF button for 10 – 20 s. If relief was not obtained after two successive applications, the patient was instructed to report to his physician immediately.

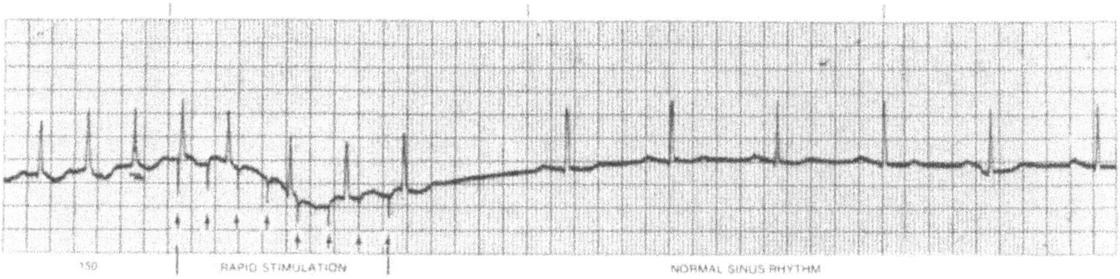

Fig. 2. Episode of tachycardia at rate of 150 bpm reverted to sinus rhythm by brief rapid atrial stimulation.

Results

The patients reported in this study ranged in age from 14 to 70 years (Table 1). Patient M. R. had the pacing system removed 13 months post-op due to persistent pericarditis. Patient E. G. died 3 months post-op of an unrelated massive cerebral hemorrhage which was confirmed at autopsy. For the 3 months following implant, this patient used the system successfully on four separate occasions.

Patient L. H. used the R – F pacemaker system successfully for a period of 12 months. Since August 1974, this patient has been in constant atrial fibrillation with propranolol and digoxin used to control ventricular rate and, therefore, has not had occasion to use the system recently. Patient R. C. presents a complex case as a result of a congenital single ventricle. Postsurgically, many episodes of tachycardia were converted to sinus rhythm with the pacemaker system. On occasion, conversion was mediated by transient atrial fibrillation which was of prolonged duration possibly due to the underlying presence of congenital heart disease. After discharge, this patient experienced one episode of SVT which was apparently converted to flutter and required cardioversion. No subsequent episodes of SVT have been experienced and, therefore, the pacemaker has not been further used. Effective management of SVT has been maintained in the 14 remaining patients in the study for periods ranging from 5 to 43 months (average 22.4 months) at the time of the last follow-up.

The usual result of brief high-rate stimulation of the atria during an episode of tachycardia was a return to sinus rhythm. Three patients occasionally developed atrial fibrillation with resulting ventricular rates of 60 bpm, 70 bpm, and 150 bpm. These fibrillatory episodes would sponta-

Table 1. R-F pacemaker patient summary

Patient	Date of implant / Months of follow-up	Age at implant	Effect of rapid stimulation [a, b]	Frequency of attack	R–F ppm [c]	Concurrent drug regimen
M. R.	7/70 [d] / 13	22	SR, B (100), AF	10/day	–	–
R. B.	2/72 / 32	46	SR	10 – 15/ week	280	Digoxin Quinidine Diazepam
B. S.	2/72 / 43	42	SR	3/week	300	Propranolol
C. S.	4/72 / 32	23	SR	2 – 4/day	300	–
L. M.	5/72 / 41	44	SR, F (60), AF (4 : 1)	2 – 3/week	300	Digoxin
B. H.	2/73 / 20	61	SR [e]	3 – 4/week	150 – 200	Propranolol
D. A.	3/73 / 30	55	SR	1/month	300	Procainamide
I. McN.	3/73 / 30	58	SR	3/month	300	Digoxin
O. C.	4/73 / 29	45	SR	7 – 10/ week	200	–
E. G. [f]	6/73 / 3	–	SR, F (70)	1/month	250 – 300	–
L. H.	8/73 / 12	67	SR	2/month	200	Procainamide Propranolol Digoxin
A. J.	11/73 / 21	52	SR	1 – 2/week	300	Digoxin
R. C. [g]	11/74 / 10	14	SR, AF (1 : 1)	–	230	–
S. P.	1/75 / 9	46	SR	1/week	300	–
J. LeC.	2/75 / 9	52	SR, F (150)	2 – 3/ month	300	–
J. S.	2/75 / 7	65	SR	1 – 2/day	150	–
T. B.	3/75 / 6	67	SR	1/day	300	–
E. B.	4/75 / 5	70	SR	1 – 3/day	220	Verapamil

neously revert to sinus rhythm within seconds or minutes. Patients M. R. and L. M. occasionally developed brief periods of atrial flutter which spontaneously reverted to sinus rhythm.

The return to sinus rhythm following application of rapid atrial stimulation may involve one of three mechanisms: (1) Rapid atrial stimulation may produce atrial fibrillation or flutter which are, in themselves, unstable rhythms and, therefore, tend to revert spontaneously to normal sinus rhythm. (2) Application of asynchronous rapid stimuli may interrupt a reentry pathway by depolarizing atrial portions of the pathway necessary to maintain rapid rhythms. (3) When an ectopic atrial focus is responsible for the tachycardia, application of rapid stimuli to the atria may result in overdrive suppression of the ectopic focus. This study was not designed to determine the specific mechanism responsible for conversion in any specific case.

Frequency of application varied from 10 per day to approximately once per month. Therefore, patient-initiated rapid atrial stimulation with the described pacing system has been used successfully in over 9800 applications by the 18 patients studied. One patient's (B. H.) attempts at conversion failed to terminate the arrhythmia on one occasion. After reporting for treatment, attempts were made to pace at several different rates (150, 180, 220, 300 ppm) using the pacemaker, but these attempts failed to revert. However, by starting pacing at 120 ppm and slowly increasing the pacing rate to 200 ppm and then switching the transmitter "OFF" resulted in a return to normal sinus rhythm. This patient has not since had an episode of SVT refractory to rapid atrial stimulation.

Several potential complications related to rapid atrial stimulation should be considered when applying this management technique. They include: (1) Ventricular stimulation and possible ventricular tachycardia or fibrillation. This may result from poor lead placement or may be due to the existence of anomalous conduction pathways bypassing normal AV conduction (as in Wolff-Parkinson-White syndrome) [5, 7]; (2) asystole following pacing; (3) patient discomfort due to pacing impulses [8, 9]. These complications could also be expected to occur with the R – F system, but we believe they can be minimized by screening through temporary external pacing and by observing the first several episodes after implantation [4]. In this study, atrial epicardial leads were applied to minimize the chances of ventricular stimulation in 14 patients. Endocardial leads were used in four patients, and it would be reasonable to assume that this is an added risk for potential inadvertent ventricular stimulation through dislodgment of the lead and,

---

[a] AF, atrial flutter; B, AV block; F, atrial fibrillation; SR, sinus rhythm.

[b] Number in parentheses is the resulting ventricular rate.

[c] ppm = most effective pacing rate (pulses per minute).

[d] Unit removed 8/71 due to refractory episodes of pericarditis.

[e] One refractory episode occurred (see text).

[f] Patient died 9/73. Autopsy was performed and showed massive cerebral hemorrhage.

[g] Patient has congenital single ventricle.

therefore, these patients will require more frequent evaluation [11]. To date, however, use of endocardial leads has not produced any untoward results.

Summary

Patient-initiated rapid atrial pacing to manage supraventricular tachycardia has been effective in the cases studied. We feel the success of this arrhythmia management technique lies with the careful screening of the patients using temporary rapid atrial stimulation to verify susceptibility to conversion and the absence of anomalous conduction pathways which may permit rapid ventricular response to rapid atrial stimulation. Applicability of this therapy depends on the severity of symptoms experienced by the patient.

Acknowledgment

The authors wish to acknowledge the following study co-investigators for screening and carefully following the patients reported in this study.

Study Co-investigators:

Dr. William Allen, Long Beach Memorial Hosp., Long Beach, California
Dr. James W. Calvin, Thoracic & Cardiovascular Medical Group, Ventura, California
Dr. T. E. Cuddy, Winnipeg General Hospital, Winnipeg, Manitoba
Dr. C. Thomas Fruehan, Upstate Medical Center, Syracuse, New York
Dr. John J. Gallagher, Duke Univ. Med. Ctr., Durham, North Carolina
Dr. Jerzy Giedwoyn, Argay Clinic, Portland, Oregon
Dr. Frank J. Indihar, St. Paul Internists, P. A., St. Paul, Minnesota
Dr. A. J. Kerwin, Toronto Western Hospital, Toronto, Ontario
Dr. Susan Lenkei, Toronto Western Hospital, Toronto, Ontario
Dr. Edgar Lichstein, City Hospital Center at Elmhurst, Elmhurst, New York
Dr. Edward N. Mercer, Montreal General Hosp., Montreal, Quebec
Dr. James Morris, Jr., Duke Univ. Med. Ctr., Durham, North Carolina
Dr. A. Glenn Morrow, Dr. David Redwood, National Inst. of Health, Bethesda, Maryland
Dr. John Ross, Jr., University of California, La Jolla, California
Dr. Eugene Shafton, University of California, San Francisco, California
Dr. David E. Uden, Toronto Western Hospital, Toronto, Ontario
Dr. Andrew G. Wallace, Duke Univ. Med. Ctr., Durham, North Carolina
Dr. Menashe B. Waxman, Toronto General Hospital, Toronto, Ontario

References

1. Bilitch, M.: A Manual of Cardiac Arrhythmias, Boston: Little, Brown, 1971, pp. 25 – 32, 75 – 82
2. Braunwald, E., Vatner, S. F., Braunwald, N. S., Sobel, B.: Carotid sinus nerve stimulation in the treatment of angina pectoris and supraventricular tachycardia, Calif. Med **112,** 41 – 50 (1970)
3. Chung, E. K.: Principles of Cardiac Arrhythmias. Baltimore: Williams & Wilkins Co., 1971, p. 117
4. Fruehan, C. T., Meyer, J. A., Klie, J. H., Johnson, L. W., Obeid, A. I., Smulyan, H., Eich, R. H.: Refractory paroxysmal supraventricular tachycardia, Amer. Heart J. **87,** 229 – 237 (1974)
5. Iwa, T., Wada, J.: Treatment of tachycardia by atrial pacing, Jap. Circulat. J. **38,** 82 – 86 (1974)
6. Lister, J. W., Cohen, L. S., Bernstein, W. H., Samet, P.: Treatment of supraventricular tachycardias by rapid atrial stimulation, Circulation **38,** 1044 – 1059 (1968)
7. Lister, W., Gosselin, A. J., Nathan, D. A., Barold, S.: Rapid atrial stimulation in the treatment of supraventricular tachycardia, Chest **63,** 995 – 1001 (1973)
8. Pittman, D. E., Makar, J. S., Kooros, K. S., Joyner, C. R.: Rapid atrial stimulation: Successful method of conversion of atrial flutter and atrial tachycardia, Amer. J. Cardiol. **32,** 700 – 706 (1973)
9. Vergara, G. S., Hildner, F. J., Schoenfeld, C. B., Javier, R. P., Cohen, L. S., Samet, P.: Conversion of supraventricular tachycardias with rapid atrial stimulation, Circulation **46,** 788 – 793 (1972)
10. Wallace, A. G., Boineau, J. P., Davidson, R. M., Sealy, W. C.: Wolff-Parkinson-White Syndrome, Amer. J. Cardiol. **28,** 509 – 515 (1971)
11. Waxman, M. B., Felderhof, C. H., Downar, E., Goldman, B. S., Morch, J. E.: Self-conversion of drug-resistant paroxysmal atrial tachycardia, Canad. Med. Ass. J. **112,** 600 – 603 (1975)
12. Williams, D., Davison, P. H.: Long-term treatment of refractory supraventricular tachycardia by patient-controlled inductive atrial pacing. Brit. Heart J. **36,** 336 – 340 (1974)
13. Wise, J. R. Jr.: Patient-activated atrial pacing in the treatment of recurrent supraventricular tachycardia, Chest **65,** 212 – 215 (1974)

Fundamentals of Orthorhythmic Pacing

F. I. ZACOUTO and L. J. GUIZE

Recurrent reentry tachycardias (junctional, ventricular, reciprocal WPW tachycardias) can be reduced by selective stimulations [1, 4, 7, 10, 25]. In some drug-resistant tachycardias, surgery is efficient [8, 10, 21]. In other cases, surgery is technically impossible because the reentry pathway is located in a dangerous region. In all these rare cases, implantation of a special pacemaker can be considered [3, 9, 24].

Furthermore, the classical demand pacemakers implanted for Adams-Stokes syndrome do not protect the patients against dangerous extrasystoles.

In order to improve electrical treatment of those arrhythmias, orthorhythmic pacing was conceived [11, 12]. An external original, programable orthorhythmic pacemaker (OP) has been realized to add increased possibilities for electrophysiologic studies to automatic antiarrhythmic stimulation [13].

Concept of Orthorhythmic Pacing

OP represents a programable demand pacing with escape intervals that adapt to the preceding cardiac cycles. Escape intervals are automatically variable in relation to each cycle length (variable hysteresis). The standby function is controlled by two parameters: instantaneous cardiac frequency, and number of consecutive detections inside the chosen threshold frequency.

Instantaneous cardiac frequency: Orthorhythmic interventions can be restricted to rapid rhythms, either spontaneous or stimulated. In Figure 1 (top panel) cycle length must be shorter than 600 ms. This adjustable interval within each heart cycle is called the "control zone"; this zone is reduced in its beginning (*shaded area*) by the refractory period (e.g., 200 ms or automatically variable depending on preceding cycle length).

Number of consecutive detections: refractory and control zones are reset by each detection or stimulation. In Figure 1 (top panel), the OP is programed to stimulate after two consecutive detections in this control zone. It is possible that up to eight consecutive detections inside the control zone may be required before release of intervention. Inversely, orthorhythmic stimulation can be released after each complex that falls within the chosen control zone.

Orthorhythmic stimulation can be represented by a single stimulus. But the coupled stimulus can consecutively be repeated twice (paired-coupled) (top panel) or up to 10 times. If a detection occurs between the consecutive stimuli, the pacemaker is inhibited and standby functions are reset.

With a fine detecting sensitivity in atria and ventricles, it is easy to stimulate all parts of the heart with an orthorhythmic system. Marking of local detection spikes on an ECG tracing in multichannel records, as realized in Savita OP, allows analysis of the functions of the system and precise electrophysiologic measurements.

Orthorhythmic Pacing in Tachycardias

OP allows automatic treatment of tachycardias [12, 15, 16, 17, 23].

The control zone may be chosen according to frequency and type of tachycardia. For example, the control zone can be set at 400 ms if the recurrent tachycardia has a rate of 180 bpm (cycle length 333 ms). Further-

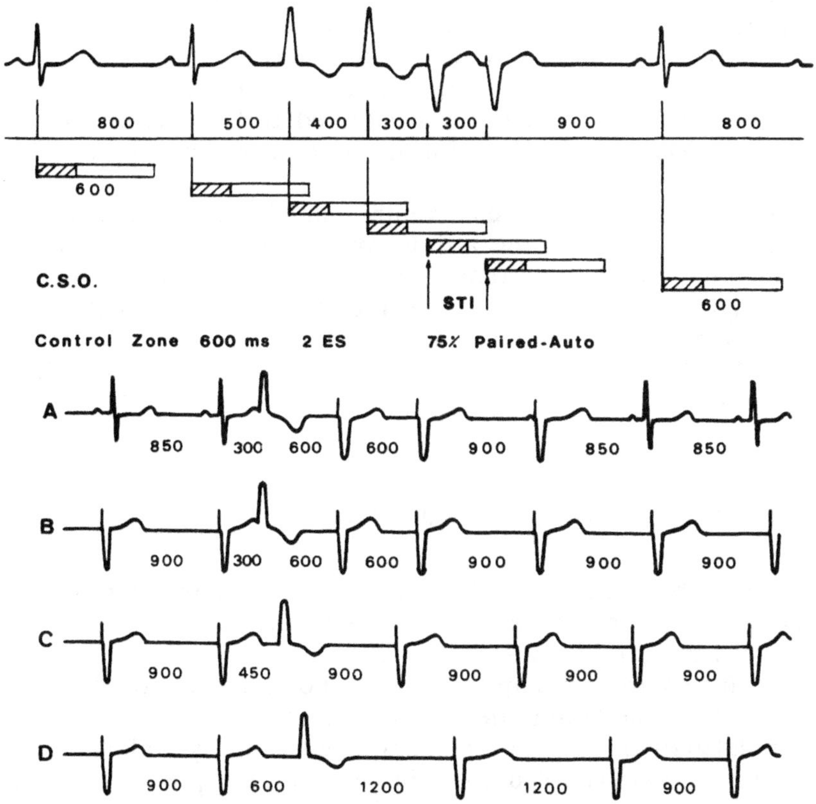

Fig. 1. *Top panel:* Principle of antitachycardia orthorhythmic system with control zone (shaded area is refractory period) and automatic R – R interval couple-paired stimulations (see text). *Bottom panel:* Schematic interventions of an implantable "variable hysteresis" demand pacemaker (see text).

more, the number of necessary consecutive detections inside the control zone can be set at eight. Thus, automatic stimulation is not released before eight complexes of the tachycardia appear.

Orthorhythmic pacing using automatically variable coupled pacing depending on a percentage of preceding cycle length could offer the following advantages: The adjustment to find the adequate reentry zone in each cycle able to break the reentry circuit is easy to obtain. We prefer to begin the setting at 100% and reduce the percentage progressively. In case of changes in the rate of recurrent tachycardias, the adjustments in percentage of preceding cycle length are more likely to remain automatically effective than adjustments made in fixed values of milliseconds [12].

The possibility of delivering up to five and more consecutive stimulations increases the efficiency of OP against tachycardias.

The number of necessary consecutive stimulations able to break a reentry circuit is related to the functional distance between the stimulating catheter and the ectopic loop. An example is shown in Figure 2 where two different ventricular tachycardias are interrupted. In the first case (top panel), the origin of the reentry circuit is in the right ventricle and the catheter situated nearly in the right ventricle detects the beginning of the ectopic QRS; a single stimulation is able to stop the tachycardia. In the second case, four consecutive stimulations were required to stop the tachycardia originating in the left ventricle. Here the electrode situated at the anterior wall of the right ventricle detects rather late during the end of the ectopic QRS complex.

To suppress ventricular tachycardias, ventricular stimulations are generally needed. Stimulations from the atrium are usually able to suppress reciprocal, junctional, WPW syndrome tachycardias (providing no severe conduction or rhythm disturbance exists in the atria). This eliminates the eventual risk of ventricular fibrillation unless a rapid AV pathway exists. Sometimes atrial tachycardias or flutter can be reduced by selective orthorhythmic stimulation [12].

Orthorhythmic Pacing in Electrophysiologic Studies

Precise marking of the intracardiac detection moment by the stimulating electrode allows correct measurement of the effective refractory periods existing in the cells around the catheter (Fig. 2).

Extension of the control zone up to 2000 ms allows delivery of coupled, paired-coupled, etc., stimulations delivered from normal or slow spontaneous or stimulated rhythms. For example, coupled orthorhythmic stimulations (delivered in R wave-coupled ms or in percentage of preceding cycle length) can be delivered automatically every eight complexes.

Thanks to these different programable functions, the external OP is an original, handy, and adaptable tool for electrophysiologists and others concerned with cardiac arrhythmias. Its applications are numerous [13]:

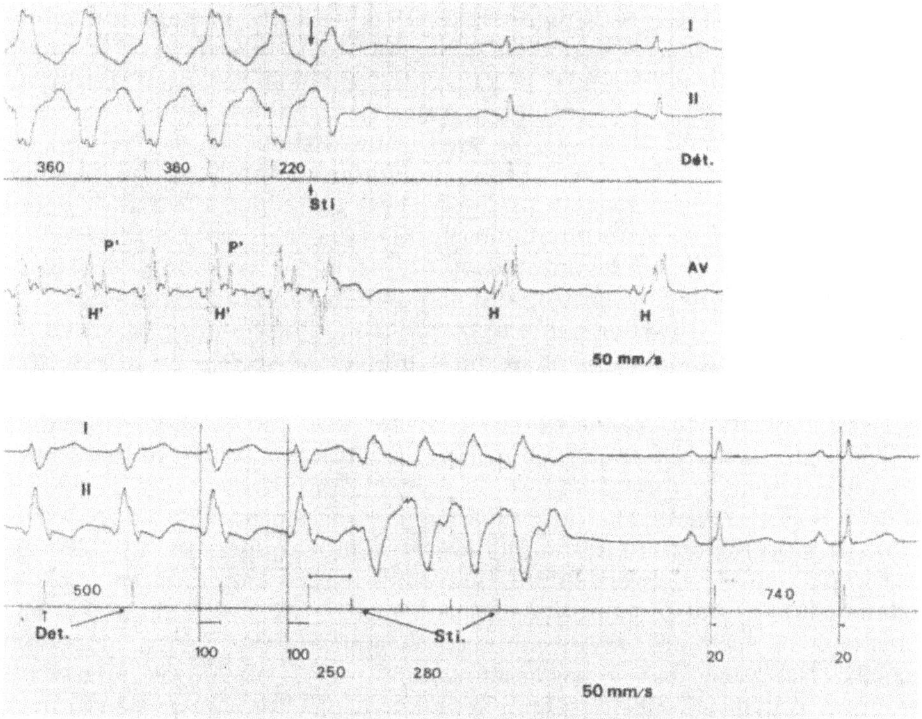

Fig. 2. *Top panel:* Reduction of right ventricular tachycardia by a single stimulus (electrode is located in right ventricle). *Bottom panel:* Four consecutive right ventricular stimulations are needed to reduce left ventricular tachycardia. Local detection (high spikes on third trace) occurs late after beginning of ectopic beats. During tachycardia, efficient refractory period of measured right ventricle is not 350 ms but only 250 ms; delay between local detection and earliest possible efficient stimulation.

Study of abnormal conduction pathways [18].
Study of conduction disturbances.
Study of refractory periods of different parts of the myocardium or conduction tissues during spontaneous and stimulated heart rhythms [5].
Study of sinus functions (automaticity and sinoatrial conduction) [22]. Repeated atrial orthorhythmic stimulations (cycle length-coupled) apparently allows separation between disturbances in automaticity and conduction [14].

Implantable Orthorhythmic Pacemaker

We have seen that the orthorhythmic concept provides a demand pacemaker able to reduce automatically recurrent tachycardias [12, 19]. The standby function is secured by a safe detection and the necessity to detect QRS complexes within the chosen control zone for a chosen number of consecutive heart cycles. Implantable OP of this type could be either adjusted for each patient in percentage of controlled preceding cycle length or used systematically for several consecutive rapid stimulations. But in all cases it is clear that the cardiologic indications remain limited and that such a device should preferably be used in the atrium to avoid ventricular fibrillation. When used in ventricular stimulation it can be useful, in some cases, to improve efficiency and safety, and to reduce the number and intensity of necessary orthorhythmic stimulations. This can be obtained by fixing epicardial electrodes located according to the proximity of reentry pathway (determined by electrophysiologic studies and/or mapping) [8].

Furthermore, it is reasonable to consider the implantation of an OP in Adams-Stokes syndrome. Such an implantable OP should be totally safe. Therefore, the escape interval for extrasystoles falling in the control zone of a cycle may be chosen, for example, to be twice the detected preceding cycle length (orthorhythmic ratio = 200%). Stimulation can be released after each detection. In this example, the control zone is restricted to 600 ms (Fig. 1 bottom panel). The orthorhythmic stimulation may be set to deliver two (or more) consecutive stimulations at identical intervals. In this way, the implanted OP delivers stimulations with temporarily different rates in relationship to the prematurity of the detected QRS complexes [9]. The functions of such an OP are shown schematically in Figure 1 (bottom panel). The pacer has a basic stimulation period of 900 ms. If a QRS complex is detected 300 ms after a spontaneous (A) or stimulated (B) beat, the pacer delivers two stimulations with an escape interval of 600 ms (positive hysteresis; intervention delay is shorter than the basic period). If no detection in the control zone occurs during those two orthorhythmic stimulations, the basic stimulation interval of 900 ms is reset.

In (C) a QRS complex is detected at 450 ms: the escape interval is 900 ms, equal to the pacing period (hysteresis zero).

In (D) a QRS complex is detected at 600 ms; the escape interval for the two following orthorhythmic stimulations is 1200 ms (negative hysteresis because the escape interval is longer than the basic period).

If a complex is detected later than 600 ms (out of control zone) the pacer may function as a classic demand pacemaker with an escape interval of 1200 ms befor reset of basic stimulation.

Such an implantable OP favors the suppression of extrasystoles. Furthermore, the return of sinus rhythm is favored by an increased negative hysteresis during two consecutive orthorhythmic stimulations when the QRS complex appears late in the cycle.

Another function of an implantable OP can be the automatic change of the basic stimulation rate (by steps) in relation to the quantity and/or prematurity of detected extrasystoles within a given sequence [2, 6, 20]. This function of automatically adapting change of frequency can be used alone or in association with variable escape interval pacing. Such an OP prevents stimulation from falling within the vulnerable period.

In patients protected against bradycardia by classical demand pacers, sudden death may result from extrasystoles. Therefore, we believe that an adequate implantable OP can increase the average life expectancy of patients with Adams-Stokes syndrome and tachyarrhythmias.

Summary

Orthorhythmic pacing realizes an automatically variable coupled stimulation dependent on the preceding cardiac cycle length. Such "variable hysteresis" stimulations are delivered according to a program which takes spontaneous (or paced) instantaneous frequency into account. The orthorhythmic pacemaker can be regulated to fire after one to eight consecutive critical beats.

One, two, three or more adjustable consecutive stimulations can be delivered by program (paired, tripled, quadruple-coupled stimulations or coupled bursts).

The orthorhythmic pacemaker also enables marking of local detection (sensed beats in atrium or in ventricle) by special spikes recorded, as pacing spikes, on a special ECG channel.

All these specific functions associated with classical demand stimulations, from 25 to 1200 beats per minute, facilitate numerous electrophysiologic studies and treatment of tachycardias:

Various aspects of normal and abnormal cardiac functions (automatism, conduction, refractory periods, accessory pathways)
Studies of sinus, atrial, junctional, and ventricular tachycardia mechanisms
Automatic treatment of reentry tachycardias, especially junctional, WPW, ventricular paroxysmal tachycardias

Implantable orthorhythmic pacers may be:

Automatic premature-coupled (single or multiple) stimulations which can be used against recurrent tachycardias
Totally safe variable hysteresis demand pacing affording protection against bradycardias and several tachyarrhythmias

References

1. Barold, S., Linhart, J. W.: Recent advances in the treatment of ectopic tachycardias by electrical pacing. Amer. J. Cardiol. **25**, 698 – 706 (1970)
2. Burchell, H. B., Merideth, J.: Management of cardiac tachyarrhythmias with cardiac pacemaker. Ann. N. Y. Acad. Sci. **167**, 546 – 551 (1969)
3. Coumel, Ph., Cabrol, C., Fabiato, A., Gourgon, R., Slama, R.: Tachycardie permanente par rhythme reciproque. I – Preuves due diagnostic par stimulation auriculaire et ventriculaire. II – Traitement par l'implantation intracorporelle d'un stimulateur cardiaque avec entrainement simultane de l'oreillette et due ventricule. Arch. Mal. Coeur **60**, 1830 – 1864 (1967)
4. Coumel, Ph., Motte, G., Gouron, R., Fabiato, A., Slama, R., Bouvrain, Y.: Les Tachycardies supra-ventriculaire par rhythme reciproque en dehors due syndrome de Wolff-Parkinson-White. Arch. Mal. Coeur **63**, 35 – 73 (1970)
5. Denes, P., Wu, D., Dhingra, R., Pietras, R. J., Rosen, K. M.: The effects of cycle length on cardiac refractory periods in man. Circulation **49**, 32 – 41 (1974)

6. De Sanctis, R. W., Kastor, J. A.: Rapid intracardiac pacing for treatment of recurrent ventricular tachyarrhythmias in the absence of heart block. Amer. Heart J. **76,** 168 – 172 (1968)
7. Durrer, D., Schoo, L., Schuilenburg, R. M., Wellens, H. J. J.: The role of premature beats in the initiation and the termination of supraventricular tachycardia in the Wolff-Parkinson-White syndrome. Circulation **36,** 644 – 662 (1967)
8. Fontaine, G., Frank, R., Guiraudon, G., Vedel, J., Grosgogeat, Y., Cabrol, C.: Surgical treatment of resistant reentrant ventricular tachycardia by ventriculotomy: a new application of epicardial mapping (abstract). Circulation **49 – 50** (suppl. III), III – 82 (1974)
9. Fontaine, G., Beneton, H., Frank, R., Guiraudon, G., Grosgogeat, Y., Facquet, J.: Prevention de la tachycardie ventriculaire apres infarctus du myocarde par pacemaker intra-corporel. Arch. Mal Coeur **68,** 961 – 968 (1975)
10. Grolleau, R., Dufoix, R., Puech, P., Latour, H.: Les Tachycardies par rythme reciproque dans le syndrome de Wolff-Parkinson-White. Arch. Mal Coeur **63,** 74 – 96 (1970)
11. Guize, L., Zacouto, F., Lenegre, J.: Un nouveau stimulateur du coer: le pacemaker orthorythmique. Presse Med. **79,** 2071 – 2072 (1971)
12. Guize, L., Zacouto, F., Meilhac, B., Le Pailleur, C., Di Matteo, J.: Stimulations endocardiaques orthorythmiques: intéret diagnostique et therapeutique. Nouv. Presse Med. **3,** 2083 – 2086 (1974
13. Guize, L. J., Zacouto, F. I.: Principle and applications of the orthorhythmic pacemaker. E.S.A.O. Proceedings **1,** 77 – 80 (1974)
14. Guize, L., Cabanis, Ch., Maurice, P.: Etude selective de la conduction sino-auriculaire par stimulations auriculaires prematurées orthorythmiques. Personal communication
15. Gurtner, H. P., Gertsch, M., Zacouto, F.: Orthorhythmischer Herzschrittmacher und salvenformige Herzstimulation. Schweiz. med. Wschr. **105,** 33 – 38 (1975)
16. Lüderitz, B., Zacouto, F., Guize, L., Steinbeck, G., Riecker, G.: Ein neues Schrittmacherprinzip zur Suppression ventrikulärer Tachykardien. Verh. dtsch. Ges. Kreisl.-Forsch. **39,** 319 – 323 (1973)
17. Lüderitz, B., Steinbeck, G., Guize, G., Zacouto, F.: Schrittmachertherapie tachykarder Rhythmusstörungen durch frequenzbezogene Intervallstimulation. Dtsch. med. Wschr. **100,** 730 – 735 (1975)
18. Motte, G., Oster, G., Coumel, Ph., Slama, R.: Tachycardies par rythme reciproque entre les voies normales et une voie auriculo-hisienne rapide. Arch. Mal. Coeur. **68,** 673 – 682 (1975)
19. Puech, P.: Tachycardies ventriculaires. In: Encyclopedie Medico-chirurgicale (Coeur-Vaisseaux). Paris: 1103 E 10, 1974
20. Sowton, E., Leatham, A., Carson, P.: The suppression of arrhythmias by artificial pacemaker. Lancet (1964) **2,** 1098 – 1100
21. Spurrell, R. A. J., Sowton, E., Deuchar, D. C.: Ventricular tachycardia in 4 patients evaluated by programmed electrical stimulation of heart and treated in 2 patients by surgical division of anterior radiation of left bundle-branch. Brit. Heart J. **35,** 1014 – 1025 (1973)
22. Strauss, H. C., Sarof, A. L., Bigger jr., J. T., Giardina, E. G.: Premature atrial stimulation as a key to the understanding of sinoatrial conduction in man. Circulation **47,** 86 – 93 (1973)
23. Theisen, K., Zacouto, F., Grohmann, H., Jahrmärker, H.: Refraktärzeitmessung bei absoluter Arrhythmie mit orthorhythmischer Serienstimulation. Klin. Wschr. **52,** 1082 – 1084 (1974)
24. Wellens, H. J.: Electrical Stimulation of the Heart in the Study and Treatment of Tachycardias. Baltimore: University Park Press, 1971
25. Wellens, H. J., Schuilenburg, R. M., Durrer, D.: Electrical stimulation of the heart in patients with ventricular tachycardia. Circulation **46,** 216 – 226 (1972)

Orthorhythmic Stimulation and Endocardial Detection as a Diagnostic Tool

K. THEISEN and H. JAHRMÄRKER

Analysis of excitation and electrical conduction in circumscribed areas of the human heart have been done mainly during open-heart surgery. Boineau et al. [2] analyzed the conduction pathway in WPW tachycardias, Fontaine et al. [5] as well as Spurell et al. [18] in recurrent ventricular tachycardias using epicardial mapping. Small silver electrodes have been used for endocardial registration for the purpose of conduction studies in congenital heart disease [9, 25].

The registration of electrical potentials in circumscribed areas of the human heart has become available by introduction of His bundle electrocardiography [17]. In a few cases this technique was used for determining the onset of excitation in the left and right Tawara fascicle [15] as well as in the right and left ventricle [3]. Monophasic action potentials have been recorded within the right atrium using suction electrodes [12] and within atria and ventricles using needle electrodes [13].

A new clinical procedure of endocardial impulse registration practicable in any part of the atria and ventricles was reported previously [19, 20]. This method may be applied as a closed-chest procedure and requires common pacemaker electrodes. Using the detection filtering device of the orthorhythmic pacemaker [1], the onset of the local excitation at the site of the endocardial electrode is recorded [19]. The apparatus allows single, paired, and coupled stimulation using up to 10 serial impulses at a variable percental distance from the preceding RR interval [28]. Endocardial detection and orthorhythmic stimulation offer new techniques for electrophysiologic studies of the human heart.

Measurement of the Functional Refractory Period (FRP) in Atrial Fibrillation

The orthorhythmic pacemaker system allows determination of the functional refractory period of the heart in atrial fibrillation [19]. The first of a series of 10 stimulation impulses is inserted at a certain percentage of the preceding RR interval. This stimulation technique assures that the impulse starts within the absolute refractory period. The following nine impulses, each at a distance of 20 ms, extend the stimulation into the relative refractory period. A potential latency period is checked by single impulse stimulation. The impulse giving a response in the series of impulses can be

[1] Cardio-Stimulateur Orthorythmique, Lab. Savita, Paris.

identified. Due to the changing RR interval and refractory period, a continuous measurement of FRP in atrial fibrillation can be achieved by serial impulses and orthorhythmic application only.

For the measurement of the functional refractory period using the coupled stimulation method, it is important to determine the onset of the local excitation at the site of the restimulating electrode. The intraventricular conduction time of the spontaneous heart action to the site of the intraventricular electrode can be measured as the interval between the beginning of the QRS complex and the detection spike. In our experiments this interval varies from 30 to 50 ms and up to 75 ms in right bundle branch block. In coupled stimulation, this value has to be deducted from the interval between the QRS and the respective response. This interval was used formerly for the estimation of the functional refractory period. The FRP is measured as the distance between the detection spike and the restimulating impulse. In coupled stimulation, this correction is not needed. These findings explain the differences of FRP values found in comparative studies of both coupled and paired stimulation [6].

In conclusion, FRP measurements in coupled stimulation experiments are valid only if endocardial detection is performed. FRP can be measured in atrial fibrillation necessitating serial impulses for continuous measurements.

Measurement of Fascicular Conduction Time

By means of endocardial detection, the onset of the local excitation within the distribution area of the right bundle and the anterior (LAB) or posterior (LPB) fascicle of the left bundle can be detected ([20] Fig. 1). The site of the detection electrode in the area of the LAB or LPB can be confirmed by stimulation experiments. Left or right axis deviation indicates the position of the electrode in the area of the respective fascicle. According to the concept of Rosenbaum [16], extrasystoles from the LPB area show left axis deviation, and extrasystoles originating in the LAB area show right axis deviation.

If the excitation in the main stem of the His bundle is recorded by means of His bundle electrocardiography and simultaneously the detection in the peripheral area of the fascicles is performed, the conduction time from the His bundle stem to the peripheral endings of the respective fascicle can be measured, termed H-DLV_{LA} and H-DLV_{LP}. These measurements make possible a more detailed analysis of the subjunctional conduction system, i.e., Tawara fascicles and peripheral Purkinje fibers.

Example. Using this method, the function of the subjunctional conduction system was studied in a patient with Jervell and Lange-Nielsen syndrome. This patient showed the characteristic abnormalities of the T-U-waves in the conventional electrocardiogram and exhibited syncopes due to recurrent ventricular tachycardias as first described by Jervell and Lange-Nielsen [8], Romano et al. [14], and Ward [26]. When coupled atrial stimu-

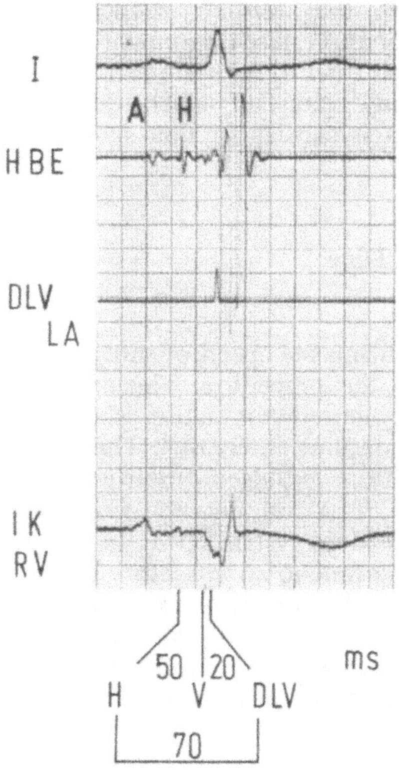

Fig. 1. Measurement of fascicular conduction time.
I is lead I, HBE is His bundle ECG recorded with a threepolar electrode catheter filtered 40–500 Hz. DLV_{LA} shows the spike of the detection representing the onset of local excitation at site of electrode. Electrode is localized endocardially on anterior wall of left ventricle (see text). IKRV is intracavitary unipolar ECG recorded from right ventricle. H-DLV is time from the beginning of His bundle detection (*H*) until arrival of excitation at peripheral parts of left anterior fascicle (DLV_{LA}). This represents conduction time in this fascicle (70 ms). V-DLV is time from beginning of QRS in the IKRV until beginning of excitation at DLV_{LA}.

lation was applied, concomitant with shortening of the coupling interval, a delay in AV conduction appeared as expected. At the same time, and at similar heart rate and coupling interval, the subjunctional conduction showed four different patterns [23] (Fig. 2).

In type 1, subjunctional conduction was normal with average values of H-V, H-DLV and V-DLV intervals. Type 2 showed left bundle branch block. Ventricles were reached via the right bundle without delay; H-V time was normal. The interval from the beginning of the excitation in the right ventricle until the onset of the excitation in the left ventricle V-DLV amounted to 100 ms. Type 3 showed, in addition to left bundle branch block, a conduction delay in the right bundle with an increase of the H-V interval to 80 ms. V-DLV was about the same as in type 2. In type 4 the conduction delay in the right bundle increased up to the amount of the conduction delay within the left bundle; therefore the QRS complex was small and did not show any signs of bundle branch block. A short interval V-DLV amounting to 40 ms excludes conduction from the right to the left ventricle as in type 2 and 3.

This spontaneously changing electrical conduction indicates an extreme lability in the function of the subjunctional conduction system in the Jervell syndrome. A conduction delay occurs in some parts up to two- to threefold of normal values, and at the same time normal conduction in other parts of the system. If there are two or three fascicles out of phase, retrograde activation of such a blocked fascicle, reentry into the His bundle stem, and beginning of a circus movement may occur [10], which was demonstrated to be the cause of ventricular tachycardias in this syndrome [21, 22].

Measurement of Intraventricular Conduction Time. Method and Example

Endocardial detection can be used for measuring the speed of intraventricular impulse propagation. Figure 3 shows the procedure. The onset of excitation is detected within the left ventricle. Paired stimulation is applied within the right ventricle, using increasing coupling intervals [2]. The intraventricular conduction time from the stimulating impulse in the right ventricle to the detection in the left ventricle ST-DLV amounts to 65 ms, and the retrograde conduction within the His-Purkinje system ST-H to 90 ms. When restimulation is done at the time of the functional refractory period, the stimulated QRS complex shows right bundle branch block in lead V_1 despite right ventricular stimulation. The explanation of this finding is given by the conduction times. Under these conditions, conduction from the right to the left ventricle amounts to 85 ms, and the retrograde conduction within the specific conduction system ST-H is increased up to more than 130 ms, the H potential being undetectable within the QRS complex. This means that left ventricular activation is faster than retrograde activation within the His-Purkinje system of the right ventricle. The earlier onset of the excitation in the left ventricle causes right bundle branch block.

The reason for this conduction pattern is due to the fact that the FRP of the peripheral Purkinje fibers is the longest of the His-Purkinje system and of similar extent as the FRP of the AV node [11]. This is the basis of the so-called gate function of the peripheral Purkinje fibers, which prevents premature activation of the myocardium in the antegrade direction and premature activation of the Purkinje system in retrograde direction. These peripheral Purkinje fibers are refractory when stimulated at the FRP of the myocardial fibers [3]. Measuring the intraventricular conduction from the right to the left ventricle under these conditions indicates myocardial conduction and allows study of pharmacologic effects on myocardial conduction [7].

Analysis of Rhythm Disturbances

Detection and orthorhythmic stimulation facilitates a differentiation of tachycardias with regard to focal or reentry genesis and allows localization

[2] Medtronic double impulse stimulator, model 5837.

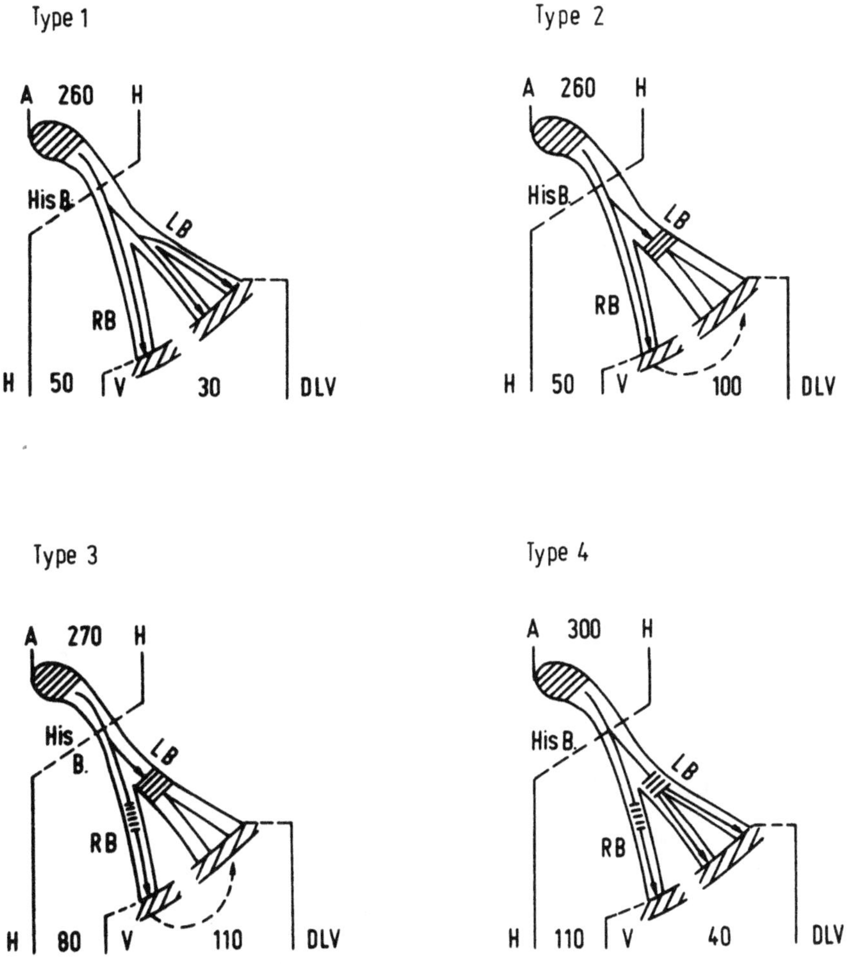

Fig. 2. Four types of subjunctional conduction measured by left ventricular endocardial detection in a patient with Jervell and Lange-Nielsen syndrome, using coupled early premature atrial stimulation (see text).

Type 1: H – V (50 ms), V – DLV (30 ms), and H – DLV (80 ms) are normal.

Type 2: Under the same stimulation conditions left bundle branch block occurs. H – V time remains unchanged with 50 ms, the right ventricle being arrived by excitation without delay. Interval from beginning of QRS complex in right ventricle (*V*) to onset of local excitation in left ventricle (*DLV*) amounts to 100 ms.

Type 3: In addition to left bundle branch block, a conduction delay in right bundle (*RB*) occurs with increased H – V interval of 80 ms. V – DLV is similar to type 2.

Type 4. Conduction delay in left and right bundle occurs to same extent. Resulting QRS complex does not show branch block pattern. V – DLV time of 40 ms is too short to allow myocardial conduction from right to left ventricle [24].

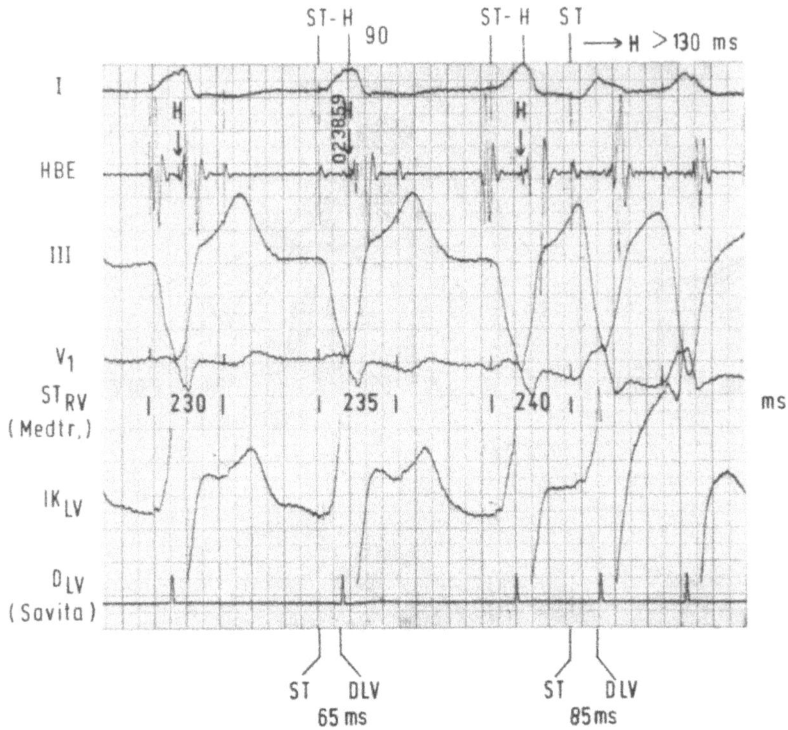

Fig. 3. Measurement of intraventricular conduction time.

Registration of lead I, His bundle electrocardiogram (*HBE*), lead III, V_1, intracavitary unipolar lead from left ventricle, and detection of onset of local excitation in left ventricle (*DLV*). STRV means right ventricular paired stimulation with increasing coupling interval. ST – DLV time (65 ms) is conduction time from right ventricular stimulating impulse to left ventricular onset of excitation. ST – H time (90 ms) is retrograde conduction time from stimulating impulse to His bundle deflection. Reexcitation of right ventricle occurs when coupling interval is extended to 240 ms, showing right bundle branch block (lead V_1). Under these conditions, ST – DLV is 85 ms, ST – H is prolonged to more than 130 ms and is not detectable within QRS complex. ST – DLV represents myocardial conduction time from right to left ventricle [24].

of their origin [20]. As an example, recordings of a patient are shown which exhibit paroxysmal tachycardias. A single stimulation impulse applied in the right ventricle induced a supraventricular tachycardia identified by His bundle recordings. A spontaneous supraventricular tachycardia of the same pattern could be interrupted by two coupled orthorhythmic pacemaker impulses applied within the right ventricle. Initiation and interruption by single or double impulses in the right ventricle suggest intra-atrial or AV nodal reentry genesis of the supraventricular tachycardia [1, 27]. The HV interval remained constant at 50 ms during both supraventricular tachycardia and sinus rhythm. The subjunctional conduction time from the entrance of the excitation in the main stem of the His bundle until the onset of local excitation in the right ventricle (H-DRV time) shortens by 20 ms from 50 to 30 ms.

Another patient exhibited ventricular tachycardia of probably focal genesis which originated from the left posterior fascicle as indicated by the electrocardiographic pattern which showed left axis deviation and right bundle branch block. In this case orthorhythmically timed single impulses applied in the area of the posterior fascicle within the left ventricle interrupted the tachycardia reproducibly but only momentarily. After two sinus beats the focus took over the pacemaker function again.

In the same patient, two different types of ventricular premature beats could be analyzed with regard to their origin by endocardial detection. In the first type of premature beat, following normal sinus action with a coupling interval of 450 ms, the conduction time from the beginning of the premature beat (V) until the detection electrode placed in the area of the left anterior fascicle ($V\text{-}DLVA_{LA}$) amounted to 30 ms and the retrograde activation of the His bundle main stem to 40 ms. The focus of a second type of premature beat showing a different configuration and a shorter coupling interval of 360 ms can be supposed to be localized more distantly in the periphery of the detected Tawara fascicle since the $V\text{-}DLV_{LA}$ interval was only 7 ms. During this premature beat the retrograde activation of the His bundle was considerably increased and not exactly detectable within the QRS complex.

Summary

Local excitation at the site of an endocardial pacemaker electrode can be recorded using the detection filtering device of the orthorhythmic pacemaker. Orthorhythmic coupled and paired stimulation can be performed additionally. This pacemaker system allows new electrophysiologic studies of the human heart: measurement of the functional refractory period in atrial fibrillation, of the conduction time in the three Tawara fascicles, and of the intraventricular conduction time. Ventricular tachycardias and ventricular premature beats may be differentiated with regard to their origin and to their focal or reentry genesis.

References

1. Bigger, Th., J., Goldreyer, B. N.: The mechanism of supraventricular tachycardia. Circulation **42,** 673 (1970)
2. Boineau, J. P., Moore, E. N., Spear, D. J. F., Sealy, W. L.: Basis of clinical ECG variations in right and left ventricular preexcitation: A unitary concept of WPW. In: Cardiac Arrhythmias, Dreifus, L. S., Likoff, W. (eds.), New York: Grune & Stratton, 1973, p. 421
3. Castellanos, A., Belfer, B., Myerburg, R. J., Castillo, C. A., Agha, A. S., Vagueiro, M. C.: Functional properties of the ventricular muscle and distal conduction system during right ventricular stimulation with special reference to the RBBB pattern in V_1, supernormal intraventricular conduction and physiological "gate". Europ. J. Cardiol. **1,** 41 (1973)
4. Castellanos, A., Castillo, C. A., Agha, A. S., Myerburg, R. J., Tessler, M.: Mechanisms of ventricular tachycardia. In: Cardiac Arrhythmias, Dreifus, L. S., Likoff, W. (eds.), New York: Grune and Stratton 1973, p. 235
5. Fontaine, G., Frank, R., Guiraudon, G., Vedel, J., Grosgogeat, Y., Cabrol, Ch.: Surgical treatment of resistant re-entrant ventricular tachycardia by ventriculotomy. A new application of epicardial mapping. Circulation **49,** Suppl. III, 82 (1974)

6. Grohmann, H. W., Theisen, K., Jahrmärker, H.: Einfach- und Doppelstimulation des menschlichen Vorhofs. Untersuchungen zur Refraktärzeitbestimmung. Verh. dtsch. Ges. Kreisl.-Forsch. **37,** 460 (1971)
7. Jahrmärker, H., Theisen, K.: Influence of Canreanoate-K on the refractory period of the human heart. In: Diuretics in Research and Clinics. International Symposium, Bürgenstock Stuttgart: Thieme 1976
8. Jervell, A., Lange-Nielsen, F.: Congenital deafmutism, functional heart disease, with prolongation of the QT-intervall and sudden death. Amer. Heart J. **54,** 59 (1957)
9. Kaiser, G. A., Waldo, A. L., Beach, P. M. et al.: Specialized cardiac conduction system: Improved electrophysiologic identification technique of surgery. Arch. Surg. **101,** 673 (1970)
10. Moe, G. K., Mendez, C.: Functional bloc in the intraventricular conduction system. Circulation **43,** 949 (1971)
11. Myerburg, R. J., Stewart, J. W., Hoffmann, B. F.: Electrophysiological properties of the canine peripheral a-v conduction system. Circulat. Res. **26,** 361 (1970)
12. Olsson, B.: In vivo recordings of action potentials in man: In: Cardiac Arrhythmias. Sandoe, E., Flensted-Jensen, E., Oelsen, K. H. (eds.) Elsinore: Astra Sweden, 1970, p. 37
13. Cabasson, J., Puech, P.: Evaluation of suction electrode recording. In: Diagnostic and Therapeutical Tools of cardiac pacing. This volume, p. 73 – 79
14. Romano, C., Gemme, G., Pongiglione, R.: Aritmie cardiache rare dell'età pediatrica. II. Accessi sincopali per fibrillazione ventricolare parossistica. Presentazione del primo case della letteratura pediatrica italiana. Clin. pediat. (Bologna) **45,** 656 (1963)
15. Rosen, K. M., Rahimtoola, S. H., Sinno, M. Z., Gunnar, R. M.: Bundle branch and ventricular activation in man. A study using catheter recordings of left and right bundle branch potentials. Circulation **43,** 193 (1971)
16. Rosenbaum, B.: Classification of ventricular extrasystoles according to form. J. Electrocardiol. **2,** 289 (1969)
17. Scherlag, B. J., Lau, S. H., Helfant, R. H., Stein, E., Berkowitz, W. D., Damato, A. N.: Catheter technique for recordings His bundle activity in man. Circulation **39,** 13 (1969)
18. Spurell, R. A. J., Sowton, E., Deuchar, D. C.: Ventricular tachycardia in 4 patients evaluated by programmed electrical stimulation of heart and treatment in 2 patients by surgical division of anterior radiation of left bundle branch. Brit. Heart J. **35,** 1014 (1973)
19. Theisen, K., Zacouto, F., Grohmann, H., Jahrmärker, H.: Refraktärzeitmessung bei absoluter Arrhythmie mit orthorhythmischer Serienstimulation. Klin. Wschr. **52,** 1082 (1974)
20. Theisen, K., Halbritter, R., Jahrmärker, H.: Messung der Leitungszeit in den Faszikeln des His-Purkinje-Systems mittels endocardialer Detektion. Klin. Wschr. **53,** 279 (1975)
21. Theisen, K., Haider, M., Jahrmärker, H.: Untersuchungen ventrikulärer Tachykardien durch Re-entry bei inhomogener Repolarisation. Dtsch. med. Wschr. **100,** 1099 (1975)
22. Theisen, K., Jahrmärker, H.: Re-entry-Mechanismus ventrikulärer Tachykardien bei inhomogener Repolarisation, unter besonderer Berücksichtigung des Jervell- und Lange-Nielsen-Syndroms sowie ähnlicher Zustände und ihrer Therapie. Dtsch. med. Wschr. **100,** 1141 (1975)
23. Theisen, K., Halbritter, R., Jahrmärker, H.: Untersuchung der subjunktionalen Erregungsleitung bei Jervell- und Lange-Nielsen-Syndrom. Verh. dtsch. Ges. Kreisl.-Forsch. **41,** 391 (1975)
24. Theisen, K., Jahrmärker, H.: Untersuchung des Erregungsablaufs am menschlichen Herzen mit endokardialer Detektion. In preparation
25. Waldo, A. L., James, Th. N.: The cardiac conduction system; electrophysiological studies during open heart surgery. Arch. intern. Med. **135,** 411 (1975)
26. Ward, O. C. J.: A new familial cardiac syndrome in children. J. Irish med. Ass. **54,** 103 (1964)
27. Wu, D., Denes, P.: Mechanisms of paroxysmal supraventricular tachycardia. Arch. intern. Med. **135,** 437 (1975)
28. Zacouto, F., Guize, L., Maurice, P., Gerbaux, A.: Orthorhythmic pacing in arrhythmias. Amer. J. Cardiol. **31,** 165 (1973)

The Use of Programmed Rate-Related Premature Stimulation in Managing Tachyarrhythmias *

B. LÜDERITZ and G. STEINBECK

Various types of supraventricular and ventricular tachycardias may be refractory to multiple drug treatment and conventional antiarrhythmic therapy. In a large number of cases electrophysiologic approaches like d-c cardioversion and cardiac pacing are effective in controlling ectopic tachycardias [2, 15, 19, 25]. Electrical pacing offers certain advantages over standard d-c cardioversion for the termination of tachycardias: (1) No general anesthesia is required. (2) Digitalis-induced arrhythmias may be abolished, a situation in which d-c cardioversion is dangerous and usually ineffective. (3) Pacing can be effected rapidly, simply, and repeatedly leaving the pacing catheter in place [2]. At the present time different modes of cardiac pacing techniques are in use in order to suppress supraventricular, junctional, and ventricular tachycardias. These are:

1. *Rapid atrial stimulation*
2. *Overdrive pacing*
3. *Coupled stimulation*
4. *Patient-initiated atrial pacing*
5. *Precisely timed single or multiple premature stimulation*
6. *Programmed rate-related interval stimulation*

Rapid Atrial Stimulation

Electrical stimulation of the right atrium using a electrode catheter may terminate atrial tachycardias and atrial flutter. Applying this method, impulses are delivered singly or repetitively at frequencies varying from 200 to 400/min. Continuous monitoring of the electrocardiogram indicates conversion of atrial flutter — frequently first to atrial fibrillation and subsequently to normal sinus rhythm. This method is an effective and safe alternative bedside treatment for terminating atrial tachycardia and flutter which does not require general anesthesia. Rapid atrial pacing seems to be an appropriate method, especially in patients receiving large doses of digitalis [9].

Overdrive Pacing

Overdriving means atrial or ventricular stimulation at frequencies above the spontaneous heart rate. This technique is an effective method, predomi-

* Supported by Deutsche Forschungsgemeinschaft.

nantly in cases of supraventricular and ventricular extrasystoles. Overdrive pacing can be performed for hours or even for several days which may be advantageous in acute myocardial infarction or following heart surgery.

Coupled Stimulation

The frequency of drug-resistant tachycardias may be reduced in some cases by coupled stimulation providing a prolongation of the electrical refractory period. Following the last QRS complex in close succession, a second ventricular contraction is prevented by the artificially induced prolongation of the refractory period. Thus, by lengthening the period of inexcitability, the heart rate is significantly reduced [17].

Patient-Initiated Atrial Pacing

Recently an artificial patient-controlled pacemaker system was described for management of supraventricular tachycardias [5, 11, 12]. This system consists of an implanted receiver connected to bipolar atrial electrodes and an external, battery-powered, patient-activated transmitter/antenna. Energy transmission between the transmitter and receiver is accomplished through radio-frequency coupling. Stimulator pulse frequency is controllable at the transmitter between 50 and 300 pulses per minute. Patient-initiated rapid atrial pacing for 10 – 20 s has been demonstrated to be effective in terminating recurrent supraventricular tachycardias with a resulting return to normal sinus rhythm. Occasionally transient episodes of atrial fibrillation or flutter precede a spontaneous return to sinus rhythm [12].

Precisely Timed Single or Multiple Premature Stimulation

It has been shown that recurrent tachycardias can be suppressed by single or multiple properly timed stimulations [25]. The termination of ectopic tachycardias by premature stimulation is best understood, if one holds responsible a reentry mechanism. This theory postulates that the premature electrical impulse creates refractoriness in a part of the reentry pathway so that the next circulating impulse dies out in the refractory area. Thereby the tachycardia is terminated. Necessary conditions for a reentrant tachycardia are: unidirectional block in one or more regions of the heart, slow passage of the impulse over an alternative pathway, delayed excitation of the tissue distal to the blocked site, and reexcitation of the tissue proximal to the site of block [22; see also 25]. Thus the perpetuation of the tachycardia demands a refractory period shorter than the time needed for conduction of the activation wave around a loop. In mathematical terms:

$$RP < \oint \frac{1}{V} \mathrm{d}l$$

i.e., the refractory period must be smaller than the circle integral of 1 over V, and V equals conduction velocity in the pathway times the differential length of the pathway (dl) [20]. A reentrant tachycardia may be terminated if the refractory period exceeds the conduction time around the loop.

Programmed Rate-Related Stimulation

Concept of Orthorhythmic Pacing: The principle of precisely timed premature stimulation is realized by programmed rate-related interval stimulation [6, 7, 10, 15, 16, 21, 26, 27]. The delivery of an electrical impulse is determined by the preceding interval of atrial or ventricular depolarization. Therefore this pacing mode is automatically frequency-dependent.

The so-called orthorhythmic pacemaker is characterized by a programmable demand pacing with escape intervals in relation to the length of the preceding cardiac cycle. Whereas conventional demand pacemakers operate at a fixed escape interval (hysteresis) the orthorhythmic system possesses a variable hysteresis, i.e., the pacemaker takes into consideration the exact time of the extrasystole and produces a response delay automatically variable as a function of the premature beat interval. The variable response delay (stimulation interval) may be identical to the premature beat interval. The ratio of these two intervals can, however, be modified. The orthorhythmic system represents an external pacemaker connected with temporary endocardial electrodes. Temporal epicardial electrodes after open heart surgery can also be used. The power source are two 9-V alkaline batteries. Orthorhythmic pacing is applicable in the atrium or in the ventricle. It can be performed with single or repeated stimulations delivered according to an adjustable program. This kind of stimulation — completed by marking the

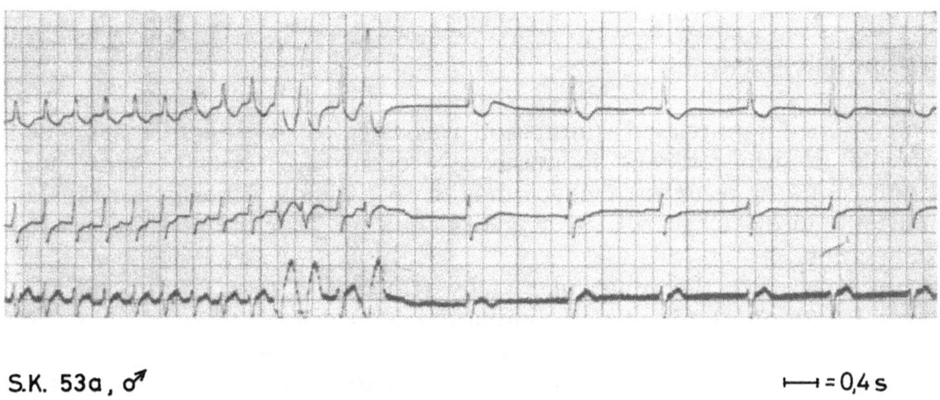

Fig. 1. Termination of supraventricular tachycardia by spontaneously occurring ventricular extrasystoles leading to retrograde conduction and thereby suppression of tachycardia followed by junctional escape rhythm.

local intracardiac detection in the atrium or in the ventricle—provides the possibility of consecutive stimulation like paired, tripled, or quadruple-coupled stimulations or impulses in very rapid coupled salvos. This on-demand stimulation coupled to the preceding cardiac depolarizations is applicable in bradycardias as well as in various types of tachycardias [8]. Figure 1 shows the termination of a supraventricular tachycardia by spontaneously occurring ventricular extrasystoles leading to retrograde conduc-

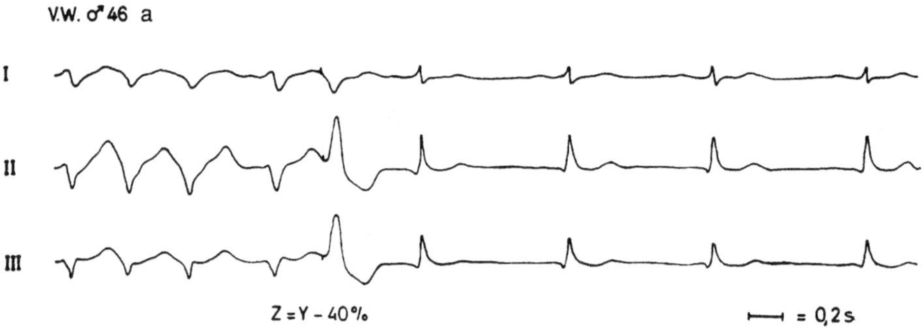

Fig. 2. Ventricular tachycardia terminated by rate-related premature stimulation. The stimulation interval is chosen as a function of the foregoing RR interval. In this case the tachycardia is terminated by a stimulation interval that is 60% shorter than the preceding RR interval.

tion and thereby termination of the tachycardia. The suppression of tachycardia by properly timed premature depolarization is obvious from Figure 2 which demonstrates the pacing mode of rate-related stimulation. The stimulation interval (Z) after which the impulse is delivered is dependent on the foregoing RR interval (Y). In this case a ventricular tachycardia is terminated by a stimulation interval that is 60% shorter than the preceding RR interval.

Results and Discussion

Programmed rate-related stimulation was effective in 54% of cases when applied in drug-resistant spontaneously occurring bursts of ventricular extrasystoles or recurrent tachycardias in 56 patients. Efficiency means an interruption of tachycardia by single or multiple programmed rate-related stimulation.

In most cases the ventricular tachyarrhythmias were terminated after several attempts of rate-related stimulation using different frequency-dependent stimulation intervals. Junctional tachycardias could be suppressed by ventricular stimulation due to retrograde penetration of the ventricular impulse and interruption of the reentry circuit.

One of the side-effects of injecting radiocontrast material into the coronary system as well as into the ventricle is the occurrence of ectopic beats, sometimes ventricular flutter or even ventricular fibrillation — either by mechanical irritation of the ventricular wall or as a consequence of sinus slowing [3; see also 4]. In order to control ventricular tachycardia, rate-related stimulation was therefore applied in patients with tachyarrhythmias occurring during diagnostic right- and left-heart catheterization and angiocardiography. The suppression of ventricular arrhythmias occurring in diagnostic heart catheterization was about half as successful (21% of 20 cases) as in spontaneously occurring drug-resistant tachyarrhythmias (54%). It may be deduced from these observations that ventricular extrasystoles and tachycardias seen during cardiac catheterization are predominantly of focal origin whereas spontaneous ventricular tachycardias might rather be caused by a reentry mechanism. Thus, the rate-related stimulation technique may contribute in some cases to the differential diagnosis of ventricular tachycardias.

On the basis of experimental evidence, stretching of Purkinje fibers leads to an increase in the depolarization rate. Single fibers of the myocardium gain transient pacemaker properties as well [14; see also 1]. These effects are completely reversible within a few seconds after extension. A similar mechanism can be assumed during cardiac catheterization.

In some cases of junctional and ventricular tachycardias two or even three coupled rate-related premature stimuli have to be delivered in close succession to terminate the tachycardia, especially in tachycardias at high rates. Ventricular tachycardias which could not be terminated by one or two stimuli were occasionally suppressed by sequential RR-related multiple stimulation. Atrial flutter was converted to atrial fibrillation and sinus rhythm by atrial interval-related multiple stimulation elicited by use of an atrial electrode catheter [7]. The efficiency of this procedure in atrial flutter depends on an adequate sensing of atrial activations which must not exceed a frequency of about 300/min in order to trigger the pacing system by sufficient voltage of depolarization. The rate-related pacing system is ineffective in atrial fibrillation.

The advantages of a pacemaker device with rate-related stimulation and additional standby stimulation function as realized in the orthorhythmic pacemaker may be illustrated in a patient with sick sinus syndrome [18]. A 53-year-old patient with coronary heart disease suffered from alternating tachycardias and bradycardias — the so-called tachycardia-bradycardia syndrome [13]. Both the sinus node recovery time and the so-called sinoatrial conduction time were conspicuously prolonged [23; see also 24]. The recurrent tachycardias were accompanied by severe angina. After termination of the tachycardia by carotid sinus massage performed by the patient himself, a short period of dizziness occurred because of sinus arrest. After several escape beats sinus rhythm reestablished. During the next onset after hospitalization, rate-related premature stimulation was applied (Fig. 3). After reduction of the tachycardia by one properly timed ventricular beat, standby stimulation was mandatory in a normofrequent mode. It is interesting that the tachycardia was terminated without a change in shape of the atrial activation pattern. Therefore it is assumed that the tachy-

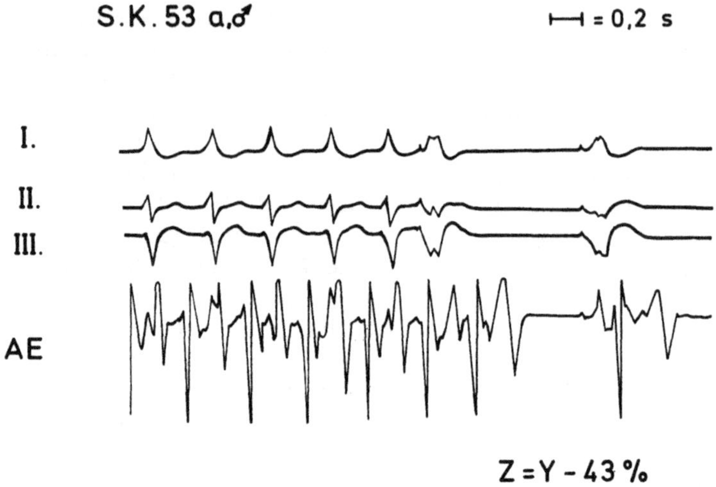

Fig. 3. Application of frequency-dependent stimulation in a patient suffering from sick sinus syndrome. Following termination of tachycardia by one properly timed premature ventricular beat, standby stimulation was mandatory in a normofrequent mode. Tachycardia was suppressed without a change in shape of atrial activation pattern (*AE*). It is assumed that the tachycardia is of junctional origin terminated by concealed retrograde penetration of the ventricular impulse.

cardia was of junctional origin interrupted by concealed retrograde penetration of the ventricular impulse. Figure 4 shows a very similar situation in the same patient. The reduction of junctional tachycardia, the normofrequent standby stimulation, and several ventricular premature beats can be seen. A new tachycardia is initiated by a ventricular extrasystole probably on a reentry basis involving ventricular and supraventricular pathways. The last rate-related impulse stops the tachycardia. Later the patient got a per-

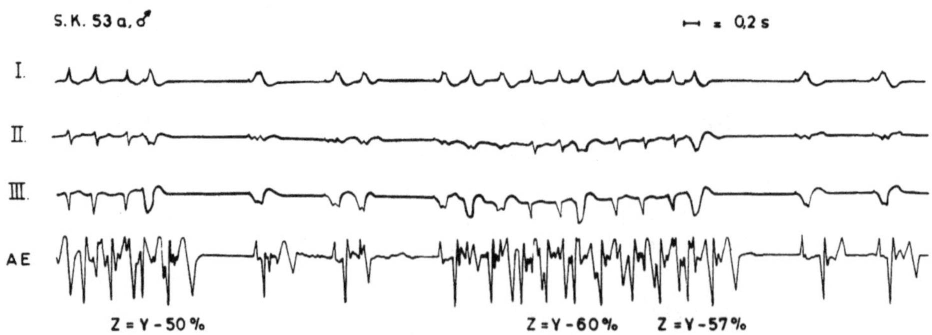

Fig. 4. Reduction of junctional tachycardia, normofrequent standby stimulation, and ventricular premature beats in a patient with sick sinus syndrome (see Fig. 3). A new tachycardia is initiated by ventricular extrasystole probably of reentry basis involving ventricular and supraventricular pathways. Last rate-related impulse stops the tachycardia.

manent standby pacemaker while onsets of junctional tachycardias were controlled by verapamil.

In conclusion: Programmed rate-related interval stimulation proved to be a low-risk method when applied in drug-resistant junctional and ventricular tachycardias or runs of ventricular extrasystoles as precursors of a tachycardia. Tachycardias that could not be terminated by single or double stimulation were sometimes successfully suppressed by sequential multiple rate-related stimulation. Orthorhythmic pacing has proved to be an alternative method for treatment of tachyarrhythmias unresponsive to conventional means. As a complication, the initiation of ventricular tachycardias due to the stimulation procedure was observed in three cases.

Summary

Termination of reentry tachycardias can be achieved by single and multiple precisely timed stimulation. To control supraventricular and ventricular tachycardias, 82 patients with recurrent tachyarrhythmias were studied. Applying a new pacemaker system, premature stimuli were elicited in the right atrium or right ventricle with automatically varying prematurity. The evaluation was performed in patients suffering from arrhythmias occurring either spontaneously or during diagnostic right- and left-heart catheterization and angiocardiography. Atrial flutter could be converted into sinus rhythm by rate-related multiple stimulations. Ventricular tachycardias which could not be terminated by one or two stimuli were occasionally suppressed by sequential RR-related multiple stimulations. Suppression of spontaneous drug-resistant ventricular arrhythmias was more than twice as successful (54%) as those occurring during diagnostic heart catheterizations (21%).

The results support the assumption that ventricular extrasystoles and tachycardias seen during cardiac catheterizations are predominantly of focal origin whereas spontaneous ventricular tachycardias may rather be caused by a reentry mechanism. The results demonstrate the significant benefit of the automatic repetitive intervention by rate-related premature stimulation while other pacing methods available do not provide automatically beat-to-beat – adapted interventions in recurrent tachycardias. This low-risk method can be an effective therapy in tachyarrhythmias when other methods have failed.

References

1. Antoni, H.: Die Entstehung ektopischer Schrittmacher durch Funktionswandel des nichtautomatischen Arbeitsmyokards. In: Herzrhythmusstörungen, Holzmann, M. (ed.) Stuttgart-New York: Schattauer, 1968
2. Barold, S. S., Linhart, J. W.: Recent advances in the treatment of ectopic tachycardias by electrical pacing. Amer. J. Cardiol. **25**, 698 (1970)
3. Benchimol, A., Mc Nally, E. M.: Atrial pacing during selective coronary angiography. Brit. Heart J. **29**, 767 (1967)

4. Desser, K. B., Benchimol, A.: Atrial pacing during selective aortocoronary saphenous vein bypass angiography. Amer. J. Cardiol. **34,** 19 (1974)
5. Goyal, S. L., Lichstein, E., Gupta, P. K., Schadda, K. D.: Refractory reentrant atrial tachycardia: successful treatment with a permanent radiofrequency triggered atrial pacemaker. Amer. J. Med. **58,** 586 (1975)
6. Guize, L., Zacouto, F., Lenegre, J.: Un nouveau stimulateur du coeur: le pacemaker orthorythmique. Presse méd. **79,** 2071 (1971)
7. Guize, L., Zacouto, F., Meilhac, B., Le Pailleur, C., Di Mattéo, J.: Stimulations endocardiaques orthorythmiques. Nouv. Presse méd. **3,** 2083 (1974)
8. Guize, L., Zacouto, F.: Principle and applications of the orthorhythmic pacemaker. E.S.A.O. Proceedings **1,** 77 (1974)
9. Gulotta, S. J., Aronson, A. L.: Cardioversion of atrial tachycardia and flutter by atrial stimulation. Amer. J. Cardiol. **26,** 262 (1970)
10. Gurtner, H. P., Gertsch, M., Zacouto, F.: Orthorhythmischer Herzschrittmacher und salvenförmige Herzstimulation. Schweiz. med. Wschr. **105,** 33 (1975)
11. Kahn, A.: Patient-initiated rapid atrial pacing to manage supraventricular tachycardia. Presented at Amer. Heart Association, 47th Scientific Session, Dallas 1974
12. Kahn, A., Citron, P.: Patient initiated rapid atrial pacing to manage supraventricular tachycardia. In this volume, p. 205 – 211
13. Kaplan, B. M., Langendorf, R., Lev, M., Pick, A.: Tachycardia-bradycardia-syndrome (so-called "sick sinus syndrome") pathology, mechanisms and treatment. Amer. J. Cardiol. **31,** 497 (1973)
14. Kaufmann, R., Theophile, K.: Automatiefördernde Dehnungseffekte an Purkinje-Fäden, Papillarmuskeln und Vorhoftrabekeln von Rhesusaffen. Pfügers Arch. ges. Physiol. **297,** 174 (1967)
15. Lüderitz, B., Zacouto, F., Guize, L., Steinbeck, G., Riecker, G.: Ein neues Schrittmacherprinzip zur Suppression ventrikulärer Tachykardien. Verh. dtsch. Ges. Kreisl.-Forsch. **39,** 319 (1973)
16. Lüderitz, B., Steinbeck, G., Zacouto, F., Riecker, G.: Ergebnisse über die Unterbrechung ventrikulärer Tachykardien durch RR-gekoppelte Intervallstimulation. Verh. dtsch. Ges. Kreisl.-Forsch. **40,** 417 (1974)
17. Lüderitz, B., Steinbeck, G., Guize, L., Zacouto, F.: Schrittmacher-Therapie tachykarder Rhythmusstörungen durch frequenzbezogene Intervallstimulation. Dtsch. med. Wschr. **100,** 730 (1975)
18. Lüderitz, B., Zacouto, F., Steinbeck, G.: Significant reduction of recurrent tachyarrhythmias by programmed rate related stimulation. Vth Int. Symp. on Cardiac Pacing, Tokyo, Excerpta Medica (in press).
19. Massumi, R. A., Kistin, A. D., Tawakkol, A. A.: Termination of reciprocating tachycardia by atrial stimulation. Circulation **36,** 637 (1967)
20. Naumann d' Alnoncourt, Ch.: Interaktion von Triamteren und Glykosiden am Arbeitsmyokard und Erregungsleitungssystem des Herzens. Inauguraldissertation, München 1976
21. Pittmann, D. E., Makar, J. S., Kooros, K. S., Joyner, C. R.: Rapid atrial stimulation: successful method of conversion of atrial flutter and atrial tachycardia. Amer. J. Cardiol. **32,** 700 (1973)
22. Sasyniuk, B. J., Mendez, C.: A mechanism for reentry in canine ventricular tissue. Circulat. Res. **28,** 3 (1971)
23. Steinbeck, G., Körber, H.-J., Lüderitz, B.: Die Bestimmung der sinuatrialen Leitungszeit beim Menschen durch gekoppelte atriale Einzelstimulation. Klin. Wschr. **52,** 1151 (1974)
24. Steinbeck, G., Lüderitz, B.: Comparative study of sinoatrial conduction time and sinus node recovery time. Brit. Heart J. **37,** 956 (1975)
25. Wellens, H. J., Schuilenburg, R. M., Durrer, D.: Electrical stimulation of the heart in patients with ventricular tachycardia. Circulation **48,** 216 (1972)
26. Zacouto, F., Guize, L., Maurice, P., Gerbaux, A.: Orthorhythmic pacing in arrhythmias. Amer. J. Cardiol. **31,** 165 (1973) Abstr.
27. Zacouto, F., Guize, L.: Fundamentals of orthorhythmic pacing. In this volume, p. 212 – 218

Future Aspects of Cardiac Pacing

R. A. J. Spurrell

Atrial or ventricular premature beats may initiate paroxysms of supraventricular tachycardia. Atrial or ventricular pacing at varying rates in order to suppress ectopic activity and recurrent bouts of ventricular tachycardia have been reported by many authors [2, 5, 10, 15].

Various pacing techniques have been used for the termination of atrial flutter and paroxysmal supraventricular tachycardia [4, 7].

As has been discussed elsewhere in this volume, in recent years programed electrical stimulation of the heart and intracardiac recordings have supported the view that a reciprocal mechanism possibly within the AV node is the basis for many paroxysmal supraventricular tachycardias [3]. It has also been shown that patients with these types of tachycardia can have their tachycardias terminated by correctly timed single or double atrial or ventricular premature beats [11].

Various workers [6, 8, 14] have made use of this characteristic of reciprocal tachycardias for the termination of supraventricular tachycardia by implanting a demand pacemaker which can be converted to a fixed rate mode externally. When this is done by the patient during an attack of tachycardia the pacemaker discharges at a rate which is slower than that of the tachycardia. Pacemaker stimuli therefore fall randomly throughout the cardiac cycle until a stimulus occurs at a suitable part of the cardiac cycle such that it produces a premature beat which terminates the tachycardia. This form of pacemaker therapy is most suitable for those patients whose tachycardias can be terminated by single ventricular premature beats. However in the author's experience, in a proportion of patients the pacing stimulus that follows the one which terminates the tachycardia may initiate a further paroxysmal tachycardia.

Recently, pacing systems for the prevention or termination of tachycardias have been developed.

In patients in whom it is found that a single ventricular premature beat can terminate the tachycardia it has been found that simultaneous atrial and ventricular pacing is an effective way of preventing attacks of tachycardia [1]. A similar principle has been used employing the technique of atrial synchronous pacing [12]. In this latter technique an implantable pacing unit was developed which was connected to an atrial sensing electrode and a right ventricular stimulation electrode. Either sinoatrial or ectopic atrial activity was sensed and the pacemaker activated such that a ventricular stimulus was induced with a short atrioventricular delay of 30 ms. In this way sinoatrial activity triggered a ventricular premature beat response, and, also, spontaneous atrial premature beats triggered ventricular

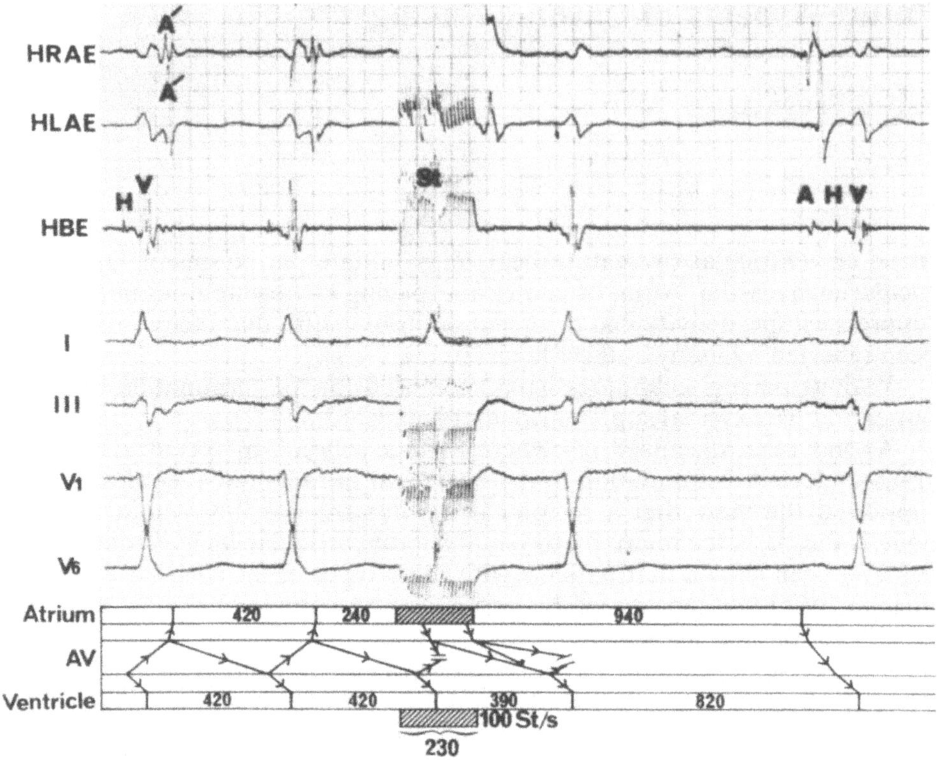

Fig. 1. Termination of supraventricular tachycardia by burst of high frequency stimulation. *HRAE* = high right atrial electrogram; *HLAE* = high left atrial electrogram; *HBE* = His bundle electrogram; *I, III*, V_1, V_6 = surface electrocardiographic leads; A^- = retrograde atrial potential as seen on atrial electrogram; *St* = stimulus artifact; *A* = antegrade atrial potential as seen on the HBE; *H* = His potential as seen on the HBE; *V* = ventricular potential as seen on the HBE; *AV* = atrioventricular junction.

premature beat responses. The ventricular premature beat was conducted retrogradely to the reciprocal circuit, presumably in the AV node, and blocked the initiation of a reciprocal supraventricular tachycardia that would have otherwise been induced by the spontaneous atrial premature beat.

For the termination of a reciprocal supraventricular tachycardia by electrical stimulation, ideally the pacemaker should be activated automatically when tachycardia occurs and then fire single or double stimuli at a preset point in the cardiac cycle when it is known that the tachycardia can be terminated. The pacemaker would then switch itself off. However it has been found that the point in the cardiac cycle where a single or double stimulus can terminate an attack varies over about 20 – 30 ms for each stimulus and so single stimuli cannot be guaranteed to consistently terminate episodes of tachycardia. To overcome this a pacing system (Devices

4270[1]) has been developed [12] which fires bursts of high-frequency stimuli at a known point in the cardiac cycle. A right atrial sensing electrode monitors atrial cycle lengths and when the cycle length is less than a preset interval — that is, when tachycardia has started — the output circuit delivers a burst of high-frequency stimuli triggered with a preset delay from the sensed intra-atrial signal. The high frequency stimuli occur at 100 stimuli per second and bursts of 100 ms duration are used when inducing single atrial premature beats, or up to 250 ms duration when inducing two atrial premature beats.

Figure 1 is a recording obtained from a patient with a reentry supraventricular tachycardia who required two atrial premature beats for termination of tachycardia. The first four beats are the last four of the tachycardia. Following the second retrograde atrial potentials as seen on the atrial electrograms, a burst of high frequency stimuli occurs in the atria with a delay of 240 ms, and a duration of 230 ms. Two atrial premature beats are induced, the tachycardia is terminated, and the fifth beat is the first beat of sinus rhythm.

This system has been used as an external system in seven patients and an overall success for immediate termination of tachycardia by the first burst of high frequency stimulation was found to be 80%. The occurrence of atrial fibrillation using this system was unusual.

The disadvantage of the above system is that it can only be used for atrial stimulation. In some patients the tachycardia can only be terminated by single or double ventricular premature beats. A different system has therefore been developed to cope with that type of situation. An electrode catheter for sensing and stimulating is positioned in the right ventricle. This is connected to a Devices 4273 miniscan. The onset of tachycardia is sensed by the sensing circuit and this leads to activation of an output circuit which induces a premature stimuli with a preset coupling time following the intraventricular endocardial potential. This delay is set so that the first stimulus occurs within the refractory period of the ventricle. One second later a further stimulus is induced but is delayed by a further 5 ms. About every second a stimulus occurs but each one is delayed by a further 5 ms. In this way 100 ms of the cardiac cycle is scanned at which time the pacemaker recycles and starts the scan again. Once the scan has occurred outside the refractory period of the ventricle, then ventricular premature beats are induced. When the tachycardia has been terminated by a suitably timed ventricular premature beat, the pacemaker is switched off and no more stimuli occur although, of course, sensing continues. If a tachycardia requires two ventricular premature beats for termination then this system can be used to scan 100 ms, of the cardiac cycle using two stimuli with a fixed coupling interval between them.

Figure 2 is a recording from a patient with a reentry supraventricular tachycardia who required two ventricular premature beats to terminate the tachycardia. The first two beats are sinus beats and the third beat is an

[1] Devices Instruments Ltd., Welwyn Garden City, Hertfordshire, England.

atrial premature beat which initiates a supraventricular tachycardia. The Devices 4273 is activated and two pacing stimuli (PS_1 and PS_2) are induced with a fixed coupling time of 230 ms between them. There is a coupling time of 255 ms between the first stimulus and the preceding spontaneous ventricular beat. Both stimuli occur within the refractory period of the ventricle and so no ventricular premature beats occur. A short time after this a second pair of stimuli occur but now the coupling time between the first stimulus and the preceding ventricular beat is delayed by 5 ms from 255 to 260 ms. The coupling time between the two stimuli remains constant

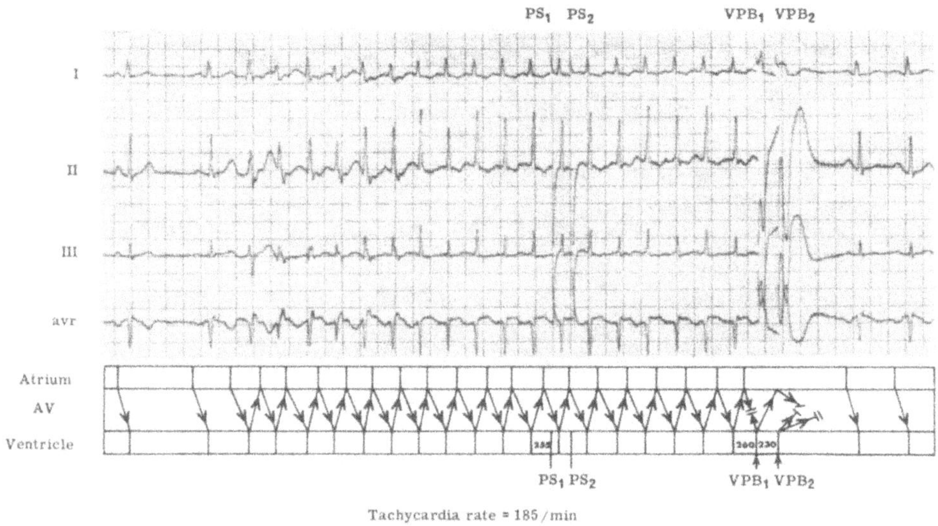

Fig. 2. Termination of supraventricular tachycardia by scanning pacemaker using two premature stimuli. *I, II, II avr* = standard electrocardiographic leads; PS_1, PS_2 = pacing stimuli 1 and 2; VPB_1, VPB_2 = ventricular premature beats 1 and 2.

at 230 ms. The second pair of stimuli now occurs outside the refractory period of the ventricle and so two ventricular premature beats are produced (VPB_1 and VPB_2); these two beats terminate the tachycardia and the last two beats are the first two beats of sinus rhythm.

The scanning system has the advantage that it can be used for either atrial or ventricular stimulation and for either single or double premature stimuli.

This system in external form has now been used with considerable success for up to 2 years in two patients with refractory drug-resistant reentry supraventricular tachycardia. Development is taking place to produce a totally implantable system.

Summary

The use of programed electrical stimulation of the heart has demonstrated that many examples of both supraventricular and ventricular tachycardia are due to a reentry or reciprocal mechanism. Tachycardias of this sort can usually be terminated by correctly timed premature beats. This characteristic has been made use of in therapy by many workers using a conventional demand pacemaker which can be activated into a fixed rate mode by the application of a magnet; pacing stimuli will then occur randomly during tachycardia but at some stage a suitably timed premature beat will occur which terminates the tachycardia. More sophisticated pacemakers have been used to induce correctly timed premature beats. The orthorhythmic pacemaker induces premature beats with coupling times that are dependent upon the preceding spontaneous cycle length, be it due to an ectopic impulse or a tachycardia. Bursts of high frequency stimulation have been used for the termination of reentry supraventricular tachycardias and more recently a system has been devised which can be used for atrial or ventricular stimulation during tachycardia. This system induces single or double premature stimuli at a preset delay following the spontaneous intracardiac potential. Every second further stimuli occur but delayed by 5 ms. This continues until 100 ms of the cardiac cycle have been scanned. At some point suitable timed premature beats will occur which terminate the tachycardia and the pacemaker then switches itself off.

Examples of such systems functioning are shown and their relative merits discussed.

References

1. Coumel, P.: Management of paroxysmal tachycardia. In: Symposium on Cardiac Arrhythmias. Sandøe, E., Flensted-Jensen, E., Olesen, K. H. (eds.) Södertälje: A. B. Astra, 1970
2. de Francis, N. A., Giordano, R. P.: Permanent epicardial pacing in the treatment of refractory ventricular tachycardia. Amer. J. Cardiol. **22,** 742, (1960)
3. Durrer, D., Schuilenburg, R. M., Wellens, H. J. J.: The role of the atrioventricular junction in the genesis of arrhythmias in the human heart. Proc. kon. ned. Akad. Wet. **72,** 515 (1969)
4. Haft, J. I., Kosowsky, B. D., Lau, S. H., Stein, E., Damato, A. N.: Termination of atrial flutter by rapid electrical pacing of the atrium. Amer. J. Cardiol., **20,** 239 (1967)
5. Hornbaker, J. H., O'Neal Humphries, J., Ross, R. S.: Permanent pacing in the absence of heart block. An approach to the management of intractable arrhythmias. Circulation **39,** 189 (1969)
6. Kitchen, J. G., Goldreyer, B. N.: Demand pacemaker for refractory paroxysmal supraventricular tachycardia. New Engl. J. Med. **287,** 596 (1972)
7. Lister, J. W., Cohen, L. S., Bernstein, W. H., Samet, P.: Treatment of supraventricular tachycardia by rapid atrial stimulation. Circulation **38,** 1044 (1968)
8. Ryan, G. F., Easley, R. M., Zaroff, L. I., Goldstein, S.: Paradoxical use of a demand pacemaker in treatment of supraventricular tachycardia due to the Wolff-Parkinson-White syndrom. Circulation **38,** 1037 (1963)
9. Sowton, E., Balcon, R., Preston, T., Leaver, D., Yacoub, M.: Long term control of intractable supraventricular tachycardia by ventricular pacing. Brit. Heart J. **31,** 700 (1969)

10. Sowton, E., Leatham, A., Carson, P.: The suppression of arrhythmias by artificial pacing. Lancet (1964), **2**, 1098.
11. Spurrell, R. A. J.: The study and management of tachycardias using intra-cardiac electrograms and programmed electrical stimulation of the heart. M. D. thesis, London, 1974
12. Spurrell, R. A. J., Sowton, E.: The use of high frequency stimulation (H.F.S.) in the management of paroxysmal supraventricular tachycardia. J. Electrocardiol. **8** (3), 287 (1975)
13. Spurrell, R. A. J., Sowton, E.: An implanted atrial synchronous pacemaker with a short atrioventricular delay for the prevention of paroxysmal supraventricular tachycardia. J. Electrocardiol. in press (1975)
14. Williams, D. O., Davison, P. H.: Long term treatment of refractory supraventricular tachycardia by patient controlled inductive atrial pacing. Brit. Heart J. **36**, 336 (1974)
15. Zipes, D. P., Festoff, B., Schaal, S. F., Cox, C., Sealy, W. C., Wallace, A. G.: Treatment of ventricular arrhythmia by permanent pacing and cardiac sympathectomy. Ann. intern. Med. **68**, 591 (1968)

Subject Index

Accessory pathway 123
— connections, concealed 158
— pathway, atrio-His 130
— —, refractory period 164
— pathways, latent 120
Acetylcholine and sinoatrial node 6, 9
—, SA node 40
Action potential, ventricular 75
Adams-Stokes attacks 99
Adrenaline and sinoatrial node 6
A – H interval 122, 132
AH interval, rate-dependent 97
Ajmaline and His-Purkinje system 136
— and WPW 169
—, MAP 76
Amiodarone and AVCS 137
— and WPW 169
—, MAP 76
Anteroseptal infarction, imitation of 115
Aprindine and HPS 136
Arrhythmias, in angiocardiography 231
—, in heart catheterization 231
A-564-1, sinoatrial conduction 62
Atrial activation pattern 55
— cycle, compensatory 48
— — length, drug effects 67
— —, noncompensatory 48
— fibrillation 188
— flutter 188
— premature depolarization, responses to 34
— stimulation, high-rate 207
— —, in (bi)fascicular block 107
— synchronous pacing, technique of 235
— tachycardia 188
— —, induced by single premature beat 177
Atrioventricular conduction system, refractory period 195
— dissociation 185
Atropine and sinoatrial conduction 50, 59
— and sinus node 49
— and WPW 169
—, AV-conduction 132
—, premature atrial stimulation 51
AV block, bradycardia-dependent 89
—, congenital 89
—, Mobitz type I 102
—, Mobitz type II 102
—, transient 125
—, unidirectional 93
—, Wenckebach period 89
—, 1st degree 102, 103
—, 2nd degree 103
AV conduction = atrioventricular conduction 88, 123
—, intracardiac electrography 87
—, different patterns 157
— disturbances 89
— —, bifascicular block 99
— —, congenital heart block 99
— —, fascicular block 99
— —, infrahisian block 89
— —, intrahisian block 89
— —, left anterior hemiblock 99
— —, left posterior hemiblock 99
— —, suprahisian block 89
— —, ventricular rate, cardiac output 99
— —, complete block 100
—, drug effects on 132, 134
—, functional dissociation 158
—, gap phenomenon 154
AVCS = atrioventricular conduction system 137
AV nodal reentry 123
— tachycardias 119
AV node, autonomous nervous system 96
— reentry 158
—, refractory period 132
AV pathway, common 128
AV tachycardia, paroxysmal 121
—, reciprocating 187

Bifascicular block, bilateral 111
— —, unilateral 114
Block, in the His-Purkinje system 153
—, intraventricular and conduction disturbance 100
Bradycardia-tachycardia syndrome 19, 33
Bypass, atrio-His 125
—, paranodal 139

Calcium and sinoatrial node 6
Carbamylcholine and tachycardia 178

Cardiac arrest 190
Carotid sinus pressure 192
Circuit of conduction 119
Circulating excitation, model of 175
Circus movement and anatomical obstacle 181
— —, within atrial muscle 177
— — tachycardia 182
CI 661, Sinoatrial conduction 63
Concealed conduction 106
— reentry 88
Conduction block, sinoatrial 53
— disturbances, inapparent 94
—, retrograde 230
— time, intra-atrial 48
— —, retrograde intraventricular 198
Congestive heart failure 99
Corrected sinoatrial recovery time 26
Coupled stimulation, method 220

D 600 and AV conduction 134
D 600, functional refractory period of AV node 133
Detection, intracardiac 230
Digitalis and sick sinus syndrome 33
— and WPW 169
Digoxin and AV conduction 134
Diphenylhydantoin and AV conduction 134
— and digitalis intoxication 68
— and WPW 169
Disopyramide and HPS 136
— and WPW 169
— (B 712), sinoatrial conduction 64
Dominant pacemaker, shift of 54

Ectopic impulse formation 183
Electrical stimulation, programmed 164
— —, ventricular vulnerability 198
Electrotonic interaction 47
Endocardial leads 209
"Entire SNRT" 29
Entrance block, sinoatrial 53
Excitability, recovery of 181
"Excitable gap" 182
Exit block, sinoatrial 9
Extrastimulus technique 152

Fascicular block, left anterior 111
— —, left posterior 111
— —, pacemaker therapy 100
— — patterns of 111
— conduction time, measurement of 220
FRP = functional refractory period 219, 220
Fusion complex 189

Gap phenomenon 96
— —, type I, type II 154

HBE = His bundle electrography 142
—, bipolar recording 142
—, clinical implications 142
—, 1st degree intra-His block 145
—, 2nd degree intra-His block, Mobitz 145
—, 2nd degree intra-His block, Wenckebach 145
—, 3rd degree intra-His block 145
—, H-V time 147
—, intra-His bundle blocks 144
—, — lesions 144
—, Mobitz 2nd degree block 146
—, morphology 143
—, position of the catheter 149
—, proximal deflection 146
—, unipolar recording 142
"High degree block" 105
His bundle, deflection of 143
— —, diseased human 143
— —, dissociation of 130
— —, distal deflection 144
— — electrocardiography, limitations of 142
— — electrography 87, 132
— — potential 142
— —, proximal deflection 144
— —, stimulation of 128 ,144
HPS = His-Purkinje system 94
His-Purkinje system, drug effects on 136
— —, reentry mechanism 194
— —, refractory period 201
Hysteresis 229
—, negative 216
—, positive 216
—, variable 212
Hypersensitive carotid sinus 47

Inferior infarction 115
Internodal tract, posterior 152
Intraventricular conduction, refractory period 200
— — time, measurement of 222
Intrinsicoid deflection 111
Impulse propagation, failure of 34
— registration, endocardial 219
— strength and ventricular fibrillation 199
Interruption of circus movement 181
Intraventricular conduction, retrograde 196
Isoproterenol and AV conduction 134

Jervell and Lange-Nielsen syndrome 220
— — syndrome, types of subjunctional conduction 223
Junctional tachycardia 119
— — and orthorhythmic pacing 232

LAFB = left anterior fascicular block, mirror-image effect 113

LAFB without QRS left axis deviation 116
LBBB = left bundle branch block, frequency-dependent 95
"Leading circle" concept 183
"Left anterior hemiblock" 114
Left axis deviation 111, 117
— — deviation without LAFB 115
— ventricular hypertrophy 116
Lenègre's disease 116
Lidocaine and AV conduction 134
— and WPW 169
Local detection 213
— reentry 201
Longitudinal dissociation 93, 129
— —, intranodal 120
LGL = Lown-Ganong-Levine syndrome 152
—, A-H interval 153, 157
—, His bundle electrography 157
—, H-V interval 153
—, P-A interval 153
— syndrome, definition 159
—, ventricular tachycardia 159

Macroreentry 201
Mahaim fibers 152
MAP = monophasic action potential 73
—, amplitude 74
— and peripheral electrocardiogram 74
—, application of 82
—, configuration 73
—, conversion of atrial arrhythmias 80
—, duration 74
—, phase 0 of 74
—, potential change 74
"Masked WPW syndrome" 152
"Maximum sinus node recovery time" 55
Mexiletine (Kö 1173), sinoatrial conduction 64
Mobitz block, atypical 108
Monophasic action potential, in man 80
Multiple microelectrode technique 178
Myocardial fibers, refractory period 201
— infarction and fascicular block 101

Nodal fibers, membrane properties 8
— pathways, functional 124

Orthorhythmic pacing 229
— — and concealed conduction 232
— —, applications of 215
— —, electrophysiologic studies 214
— — in tachycardias 213
— —, measurement of refractory period 214
— —, fundamentals of 212
— pacemaker, implantable 215
— stimulation, endocardial detection 219

Overdrive pacing 227
— suppression 9
Oxprenolol and AV conduction 134
Oxyfedrin and AV conduction 134

Pacemaker cell, microelectrode studies 48
— —, transmembrane potentials 47
— fibers, dominant 5
— —, latent 5
— implantation, age of patients 14
—, patient-controlled 205
— shift 6, 41, 54
— —; compensatory, noncompensatory cycles 55
Pacing, orthorhythmic 231
—, patient-initiated 228
Paired stimulation 222
"Peri-infarction block" 115
Pindolol and AV conduction 134
Postreturn cycle 34
— —, drug effects 34
Potassium and sinoatrial node 7
PQ interval and fascicular block 101
Practolol and AV conduction 134
Preautomatic interval 25
Pre-excitation, retrograde 123
— syndrome 152
Premature atrial stimulation 33
— — stimulation, technique 36, 42
— — stimulation technique, limitations of 43
— stimulation 228
— ventricular beats 194
Procainamide and HPS 136
— and WPW 169
Propafenone and HPS 136
—, SA conduction 60
Propranolol and AV conduction 134
— and WPW 169
"Pseudoblock" 106
Purkinje fiber 7
— fibers, junction of, local reentry 202

QRS, left axis deviation 114
Quinidine and HPS 136
— and WPW 169

Rabbit, right atrial preparation 39
Radiocontrast material, arrhythmias due to 230
Radiofrequency pacemaker 206, 228
— —, effect of 207
Rapid atrial pacing, patient initiated 205
— — stimulation 46
— — stimulation, complications 209
— — stimulation, mechanism 209
Reciprocal supraventricular tachycardia, termination of 236

Reciprocating tachycardias, intranodal 121
— tachycardia, junctional 121
Reentrant mechanism 175
Reentry circuit, junctions of 127
—, intranodal 121, 130
—, localized 189
— mechanism 119
—, supraventricular tachycardia 236
— tachycardia 228
— tachycardias, recurrent 212
—, within AV node 176
—, — SA node 176
Refractory period, functional 94
Retrograde intraventricular conduction, rate dependency 198
— penetration, concealed 187
"Retrograde preexcitation syndromes" 158
Return cycles, biphasic pattern after atropine 60
— cycle, compensatory 34
— —, noncompensatory 34
Rhythm disturbances, analysis of 222
Right atrium, refractory period 195
— axis deviation 111
— ventricle, extrasystolic stimulation 194
— —, refractory period 195, 196
— —, vulnerability 196
R 818, Sinoatrial conduction 63

SACT = Sinoatrial conduction time
— and spontaneous cycle length 69
—, antegrade 42
—, diphenylhydantoin, digitalis intoxication 62
—, limitations of 49
—, pharmacologic intervention 41
SA node = sinoatrial node, electrophysiology 5
—, microelectrode studies 43
—, parasympathetic influences 31
Scanning pacemaker 238
Short P-R interval and normal QRS complex 152
Sick sinus node 10
— — syndrome and arrhythmias 16
— — syndrome and ischemic heart disease 14
— — syndrome and orthorhythmic pacing 232
— — syndrome, asymptomatic 15
— — syndrome, AV block 18
— — syndrome, clinical aspects 12
— — syndrome, course 22
— — syndrome, diagnosis 13, 21
— — syndrome, diseases associated with 14
— — syndrome, disturbances of impulse conduction 17
— — syndrome, disturbances of impulse formation 17
— — syndrome, ECG criteria 18
— — syndrome, ECG magnetic tape recording 26
— — syndrome, escape beats after atropine 31
— — syndrome, etiology 13
— — syndrome, general symptoms 17
— — syndrome, history of symptoms 16
— — syndrome, incidence of syncope 16
— — syndrome, pacemaker implantation 13
— — syndrome; pacemaker implantation, atrial rhythm 20
— — syndrome, pacemaker therapy 12, 19
— — syndrome pharmacotherapy 23
— — syndrome, prognosis 22
— — syndrome, progression of 22
— — syndrome, sinus bradycardia 18
— — syndrome, supraventricular tachyarrhythmia 18
— — syndrome, symptoms 15, 22
— — syndrome, therapy 23
— — syndrome, ventricular tachyarrhythmia 18
Sinoatrial block 19
— —, animal experiments 52
— —, 1st degree of 52
— —, mechanism of 52
Sinoatrial conduction 33, 46
— —, estimation of 36
— —, limitation of estimation 66
— —, retrograde 28, 39
"Sinoatrial conduction time" 37, 55
— —, -time, -velocity 37
— — time, drug effects 58
— disease 46, 49
— node 47
— — and ectopic impulse 8
— —, entrance block 9
— —, prepotential 5
— —, exit block 49
— — function 5
Sinus automaticity, depression of 39
— node, action potential 43
— —, action potential duration 38
— — automaticity 38
— — automaticity, drug effects 58
— — automaticity, suppression by atrial pacing 25
— — dysfunction 33
— — dysfunction, atropine effect 59
— — dysfunction, pathophysiology 42

— —, exit block 49
— — function, drug effects 58
— —, impulse conduction 12
— —, impulse formation 12
— — recovery time 9, 46
— — recovery time, drug effects 58
— — reentry 185
— — response 48
— — return cycle 40
— nodal exit block and arterial pressure 30
— tachycardia, reciprocating, paroxysmal 185
Slowed conduction 120
SNRT = sinus node recovery time, and sick sinus syndrome 25
— and arterial pressure 29
— and pacing rate 26
— at low stimulation rates 27
—, AV nodal escape systoles 29
—, effect of atropine 27
—, paradoxical atropine effect 50
—, paradoxical prolongation following atropine 28
Sodium and sinoatrial node 7
Split His 142
Spread of activation, maps of 179
Stimulation, automatic antiarrhythmic 212
—, — orthorhythmic 232
—, coupled 228
—, programmed-rate-related 229
—, rapid atrial 227
—, rate-related 227
—, sequential RR-related 231
Subjunctional conduction 221
— — time 224
Suction electrode 73
— —, cardiac arrhythmias 75
— —, perisinusnodal region 73
— —, pharmacologic studies 76
— —, right atrial potential 73
— — technique 80
— —, ventricular repolarization 76
Supraventricular reentry tachycardias, drug effects 138
— tachycardias 185
— tachycardia, aberration of 191
SVT = supraventricular tachycardia 205
—, drug therapy 205
—, electrical stimulation 205
—, manual neural stimulation 205
—, surgical intervention 205

Tachyarrhythmias, clinical features 185
—, electrocardiographic diagnosis 191
—, recurrent 232
Tachycardia, AV nodal 125
— -bradycardia syndrome 231
—, idioventricular 189
—, intranodal reciprocating 129
—, parasystolic 185
—, slow ventricular 189
—, supraventricular 125, 205
—, — paroxysmal 185
Tachycardias, drug-resistant 212, 230
—, focal 231
—, junctional 130
—, reciprocal 235
"Torsade de pointes" 189
Trifascicular block 114

Unidirectional block 120, 180

VA conduction, retrograde 123
Ventricular conduction, aberrant 187
— myocardium, vulnerability 195
— —, vulnerable period 194
— premature beats, types of 225
— stimulation, extrasystolic 202
— tachycardia, paroxysmal 189
— tachycardias 185
Verapamil and AV conduction 134
— and LGL 156
—, sinoatrial conduction 61
—, sinus node function 68
— and WPW 169
Vulnerability, to electrical stimulation 200

WPW = Wolff-Parkinson-White syndrome, Rosenbaum's classification 164
—, accessory pathway 164, 165
—, atrial fibrillation 168
—, circus-movement tachycardia 167
—, "concealed" accessory pathway in tachycardia 167
—, drug effects 168
—, drug effects on accessory pathway and AV node 169
—, electrophysiology 164
—, indications for stimulation studies 169
—, mechanism of tachycardia 166
—, surgical interruption of accessory pathway 169
— syndrome and cardiac abnormalities, atrial fibrillation 168
— —, concealed 121
—, type of tachycardias 167
—, VA conduction 165, 166
—, —, His-AV node pathway 165
"Wavelength" 182
Wenckebach period, atypical 104

GPSR Compliance
The European Union's (EU) General Product Safety Regulation (GPSR) is a set of rules that requires consumer products to be safe and our obligations to ensure this.

If you have any concerns about our products, you can contact us on

ProductSafety@springernature.com

In case Publisher is established outside the EU, the EU authorized representative is:

Springer Nature Customer Service Center GmbH
Europaplatz 3
69115 Heidelberg, Germany

www.ingramcontent.com/pod-product-compliance
Lightning Source LLC
Chambersburg PA
CBHW061206240926
51846CB00006B/1123
* 9 7 8 3 6 4 2 6 6 3 5 8 1 *